Single Agents in Cancer Chemotherapy

Single Agents in Cancer Chemotherapy

Robert B. Livingston and Stephen K. Carter

National Cancer Institute
Bethesda, Maryland

IFI/PLENUM • NEW YORK-WASHINGTON-LONDON • 1970

ISBN-13: 978-1-4684-1380-9   e-ISBN-13: 978-1-4684-1378-6
DOI: 10.1007/978-1-4684-1378-6

Softcover reprint of the hardcover 1st edition 1970

Library of Congress Catalog Card Number 76-139580
SBN 306-65153-X

IFI/Plenum Data Corporation is a subsidiary of
Plenum Publishing Corporation
227 West 17th Street, New York, N. Y. 10011

United Kingdom edition published by Plenum Press, London
A Division of Plenum Publishing Company, Ltd.
Donington House, 30 Norfolk Street, London W.C. 2, England

Foreword

The clinical trials program of anti-tumor drugs was started
by the National Cancer Institute in 1955. In the past 15 years,
this national network has collected a large body of data on all
of the recognized anti-tumor drugs as well as upon new,
experimentally promising agents. While the most important of
these studies have been published, there has remained a wealth
of data not generally available to the scientific community.
Drs. Carter and Livingston have not only succeeded in organizing
this large corpus, they have in addition analyzed and interpreted
the clinical data in a way that will be highly useful for years
to come. From a perusal of this volume it becomes apparent
that some drugs are more active against certain tumors than had
been realized; that the evidence for the activity of certain
drugs against specific tumors is sometimes tenuous; surprisingly,
that some highly active agents have never been tried against some
of the fairly common tumors. Their monumental work has provided
not only access to the hard data, it has also shown the need for
research to fill in important gaps in our knowledge. The authors
and the IFI/Plenum Press are to be congratulated for this useful
and important work.

C. Gordon Zubrod, M.D.
Scientific Director for Chemotherapy
National Cancer Institute
National Institutes of Health
Bethesda, Maryland

v

Acknowledgment

The authors wish to thank Dr. C. Gordon Zubrod and
Dr. Oleg Selawry for their encouragement and advice during the
preparation of this book. We wish also to express our gratitude
to Mrs. Martha Harshman for her dedicated efforts in the
preparation of the manuscript.

Abbreviations

ALL-AUL	acute lymphocytic and undifferentiated leukemias
AML-AMoL	acute myelocytic and monocytic leukemias
ara-C	cytosine arabinoside
BCNU	bis-chlorethyl nitrosourea
CF	citrovorum factor (leucovorin)
CLL	chronic lymphocytic leukemia
CML	chronic myelocytic leukemia
CR	complete remission (or response)
CSF	cerebrospinal fluid
CTX	cyclophosphamide
DNA	deoxyribonucleic acid
DNR	daunorubicin (daunomycin, rubidomycin)
DTIC	dimethyl triazeno imidazole carboxamide
eod	every other day
FUDR	5-fluoro-2'deoxyuridine
gm	grams
HN_2	mechlorethamine
HU	Hydroxyurea
IM	intramuscular(ly)
IV	intravenous(ly)
kg	kilograms
M_1	refers to a bone marrow rating of "1", which in most studies implies that the proportion of blasts is $\leq 5\%$ in a setting of normal cellularity
m^2	meters squared (of body surface area)
mcg	micrograms
mg	milligrams
mo	month
M-protein	myeloma protein
MST	median survival time
MTX	methotrexate
PO	per os (orally)
PR	partial remission (or response)
q	every
RNA	ribonucleic acid
S phase	phase of DNA synthesis in cell cycle

TG	thioguanine
UM	uracil mustard
WBC	white blood cell (count)
wk	week
↓	decrease
↑	increase
5-FU	5-fluorouracil
6 CP	6-chloropurine
6 MP	6-mercaptopurine
6 MPR	6-mercaptopurine riboside
ALGB	Acute Leukemia Group B
CCGA	Children's Cancer Group A (formerly Acute Leukemia Group A)
COG	Central Oncology Group (formerly Central Drug Evaluation Program
ECOG	Eastern Cooperative Oncology Group (formerly Eastern Solid Tumor Group)
MWCCG	Midwestern Cancer Chemotherapy Group
PVACCG	Pacific Veterans Administration Cancer Chemotherapy Group
SECCG	Southeastern Cancer Chemotherapy Group
SWCC(S)G	Southwest Cancer Chemotherapy Study Group
VACCG	Veterans Administration Cancer Chemotherapy Group
VAL	Veterans Administration Lung Group
WCCG	Western Cancer Chemotherapy Group
Eastern CDEP	Eastern Clinical Drug Evaluation Program

Contents

Introduction

This book was written to fill a gap in the literature of chemotherapy: to our knowledge, there has previously been no comprehensive review of reported results for the commonly used antineoplastic agents. We have attempted to do this, and hope that the work will prove useful to physicians in at least three respects: (1) to aid in the choice of a drug, and of an appropriate dose schedule, in a given clinical situation; (2) as a bibliography of clinical experience to date with each agent; and (3) to aid in the rational design of potentially useful drug combinations. Clearly, such efforts should be predicated on the fullest possible knowledge of results with each drug used alone. It is our feeling that this third objective will become more and more important as the trend continues in cancer chemotherapy away from the use of single agents and toward the use of combinations.

It is important to note what is _not_ included in this book: results of combination chemotherapy; reports of the use of drugs as adjuvants to surgery or radiation therapy; and most reports of the use of drugs in regional perfusion, with the exception of methotrexate for head and neck cancer. These have been omitted, largely because in each case, it is quite difficult to assess the contribution of a specific drug to the overall results obtained. Foreign-language reports have been omitted, for the most part. Finally, there is a great mass of unpublished data in this field, most of which is not included. It is quite possible that such information may, at times, refute that which is in the literature, and we welcome communications to this effect which might be incorporated into future revisions. Indeed, we hope to stimulate the independent publication of such data as this is the only way in which it can become generally useful. A few commercially available agents in cancer chemotherapy have not been included, as they were considered of minor importance and it has not been our intent to be encyclopedic.

An understanding of the plan of the chapters should make them easier to use. The bulk, both in content and in value, lies in the tables, which are arranged for each drug according to tumor

1

type or site. Available information has always been included with
respect to the following tumors: breast, colorectal, lung,
melanoma, lymphoma, acute lymphocytic and undifferentiated
leukemia, and acute myelocytic and monocytic leukemia. Other tumors
are included if they have been reported to be responsive to the
drug, or if an adequate trial has been reported for the drug in
that tumor type. Caveats are in order with respect to the columns
headed "# Pts Evaluated" and "# Pts Responding". First, the
number of patients evaluated was often not equal to the total
number treated. What constitutes an "evaluable" patient is not
yet a standardized concept, and differences in this concept
among various investigators often account largely for apparent
differences in response rate. Secondly, with respect to what
constitutes a meaningful "objective response", this has not been
entirely consistent either, especially in the older reports.
In general, an effort has been made to include only those
responses which constituted >50% tumor regression on the basis of
measurable lesions; exceptions have been cited where possible.
In the case of the acute leukemias, it should be noted that there
is variability, especially in the criteria of what is required
for "complete response" (CR). Some groups and investigators
regard the attainment of an M_1 marrow as equivalent to CR; others
have set more stringent requirements, (e.g., return to normal
hemoglobin level). Again, where possible, we have tried to note
where varying criteria seemed to account for variations in the
CR rate.

Dose schedules used are separately listed for each entry in
the tables. These are followed in some cases by "Remarks",
which include such things as survival data, comparison with other
drugs, and unusual or fatal toxicity, if these were part of the
original report. Also included is the name of the cooperative
group performing the study, where such was the case. Abbreviations
used for the group names (and others) may be found at the end of
the book.

Preceding the tables in each chapter are a list of synonyms
for the drug, its structure, recommended dosage(s) (which may or
may not conform to the package insert), and a brief summary of
toxicity and mechanism of action. The section entitled "Role
in Cancer Therapy" attempts to summarize the results reported in
the tables, and analyze the clinical data in greater depth where
pertinent.

Robert B. Livingston, M.D.
Stephen K. Carter, M.D.
National Cancer Institute
Bethesda, Maryland

Mechlorethamine

Synonyms: Nitrogen mustard, HN$_2$, Mustargen.

Structure:

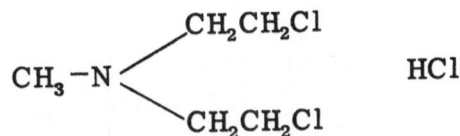

$$CH_3-N\diagdown \begin{matrix} CH_2CH_2Cl \\ CH_2CH_2Cl \end{matrix} \qquad HCl$$

Dosage: 0.4 mg/kg x 1, IV, repeated as tolerated (usually 3-6
              wks), or 0.4 mg/kg x 1, IV, off 2-3 wks (until bone
              marrow recovery), then 0.1 mg/kg/wk as tolerated.

Toxicity: I.   Gastrointestinal
                   A.   Nausea, vomiting, and anorexia - vomiting
                        usually stops within 8 hours, but nausea and
                        anorexia may persist for 24 hours.

              II. Hematological - major dose-limiting toxicity
                   A.   Leukopenia
                   B.   Thrombocytopenia

Mechanism of Action: HN_2 is an alkylating agent. Like other
              nitrogen mustards, it reacts with (alkylates)
              nucleophilic substances within the cell, including
              a number of biologically important groups, e.g.,
              phosphate, amino, sulfhydryl, hydroxyl, imidazole,
              and carboxyl. This takes place through formation
              of the highly reactive, electrophilic ethylenimonium
              derivative from the tertiary amine in neutral or
              alkaline aqueous solution, according to the following
              general reaction:

$$R-N\begin{matrix} CH_2CH_2Cl \\ \\ CH_2CH_2Cl \end{matrix} \rightarrow R-\overset{+}{N}\begin{matrix} CH_2 \\ | \\ CH_2 \\ \\ CH_2CH_2Cl \end{matrix} \quad + Cl-$$

              Internal cyclization of a bis (β-chloroethyl) grouping
              is necessary to the biological activity of the
              mustard derivatives.

                          Role in Cancer Therapy

     HN_2 has been in clinical use against cancer for more than
twenty years. Hundreds of papers have been published describing
its application. Our review, however, utilizes only a small fraction
of the published reports, because the following limitations were
imposed: (1) only reports dealing with the systemic, intravenous
use of the compound alone were included; and (2) some quantification
of objective response was required as a prerequisite to inclusion,
with a few exceptions. (These exceptions seemed relevant to a
discussion of the drug).

HN$_2$ appears to be the alkylating agent of choice at present for the treatment of advanced Hodgkin's disease. Its use has been reported in 682 patients, with an overall response rate of 63% and CR in 12/95 = 13% of those evaluated. This compares with an overall reported response rate of 54% for CTX, and a reported CR rate of 12%. In six studies which directly compared the two agents,[19,20,26,27,30,32] HN$_2$ produced responses in 83/123 = 68%, and CTX in 66/115 = 57%. Seven of 60 (12%) treated with HN$_2$, and 5 of 61 (8%) treated with CTX were recorded as CR in these series. More important than its ability to produce a slightly higher response rate is the apparent superiority of HN$_2$ over CTX as regards the survival of patients with Hodgkin's disease. Sullivan[26] found that children with this diagnosis who received HN$_2$ as initial therapy had a MST of 30.9 months, while those initially treated with CTX had a MST of 20.8 months. In a large study of the ECOG, Gold et al[30] found that HN$_2$-treated patients had a median survival of 17 months, vs only 7 months for Hodgkin's patients who received CTX. They speculated that the relatively less immunosuppressive effect of HN$_2$ might help account for this difference.

Against lymphosarcoma, the overall reported response rate for HN$_2$ (49% of 154), is less than that reported for CTX (63% of 276). However, Gold et al[30] found the MST to be much superior for HN$_2$-treated patients, relative to those treated with CTX (19 months and 8 months, respectively). Only in reticulum cell sarcoma did these authors find the MST to be longer for patients who received CTX, and here HN$_2$ appears clearly inferior on the basis of response rate also (3 of 17 = 18%, vs 56% of 219 patients treated with CTX).

The other major tumor category, other than lymphomas, in which HN$_2$ may have a role to play as the preferred alkylating agent is well-differentiated carcinoma of the lung. The VA Lung Group[29] found that HN$_2$ caused statistically significant prolongation of life in patients with squamous cell bronchogenic carcinomas, with no effect on MST in patients with the "oat-cell" or undifferentiated, small-cell histologic type. In the former group, the MST from the time of randomization into the study was ~3.2 months for a placebo-treated control group and ~6 months for the HN$_2$-treated patients. These findings with respect to HN$_2$ correlate well with those in a much earlier study by Hatch et al,[13] who, in an analysis of 198 cases of lung cancer, stated that "epidermoid carcinoma and adenocarcinoma responded best" to HN$_2$ therapy. The VA Lung Group study found that CTX, on the other hand, was most effective in prolonging the lifespan of patients with undifferentiated small-cell bronchogenic carcinoma, and had no beneficial effect on those with squamous cell types.

The results obtained in both lymphomas and lung cancer might be used to support a contention that HN$_2$ is relatively more

effective against "slowly" growing tumors, and CTX relatively
more effective against "rapidly" growing ones. Further support
for this proposition rests in the lack of observed activity for
HN_2 against acute leukemia,[1,3,5] vs the significant activity
of CTX, at least against ALL-AUL.

The overall reported response rate for HN_2 of 12% in 50
cases of colorectal carcinoma is comparable to the 16% of 43
reported for CTX. As single agents, both appear here inferior
to 5-FU.

Although it has activity in other forms of cancer, HN_2 has
been largely supplanted by newer alkylating agents in these types,
since it is more difficult to administer, requiring the parenteral
route and care in preparation, and is more poorly tolerated by
patients, at least in terms of immediate toxicity.

Tumor Type or Site

Breast

Ref #	# Pts Evaluated	# Pts Responding	% Response	Dose Schedule and Remarks
1	2	0		0.4 mg/kg/day x 4, repeated when possible.
16	37	7	19	HN_2, 0.1 mg/kg/day x 4; off 2 wks, then 0.1 mg/kg/wk, up to 3 mo as tolerated -- vs Thio-TEPA, 0.2 mg/kg/day x 4; off 2 wks, then 0.2 mg/kg/wk, up to 3 mo as tolerated. Response = decrease in total measured tumor mass. Thio-TEPA→3/39. Mean duration response 36 days for HN_2, MST 5 mo. ECOG study.
18	53	25		0.6 mg/kg over 3 days (on "alternate days"). Repeated at 2 mo intervals in responders. Selected patients. Mean response duration = 5.3 mo.
30	6	1		0.4 mg/kg x 1, IV, then 0.1 mg/kg/wk as tolerated (HN_2) -- vs 0.15 mg/kg/wk, PO (uracil mustard) -- vs 15 mg/kg/wk, IV (CTX). CTX→4/9. ECOG study.
	98	33	34	Total.

Colorectal

Ref #	# Pts Evaluated	# Pts Responding	% Response	Dose Schedule and Remarks
1	7	0		0.4 mg/kg/day x 4, repeated when possible. "GI" carcinomas.

Colorectal (cont.)

Ref #	# Pts Evaluated	# Pts Responding	% Response	Dose Schedule and Remarks
7	11	0		0.1 mg/kg/day x 4. "GI tract" cancer.
17	24	5		0.6 mg/kg over 3 days, repeated q ~8 wks if possible. No details as to response.
30	8	1		0.4 mg/kg x 1, IV, then 0.1 mg/kg/wk as tolerated (HN_2) -- vs 0.15 mg/kg/wk, PO (uracil mustard) -- vs 15 mg/kg/wk, IV (CTX). CTX→0/7. ECOG study.
	$\overline{50}$	$\overline{6}$	12	Total.
Melanoma				
1	7	3		0.4 mg/kg/day x 4, repeated when possible. No details as to response.
3	1	0		0.1 mg/kg/day x 4-6, repeated at 2 or 3 mo intervals or longer.
4	2	0		0.1 mg/kg/day x 4, or 0.2 mg/kg/day x 2. Repeated at time of relapse (in those who had response) if possible.
7	5	0		0.1 mg/kg/day x 4.
15	5	0		HN_2, 0.2 mg/kg/day x 2 -- vs DON, 0.2 mg/kg/day x 30, PO.

Melanoma (cont.)

Ref #	# Pts Evaluated	# Pts Responding	% Response	Dose Schedule and Remarks
16	14	0		HN_2, 0.1 mg/kg/day x 4; off 2 wks, then 0.1 mg/kg/wk, up to 3 mo as tolerated -- vs Thio-TEPA, 0.2 mg/kg/day x 4; off 2 wks, then 0.2 mg/kg/wk, up to 3 mo as tolerated. Thio-TEPA →2/16 transient responses. MST = 2.7 mo for HN_2-treated patients. ECOG study.
	$\overline{34}$	$\overline{3}$	9	Total.

Lung

1	30	12		0.4 mg/kg/day x 4, repeated when possible.
3	4	2		0.1 mg/kg/day x 4-6, repeated at 2 or 3 mo intervals or longer. 1 "good" response.
4	7	5		0.1 mg/kg/day x 4, or 0.2 mg/kg/day x 2. Repeated at time of relapse (in those who had response) if possible. Anaplastic carcinoma. 3 "good", 2 "fair". Mean response duration = 3 wks.
4	10	8		0.1 mg/kg/day x 4, or 0.2 mg/kg/day x 2. Repeated at time of relapse (in those who had response) if possible. Epidermoid carcinoma. 3 "good", 5 "fair". Mean duration = 3 mo.

Lung (cont.)

Ref #	# Pts Evaluated	# Pts Responding	% Response	Dose Schedule and Remarks
7	26	1		0.1 mg/kg/day x 4.
9	5	0		0.2-0.6 mg/kg as single injection, repeated when possible.
12	10	7		0.4-1.5 mg/kg per course as tolerated, IV. Undifferentiated small cell.
12	22	1		0.4-1.5 mg/kg per course as tolerated, IV. "Other types".
13	-	-		0.1 mg/kg/day x 4, IV; repeat q 8 wks as tolerated. See discussion.
15	34	4	12	HN_2, 0.2 mg/kg/day x 2 -- vs DON, 0.2 mg/kg/day x 30, PO. DON→0/18. VACCG study.
16	46	9	20	HN_2, 0.1 mg/kg/day x 4; off 2 wks, then 0.1 mg/kg/wk, up to 3 mo as tolerated -- vs Thio-TEPA, 0.2 mg/kg/day x 4; off 2 wks, then 0.2 mg/kg/wk, up to 3 mo as tolerated. DON→4/42 = 9.5%. MST 2 mo. Patients without prior x-ray therapy. ECOG study.
16	15	0		HN_2, 0.1 mg/kg/day x 4; off 2 wks, then 0.1 mg/kg/wk, up to 3 mo as tolerated -- vs Thio-TEPA, 0.2 mg/kg/day x 4; off 2 wks, then 0.2 mg/kg/wk, up to 3 mo as tolerated. DON→0/14. MST 3.5 mo. Patients with prior x-ray therapy. ECOG study.

Lung (cont.)

Ref #	# Pts Evaluated	# Pts Responding	% Response	Dose Schedule and Remarks
18	45	10		0.6 mg/kg over 3 days (on "alternate days"). Repeated at 2-mo intervals in responders. Selected patients. Mean response duration = 4.6 mo.
20	53	6	11	HN_2, 0.4 mg/kg, then off drug 3-6 wks, followed by (a) no maintenance or (b) chlorambucil 0.2 mg/kg/day, PO as tolerated. CTX→11/70 = 16%. VACCG study.
22	48	16	33	10 mg/day, on alternate days x 4 (HN_2) -- vs 400 mg/day, PO to total 5 gm if tolerated (CTX). CTX→29/51. All patients on steroids.
29	-	-		0.4 mg/kg x 1, repeat q 6 wks. See discussion. VA Lung Group study.
30	36	0	0	0.4 mg/kg x 1, IV, then 0.1 mg/kg/wk as tolerated (HN_2) -- vs 0.15 mg/kg/wk, PO (uracil mustard) -- vs 15 mg/kg/wk, IV (CTX). CTX→3/30 = 10%. ECOG study.
	$\overline{391}$	$\overline{81}$	21	Total.

"Acute Leukemia"

1	12	2		0.4 mg/kg/day x 4, repeated when possible. Response not defined.

"Acute Leukemia" (cont.)

Ref #	# Pts Evaluated	# Pts Responding	% Response	Dose Schedule and Remarks
3	12	0		0.1 mg/kg/day x 4-6, repeated at 2 or 3 mo intervals or longer. 7 AML, 2 AMoL, 3 ALL.
5	5	0		0.1 mg/kg/day x 4.
	29	2	7	Total.

Hodgkin's Disease

Ref #	# Pts Evaluated	# Pts Responding	% Response	Dose Schedule and Remarks
1	126	93	74	0.4 mg/kg/day x 4, repeated when possible. Median duration remission ~1.7 mo.
2	31	20		0.1 mg/kg/day x 5.
3	32	17		0.1 mg/kg/day x 4-6, repeated at 2 or 3 mo intervals or longer. Only "good" responses included. Usual remission duration = 2.5 mo.
6	16	9		Varied. Patients had no previous x-ray treatment.
6	14	5		Varied. Patients had responded to previous x-ray treatment.
6	13	3		Varied. Patients refractory to x-ray treatment.
7	4	1		0.1 mg/kg/day x 4.

Hodgkin's Disease (cont.)

Ref #	# Pts Evaluated	# Pts Responding	% Response	Dose Schedule and Remarks
8	50	39	78	4-5 mg on day 1, repeated and/or increased by incremental amounts of 1 mg over 4 to 6 injections, in 5-10 days. 13/31 "radio-resistant" patients had good responses. 35% had responses >50 days (up to 331 days).
9	23	22		0.2-0.6 mg/kg as single injection, repeated when possible.
10	57	20	35	0.1 mg/kg/day x 4. Only "good" responses included.
15	21	17		HN_2, 0.2 mg/kg/day x 2 -- vs DON, 0.2 mg/kg/day x 30, PO. DON→1/11. VACCG study.
16	9	8		HN_2, 0.1 mg/kg/day x 4; off 2 wks, then 0.1 mg/kg/wk, up to 3 mo as tolerated -- vs Thio-TEPA, 0.2 mg/kg/day x 4; off 2 wks, then 0.2 mg/kg/wk, up to 3 mo as tolerated. Mean duration response = 81 days. Thio-TEPA→7/11, with mean response = 44 days.
19	17	13		0.4 mg/kg x 1, IV, then 0.1 mg/kg/wk as tolerated (HN_2) -- vs 0.15 mg/kg/wk, PO (uracil mustard) -- vs 15 mg/kg/wk, IV (CTX). 3 CR. CTX→9/20, with 3 CR.
20	31	22	71	0.2 mg/kg/day x 2, repeat monthly (HN_2) -- vs 8 mg/kg/day x 5, IV; repeat monthly (CTX). 2 CR. CTX→22/33, all PR.

Hodgkin's Disease (cont.)

Ref #	# Pts Evaluated	# Pts Responding	% Response	Dose Schedule and Remarks
21	89	50	56	HN_2, 0.4 mg/kg, then off drug 3-6 wks, followed by (a) no maintenance or (b) chlorambucil 0.2 mg/kg/day, PO as tolerated. Patients maintained on chlorambucil (16) had mean duration response = 36 wks. Unmaintained patients = 12 wks.
26	12	9		0.4 mg/kg x 1, IV (HN_2) - unmaintained. 2 CR. CTX→5/8 responses. See discussion.
27	19	11		0.4 mg/kg HN_2 x 1, then daily chlorambucil PO -- vs 40 mg/kg CTX, IV "loading", then daily CTX PO maintenance. Median response duration = 10 mo. Chlorambucil maintenance. CTX→11/18, with median response duration = 8 mo (maintained).
28	27	22	82	0.2 mg/kg x 2 or 0.1 mg/kg x 4 (HN_2) -- vs 0.15-0.2 mg/kg/wk, IV x 6 (Vinblastine). Median response duration = 2.4 mo (unmaintained). VLB→20/27, with median response duration = 2.4 mo (unmaintained).
30	26	17		0.4 mg/kg/x 1, IV then 0.1 mg/kg/wk as tolerated (HN_2) -- vs 0.15 mg/kg/wk, PO (uracil mustard) -- vs 15 mg/kg/wk, IV (CTX). MST = 17 mo. CTX→10/19, with MST = 7 mo.

Hodgkin's Disease (cont.)

Ref #	# Pts Evaluated	# Pts Responding	% Response	Dose Schedule and Remarks
31	35	14		0.2 mg/kg/day x 2, IV, then 0.15 mg/kg q 2 wks x 6 mo. 5 CR. 4-drug combination ("MOPP")→ 21 CR, 10 PR of 44 (48% CR, 71% response).
32	18	11		0.2-0.4 mg/kg, IV x 1 (HN$_2$); off 2-6 wks, then chlorambucil, 0.2 mg/kg/day, PO. Median response duration = 20 wks for both CTX and HN$_2$-treated patients. CTX→9/17 responses.
	682	432	63	Total.

Lymphosarcoma

Ref #	# Pts Evaluated	# Pts Responding	% Response	Dose Schedule and Remarks
1	44	23		0.4 mg/kg/day x 4, repeated when possible. Usually <1 mo duration.
3	11	3		0.1 mg/kg/day x 4-6, repeated at 2 or 3 mo intervals or longer. Only "good" responses included.
7	7	1		0.1 mg/kg/day x 4.
9	15	13		0.2-0.6 mg/kg as single injection, repeated when possible.
10	10	4		0.1 mg/kg/day x 4. Only "good" responses included.

Lymphosarcoma (cont.)

Ref #	# Pts Evaluated	# Pts Responding	% Response	Dose Schedule and Remarks
15	12	2		HN$_2$, 0.2 mg/kg/day x 2 -- vs DON, 0.2 mg/kg/day x 30, PO. DON→0/7. VACCG study.
20	17	9		0.2 mg/kg/day x 2, repeat monthly (HN$_2$) -- vs 8 mg/kg/day x 5, IV; repeat monthly (CTX). 0 CR. CTX→12/17, with 1 CR.
27	18	8		0.4 mg/kg HN$_2$ x 1, then daily chlorambucil PO -- vs 40 mg/kg CTX, IV "loading", then daily CTX PO maintenance. Median remission duration = 7.5 mo. (Chlorambucil maintenance). CTX→9/19, median remission duration 3.0 mo. (CTX maintenance).
30	20	12		0.4 mg/kg x 1, IV, then 0.1 mg/kg/wk as tolerated (HN$_2$) -- vs 0.15 mg/kg/wk, PO (uracil mustard) -- vs 15 mg/kg/wk, IV (CTX). MST = 18 mo. CTX→13/17 responses, with MST = 8 mo. ECOG study.
	$\overline{154}$	$\overline{75}$	49	Total.

Reticulum-cell Sarcoma

3	5	1		0.1 mg/kg/day x 4-6, repeated at 2 or 3 mo intervals or longer. Only "good" responses included.

Reticulum-cell Sarcoma (cont.)

Ref #	# Pts Evaluated	# Pts Responding	% Response	Dose Schedule and Remarks
7	1	1		0.1 mg/kg/day x 4.
27	5	0		0.4 mg/kg HN_2 x 1, then daily chlorambucil PO -- vs 40 mg/kg CTX, IV "loading", then daily CTX PO maintenance. CTX 5/7.
30	6	1		0.4 mg/kg x 1, IV, then 0.1 mg/kg/wk as tolerated (HN_2) -- vs 0.15 mg/kg/wk, PO (uracil mustard) -- vs 15 mg/kg/wk, IV (CTX). MST = 3 mo. CTX→4/10 responses, with MST = 5 mo. ECOG study.
	$\overline{17}$	$\overline{3}$	18	Total.

Lymphosarcoma + Reticulum-cell Sarcoma

Ref #	# Pts Evaluated	# Pts Responding	% Response	Dose Schedule and Remarks
19	14	8		0.4 mg/kg x 1, IV then 0.1 mg/kg/wk as tolerated (HN_2) -- vs 0.15 mg/kg/wk, PO (uracil mustard) -- vs 15 mg/kg/wk, IV (CTX). 2 CR. CTX→5/11, all PR.
26	11	1		HN_2, 0.4 mg/kg x 1 - unmaintained -- vs CTX, 7.5 mg/kg/day x 6, IV; then 2.5 mg/kg/day PO, as tolerated. PR. CTX→6/16, with 1 CR.
	$\overline{26}$	$\overline{9}$	35	Total.

Ovary

Ref #	# Pts Evaluated	# Pts Responding	% Response	Dose Schedule and Remarks
3	1	0		0.1 mg/kg/day x 4-6, repeated at 2 or 3 mo intervals or longer.
14	8	4		0.1-0.2 mg/kg x 2-3 (HN_2). Chlorambucil maintenance as tolerated (most patients). 2 "good", 2 "fair".
	$\overline{9}$	$\overline{4}$	45	Total.

Prostate

Ref #	# Pts Evaluated	# Pts Responding	% Response	Dose Schedule and Remarks
4	3	2		0.1 mg/kg/day x 4, or 0.2 mg/kg/day x 2. Repeated at time of relapse (in those who had response) if possible.
7	3	0		0.1 mg/kg/day x 4.
	$\overline{6}$	$\overline{2}$	33	Total.

Stomach

Ref #	# Pts Evaluated	# Pts Responding	% Response	Dose Schedule and Remarks
4	2	1		0.1 mg/kg/day x 4, or 0.2 mg/kg/day x 2. Repeated at time of relapse (in those who had response) if possible. About 1 mo duration, obtained twice.

Stomach (cont.)

Ref #	# Pts Evaluated	# Pts Responding	% Response	Dose Schedule and Remarks
18	18	5		0.6 mg/kg over 3 days (on "alternate days"). Repeated at 2-mo intervals in responders. Each of >3 mo duration. Selected patients.
	$\overline{20}$	$\overline{6}$	30	Total.
Cervix				
3	1	0		0.1 mg/kg/day x 4-6, repeated at 2 or 3 mo intervals or longer.
9	2	0		0.2-0.6 mg/kg as single injection, repeated when possible.
25	5	0		0.4 mg/kg q 2-4 wks.
30	4	0		0.4 mg/kg x 1, IV then 0.1 mg/kg/wk as tolerated (HN$_2$) -- vs 0.15 mg/kg/wk, PO (uracil mustard) -- vs 15 mg/kg/wk, IV (CTX). CTX→1/10 responses. ECOG study.
	$\overline{12}$	$\overline{0}$		Total.
CLL				
1	41	22		0.4 mg/kg/day x 4, repeated when possible. Response not defined.

CLL (cont.)

Ref #	# Pts Evaluated	# Pts Responding	% Response	Dose Schedule and Remarks
3	14	5		0.1 mg/kg/day x 4-6, repeated at 2 or 3 mo intervals or longer. "Good" responses.
5	17	3		0.1 mg/kg/day x 4. "Good" responses of >6 mo duration.
10	10	2		0.1 mg/kg/day x 4. "Good" responses.
	82	32	39	Total.
CML				
1	17	8		0.4 mg/kg/day x 4, repeated when possible. Response not defined.
3	11	7		0.1 mg/kg/day x 4-6, repeated at 2 or 3 mo intervals or longer. "Good" responses.
5	16	11		0.1 mg/kg/day x 4. "Good" responses of 1-4 mo duration.
	44	26	59	Total.

Multiple Myeloma

Ref #	# Pts Evaluated	# Pts Responding	% Response	Dose Schedule and Remarks
1	7	1		0.4 mg/kg/day x 4, repeated when possible. Response not defined.
3	2	0		0.1 mg/kg/day x 4-6, repeated at 2 or 3 mo intervals or longer.
	9	1	11	Total.

Head and Neck

4	2	0		0.1 mg/kg/day x 4, or 0.2 mg/kg/day x 2. Repeated at time of relapse (in those who had response) if possible.
7	13	0		0.1 mg/kg/day x 4.
18	41	5	12	0.6 mg/kg over 3 days (on "alternate days"). Repeated at 2 mo intervals in responders. Mean duration response = 4.5 mo.
	66	5	7.5	Total.

Pancreas

3	1	1		0.1 mg/kg/day x 4-6, repeated at 2 or 3 mo intervals or longer.
7	2	0		0.1 mg/kg/day x 4.
	3	1	33	Total.

References

(1)   Rhoads, C. Report on a cooperative study of nitrogen mustard
       (HN$_2$) therapy of neoplastic disease. Trans Assoc Amer Phys
       60: 110, 1948.

(2)   Zanes, R., Doan, C., and Hoster, H. Studies in Hodgkin's
       syndrome. VII. Nitrogen mustard therapy. J Lab Clin Med
       33: 1002, 1948.

(3)   Wintrobe, M., and Huguley, C. Nitrogen-mustard therapy for
       Hodgkin's disease, lymphosarcoma, the leukemias, and other
       disorders. Cancer 1: 357, 1948.

(4)   Karnofsky, D., Abelmann, W., Craver, L., et al. The use of
       the nitrogen mustards in the palliative treatment of
       carcinoma. Cancer 1: 634, 1949.

(5)   Burchenal, J., Myers, W., Craver, L., et al. The nitrogen
       mustards in the treatment of leukemia. Cancer 2: 1, 1949.

(6)   Erf, L., and Bauer, R. The clinical effect of nitrogen
       mustard on Hodgkin's disease. Amer J Clin Path 19: 372,
       1949.

(7)   Ariel, I., and Kanter, L. Nitrogen mustard therapy. Amer
       J Surg 77: 509, 1949.

(8)   Dameshek, W., Weisfuse, L., and Stein, T. Nitrogen mustard
       therapy in Hodgkin's disease. Analysis of fifty consecutive
       cases. Blood 4: 338, 1949.

(9)   Bierman, H., Shimkin, M., Mettier, S., et al. Methyl-bis
       (β-chloroethyl) amine in large doses in the treatment of
       neoplastic diseases. Calif Med 71: 117, 1949.

(10)   Spurr, C., Smith, T., Block, M., et al. The role of
       nitrogen mustard therapy in the treatment of lymphomas and
       leukemias. Amer J Med 8: 710, 1950.

(11)   Gellhorn, A., and Collins, V. A quantitative evaluation of
       the contribution of nitrogen mustard to the therapeutic
       management of Hodgkin's disease. Ann Intern Med 35: 1250,
       1951.

(12)   Levine, B., and Weisberger, A. The response of various types
       of bronchogenic carcinoma to nitrogen mustard. Ann Intern
       Med 42: 1089, 1955.

(13)   Hatch, H., Bradford, J., and Ochsner, A.   Nitrogen mustard
       in treatment of advanced carcinoma of the lung. Analysis of
       198 cases. JAMA 160: 1129, 1956.

(14)   Coonrad, E., and Rundles, R.   Mustard chemotherapy in ovarian
       carcinoma. Ann Intern Med 50: 1449, 1959.

(15)   VACCSG. A clinical study of the comparative effect of
       nitrogen mustard and DON in patients with bronchogenic
       carcinoma, Hodgkin's disease, lymphosarcoma and melanoma.
       J Nat Cancer Instit 22: 433, 1959.

(16)   Zubrod, C., Schneiderman, M., Frei, E., et al. Appraisal of
       methods for the study of chemotherapy of cancer in man:
       comparative therapeutic trial of nitrogen mustard and
       triethylene thiophosphoramide.   J Chronic Dis 11: 7, 1960.

(17)   Hurley, J., and Ellison, E.   Chemotherapy of solid cancer
       arising from the gastro-intestinal tract.   Ann Surg 152:
       568, 1960.

(18)   Hurley, J., Ellison, E., Riesch, J., et al.   Chemotherapy of
       solid carcinoma.   JAMA 174: 1696, 1960.

(19)   Laszlo, J., Grizzle, J., Jonsson, U., et al.   Comparative
       study of mannitol mustard, cyclophosphamide, and nitrogen
       mustard in malignant lymphomas.   Cancer Chemother Rep 16:
       247, 1962.

(20)   Spear, P., and Patno, M.   A comparative study of the
       effectiveness of HN_2 and cyclophospahmide in bronchogenic
       carcinoma, Hodgkin's disease, and lymphosarcoma.   Cancer
       Chemother Rep 16: 413, 1962.

(21)   Scott, J.   The effect of nitrogen mustard and maintenance
       chlorambucil in the treatment of advanced Hodgkin's disease.
       Cancer Chemother Rep 27: 27, 1963.

(22)   Barran, K., Helm, W., and King, D.   Bronchial carcinoma
       treated with nitrogen mustard and cyclophosphamide.   Brit
       Med J 2: 685, 1965.

(23)   Boggs, D., Sofferman, S., Wintrobe, M., et al.   Factors
       influencing the duration of survival of patients with chronic
       lymphocytic leukemia.   Amer J Med 40: 243, 1966.

(24)   Decker, D., Malkasian, G., Mussey, E., et al.   Cyclophosphamide:
       evaluation in recurrent and progressive ovarian cancer.
       Amer J Obstet Gynec 97: 656, 1967.

(25) Smith, J., Rutledge, F., Burns, B., et al. Systemic
      chemotherapy for carcinoma of the cervix. Amer J Obstet
      Gynec 97: 800, 1967.

(26) Sullivan, M. Cyclophosphamide therapy for children with
      generalized lymphoma and Hodgkin's disease. Cancer
      Chemother Rep 51: 393, 1967.

(27) Jacobs, E., Peters, F., Luce, J., et al. Mechlorethamine
      HCl and cyclophosphamide in the treatment of Hodgkin's
      disease and the lymphomas. JAMA 203: 392, 1968.

(28) Ezdinli, E., and Stutzman, L. Vinblastine vs nitrogen
      mustard therapy of Hodgkin's disease. Cancer 22: 473, 1968.

(29) Green, R., Humphrey, E., Close, H., et al. Alkylating agents
      in bronchogenic carcinoma. Amer J Med 46: 516, 1969.

(30) Gold, G., Shnider, B., Salvin, G., et al. The use of
      mechlorethamine, cyclophosphamide, and uracil mustard in
      neoplastic disease: a cooperative study. J Clin Pharmacol
      New Drugs 10: 110, 1970.

(31) Moores, R. Comparison of combination therapy vs nitrogen
      mustard in Hodgkin's disease. Proc Amer Assoc Cancer Res
      11: 58 (#227), 1970.

(32) Papac, R., and Wood, D. Long term results achieved with the
      use of alkylating agents in malignant lymphoma and
      Hodgkin's disease. Acta Un Int Contra Cancer 20: 377, 1964.

Cyclophosphamide

Synonyms: Cytoxan, CTX; Endoxan, Procytox.

Structure:

$$O \quad CH_2CH_2-Cl$$
$$\overset{\displaystyle O}{\underset{\displaystyle N-H}{\overset{\parallel}{P}}}-N-CH_2CH_2-Cl$$

. H_2O

Dosage: 1. 1 to 1.5 gm/m^2 (30-50 mg/kg) as a single rapidly
                administered infusion, IV; repeated as soon as WBC
                returns toward normal (usually 17 to 21 days).
                a. Recommended in bronchogenic carcinoma; may be
                    used in other solid tumors and in lymphoma.
            2. 2 to 7.5 mg/kg/day, IV or PO (often 5 mg/kg/day x
                10, then dose adjusted according to toxicity and
                response); continuous low-dose therapy.
                a. Recommended in acute lymphocytic leukemia and
                    chronic lymphocytic leukemia; may be used in
                    lymphoma.
            3. 10 mg/kg/day ($^\sim$250 mg/m^2/day), IV or PO, to WBC
                <1500 mm^3. (Often a course consists of 10 mg/kg
                daily for 10 days).
                a. Recommended in childhood solid tumors.

Toxicity: I. Gastrointestinal
                A. Anorexia, nausea and vomiting
                B. Stomatitis, diarrhea - uncommon

           II. Genitourinary
                A. Sterile, hemorrhagic cystitis - common and may
                    be dose-limiting; may be largely prevented
                    by maintaining the patient's hydration.

          III. Hematological
                A. Leukopenia - most common dose-limiting side
                    effect
                B. Anemia
                C. Thrombocytopenia - usually less severe than
                    leukopenia

           IV. Dermatological
                A. Alopecia - common
                B. Transverse ridging of nails, skin
                    hyperpigmentation

Mechanism of Action: CTX is an alkylating agent. Like other
            nitrogen mustards, it reacts with (alkylates)
            nucleophilic substances within the cell, including
            a number of biologically important groups, e.g.,
            phosphate, amino, sulfhydhyl, hydroxyl, imidazole, and
            carboxyl. This takes place through formation of the
            highly reactive electrophilic ethylenimonium
            derivative from the tertiary amine in neutral or
            alkaline aqueous solution, according to the following
            general reaction:

$$R-N\begin{array}{l} CH_2CH_2Cl \\ \\ CH_2CH_2Cl \end{array} \rightarrow R-\overset{+}{N}\begin{array}{l} CH_2 \\ \diagdown \\ CH_2 \\ \\ CH_2CH_2Cl \end{array} \quad +Cl^-$$

Internal cyclization of a bis-(β-chloroethyl) grouping is necessary to the biological activity of the mustard derivatives.

In the case of CTX, a cyclic phosphamide has been substituted for the N-methyl of mechlorethamine (HN_2, the prototype nitrogen mustard). The bis-(β-chloroethyl) portion of the molecule cannot be ionized until the cyclic group is cleaved enzymatically at the phosphorus-nitrogen linkage. Thus, CTX is relatively inert in vitro; it is the metabolites of this compound which account for its biological effects. Originally, it was felt that the high phosphatase and phosphamidase activity in certain neoplastic tissues might "activate" CTX selectively at its desired sites of action. However, such "activation" probably takes place primarily in the liver.[2] Efforts to identify the metabolite(s) responsible for the antitumor effect of CTX are currently under way. If successful, they may result in the ultimate development of an agent with an improved therapeutic index.

Role in Cancer Therapy

CTX has been in widespread clinical use for ten years. It has proven to be one of the most useful agents in the chemotherapist's armamentarium, with activity against a broad spectrum of tumors.

In the treatment of disseminated breast carcinoma, objective tumor regression has been reported in 32% of 189 patients. Very limited experience with CTX given by intermittent, rather than daily schedules, indicates the response rate is similar by either method. The high-dose intermittent schedule[70] has not, however, received adequate evaluation. CTX appears comparable to 5-FU and MTX, and somewhat superior to prednisone or either vinca alkaloid used alone, in the response rate obtained; in a single comparative study with 5-FU,[54] CTX produced regressions in 7/32 (22%), and 5-FU in 11/30 (37%), with comparable durations of response.

CTX has been reported to produce responses in a few patients with carcinoma of the colon (16% of 43 cases). Although it is not generally considered an active agent against this tumor type, no definitive evaluation has been published.

On the basis of the published data, CTX appears to be an agent with some potential against malignant melanoma. The reported response rate of 26% is at least comparable to that achieved with imidazole carboxamide dimethyl triazeno (DTIC - an investigational drug) or hydroxyurea used alone. Here, too, a definitive trial is lacking, with only 31 treated cases in the literature.

CTX is quite possibly the most effective single drug in the treatment of lung cancer. Of 509 reported cases who received the agent, 33% had an objective response. Response rates in patients with lung cancer are, however, difficult to evaluate, since objective criteria for response often cannot be adequately applied to an analysis of therapeutic results. Perhaps more meaningful is the single major criterion of improvement in survival applied by the VA Lung Group in its studies. Here, intermittent IV CTX has been shown to produce a significant increase in median survival relative to placebo treatment.[76] This increase in survival is accounted for by the drug's effect on undifferentiated, small cell ("oat cell") tumors. The specificity for this histologic type corroborates the earlier reported findings of McLean,[55] and may explain why such studies as that of Barran et al[51] were unable to show an increase in survival time with CTX treatment. HN_2, on the other hand, appears most effective in the relatively well differentiated squamous cell bronchogenic carcinomas, with little effect on MST in patients with the "oat cell" type.[76] The best MST yet reported for patients with inoperable lung cancer who received chemotherapy is from the series of Bergsagel et al,[70] using single, high doses of CTX on an intermittent schedule in a total dose per injection (1.5 gm/m^2) roughly equivalent to that received in each five-day monthly course as reported by the VA Lung Group (40 mg/kg). CTX appears clearly less effective against this tumor type on a low-dose, chronic daily schedule: no positive effect on MST could be shown with this type of regimen.[76]

The use of CTX has been reported in 452 patients with Hodgkin's disease, with an overall response rate of 54% and CR in 12% of those evaluated. The overall response rate is somewhat lower than that reported for HN_2; in six studies which directly compared the two agents in Hodgkin's disease,[19,20,34,65,73,78] CTX produced responses in 66/115 = 57%, and HN_2 in 83/123 = 68%. Five of 61 (8%) treated with CTX, and 7/60 (12%) treated with HN_2 were recorded as CR in these series.

Aside from the fact that it produces a slightly lower response rate, CTX also appears to be markedly inferior to HN_2 when the survival times of patients with Hodgkin's disease who received either agent are compared. Sullivan[65] found that children with Hodgkin's disease who received CTX as initial therapy had a MST of 20.8 months, while those initially treated with HN_2 had a MST of

30.9 months. In a large study by the ECOG, Gold et al[78] found that CTX-treated patients with Hodgkin's disease had a MST of 7 months, while those treated with HN_2 survived a median of 17 months. These authors speculated that the apparent detrimental effect of CTX on survival might be related to its potent immunosuppressive qualities: ..."suppression of immune response may be a factor in the early favorable and later unfavorable reaction of patients treated with CTX." They cited the suggestion of Santos et al[3] that CTX (and several antimetabolites) can eliminate or markedly impair the serologic responses to foreign antigens, while HN_2 does not notably interfere with the development of certain circulating antibodies. Gold et al concluded that HN_2 appeared to be the alkylating agent of choice in the therapy of advanced Hodgkin's disease.

In lymphosarcoma, CTX has produced responses in 63% of 276 reported cases, with CR in 18/107 (17%) evaluated in American studies. In terms of response rate alone, CTX appears somewhat superior to HN_2 against this tumor type. However, again the apparent effect on MST is in favor of HN_2: the study of Gold et al[78] showed that patients treated with CTX survived a median of 8 months from start of therapy, vs 19 months for those who received HN_2 (in this series, response rates were essentially identical). In general, the duration of CTX-induced responses in patients with lymphosarcoma has been relatively short: 3 to 6 months. An exception to this is offered by the study of Mendelson et al,[79] who reported a median duration of CR (in 4 patients) of 22 months. Their dose schedule differed from that used by others in that they chose a high-dose, widely-spaced regimen (1.5 gm/m^2 q 3 weeks). It is an intriguing possibility that their use of such a schedule allowed for recovery of host immune response mechanisms between exposures to the drug, and that the latter was related to the unusually long duration of response. Further studies may elucidate the answer.

Against reticulum-cell sarcoma, 56% of 219 patients receiving CTX had reported responses, with a 15% CR rate in American studies. The study of Gold et al[78] showed a slightly longer MST for CTX-treated patients with reticulum-cell sarcoma (and a higher response rate) than for those receiving HN_2. The comparative study of Jacobs et al[73] also indicated superiority for CTX over the sequential combination of HN_2 and chlorambucil in a small number of patients. It thus appears that, for this most undifferentiated lymphoma, CTX is the alkylating agent of choice, with activity as a single agent equalled only by vincristine.

CTX is unique among the alkylating agents as an agent of proven, although modest, effectiveness against ALL-AUL, when used alone. In previously untreated patients, its use yields a 40% CR rate,[64] comparable to 6 MP and inferior only to vincristine

and to prednisone. Used against patients with disease refractory
to other agents, it is much less effective, with an overall CR
rate of only 9%. However, if only patients treated on a daily
schedule, rather than weekly, are considered, the CR rate in
refractory patients becomes 12%, with 24% of 117 patients in two
large group studies attaining M_1 marrow status. It is of interest
(and contrary to what results in animal leukemia systems predicted)
that daily treatment appears twice as effective as weekly dosing in
producing CR.

Unlike other agents of comparable activity in ALL-AUL, CTX
has been little exploited in attempts at combination chemotherapy
for induction. In a single large study reported by Fernbach
et al[62,63] which compared the combination of CTX and prednisone
with that of 6 MP and prednisone for the initial therapy of such
patients, there was no statistically significant difference in
the response rates obtained, or in the duration of response. The
use of CTX in combination with other agents against relatively far-
advanced ALL-AUL has not been reported for any series of meaningful
size.

Against AML-AMoL, CTX alone appears to be an agent of no
value. It may, however, be of use in combination with cytosine
arabinoside and other drugs (SWCCSG-unpublished data).

CTX demonstrates an overall response rate of 29% in 413
reported cases of multiple myeloma. As in lung cancer, probably
a more meaningful figure is obtained by comparing the MST of
treated patients with that of a control group. Significant
prolongation of life for CTX-treated patients vs controls receiving
placebo has been demonstrated,[30,39] although there is also marked
variation in the results reported by various investigators. In a
single study designed to compare the efficacy of CTX and melphalan,[75]
the results with each of the two agents appeared virtually identical.
Unlike melphalan, CTX has not received a trial against multiple
myeloma on an intermittent dose schedule.

CTX does not appear to have a therapeutic advantage in CLL
or CML over more commonly employed alkylating agents (chlorambucil
and busulfan, respectively), although it has demonstrable activity.

In a total of 77 patients with head and neck cancer, CTX has
been reported to produce a 36% response rate. However, 56 of these
patients were included in a single British study. The published
experience otherwise is too small to draw definite conclusions.

A large number of patients with uterine and cervical carcinoma,
primarily the latter, have been treated with CTX. The series of
Smith et al[80] is representative, and the largest; using a schedule
of 5-day, monthly intravenous courses in most patients, these

authors obtained an objective response in 20%. CTX is probably
as active in this tumor type as any other single agent.

Ovarian carcinoma is quite responsive to CTX, as it is to
other alkylating agents (see melphalan and chlorambucil).
Forty-four percent of 262 evaluated patients had objective
evidence of tumor regression, and there is some evidence that
patients with disseminated disease have their lifespan prolonged
by treatment with CTX.[71] In the series showing only 3 responses
in 40 evaluable patients,[81] it appears that only "poor risk"
patients received the drug alone; those who were felt to be
suitable candidates were treated with CTX + radiotherapy, with
9/22 responses.

In a small number of patients with carcinoma of the
prostate, kidney, and bladder, CTX has had reported activity
sufficient to justify consideration of trials aimed at
delineating its clinical usefulness.

In the group of "childhood" solid tumors, CTX has shown
marked effectiveness against rhabdomyosarcoma, with a clear
advantage demonstrated for use of an intermittent rather than
daily dose schedule. It is also active against neuroblastoma,
Ewing's sarcoma, and, to a lesser extent, retinoblastoma, Wilms'
tumor, and possibly osteogenic sarcoma. An important recent
study by Finklestein et al of Children's Cancer Study Group A[77]
reported increased effectiveness for the drug when administered
at 10 mg/kg/day to a median WBC of $1500/mm^3$ (usually about 10
days), with such high-dose courses repeated at approximately
monthly intervals. Of special interest was the observation
that some patients who had failed to respond, or become refractory,
at lower dosages of CTX had regressions on this regimen. Toxicity
was significant, but tolerable. (Note: the use of this schedule
in adults would almost certainly necessitate downward dose
modification, if kept on a mg/kg basis).

Tumor Type or Site

Breast

Ref #	# Pts Evaluated	# Pts Responding	% Response	Dose Schedule and Remarks
8	6	0		0.8–9.3 mg/kg/day, IV or PO, x 5 to 35 days (Majority received total dose in 5 days). Phase I study.
9	1	1		Varied; "optimal dose is between 2.5 and 3.0 mg/kg/day."
10	13	2		Varied. ECOG.
13	8	3		(1) ~7.5 mg/kg/day x 6, IV, then 6–20 mg/kg (usually 10 mg/kg)/wk or q 2 wks. (2) 45–100 mg/kg x 1, IV, then 75 to 100% of initial dose "as soon as peripheral blood count began to show a rebound from its lowest point", usually in 19–23 days, and again as tolerated.
16	10	1		100–200 mg/day, IV, to toxicity or response, then PO maintenance as tolerated.
17	20	6	30	200 mg/day, IV, to WBC of 2000, then 100–200 mg/day, PO. Four responses >6 mo duration.
18	15	6		10–20 mg/kg/day, IV, to total of 40 mg/kg, then 100–250 mg/day, PO as tolerated. All PR; 3 "good" responses.
21	12	3		30–40 mg/kg in 5–10 days, IV, then 50–150 mg/day, PO as tolerated. Two responses >2 mo duration.

Breast (cont.)

Ref #	# Pts Evaluated	# Pts Responding	% Response	Dose Schedule and Remarks
40	16	1		15 mg/kg/wk x 4, IV (as tolerated), then q 2-3 wks. Response of 4.5 mo duration.
53	24	15	62.5	100 mg on day 1, then 200 mg/day, IV, to WBC of 2000; then 50-100 mg/day, PO as tolerated. Scottish study.
54	32	7	22	40 mg/kg over 8 days, IV, or 20 days, PO; then 2 mg/kg/day x 18-24 days per month, PO. Mean response duration = 7.1 mo. Comparison study with 5-FU, which →11/30.
70	3	3		$1 \rightarrow 2.5$ gm/m^2 x 1, IV, repeated as soon as WBC returns toward normal (17-21 days; nadir reached between days 9 and 12). 1-1.5 gm/m^2= "optimal" dose.
74	20	8	40	3 mg/kg/day, PO. 5/14 postmenopausal; 3/6 premenopausal. Median remission duration = 6 mo.
78	9	4		CTX, 15 mg/kg/wk, IV; HN_2, 0.2 mg/kg/day x 2, IV, off 2 wks, then 0.1 mg/kg/wk; UM, 0.15 mg/kg/wk, PO. Uracil mustard →2/6; HN_2→1/6 (comparison). ECOG study.
	$\overline{189}$	$\overline{60}$	32	Total.
	36	11	31	Total, intermittent regimens.

Colorectal

Ref #	# Pts Evaluated	# Pts Responding	% Response	Dose Schedule and Remarks
12	2	1		Varied. "Moderate" response.
13	16	2		(1) ~7.5 mg/kg/day x 6, IV, then 6–20 mg/kg (usually 10 mg/kg)/wk or q 2 wks. (2) 45–100 mg/kg x 1, IV, then 75 to 100% of initial dose "as soon as peripheral blood count began to show a rebound from its lowest point", usually in 19–23 days, and again as tolerated. Two responses, both in carcinoma of the colon, among 16 patients with "GI tract" carcinoma.
14	16	4		Not given (for individual agents). Mean response duration = 3.5 mo. 1/16 drug deaths. $HN_2 \rightarrow 3/26$ responses; $5\text{-}FU \rightarrow 35/104$ responses. "Response" = both subjective and objective improvement (latter not defined) for $\geq$ 3 mo.
16	2	0		100–200 mg/day, IV, then PO maintenance as tolerated, to response or limiting toxicity.
78	7	0		CTX, 15 mg/kg/wk, IV; HN_2, 0.2 mg/kg/day x 2, IV, off 2 wks, then 0.1 mg/kg/wk; UM, 0.15 mg/kg/wk, PO. Uracil mustard $\rightarrow$ 0/5; $HN_2 \rightarrow$ 1/8 PR. (Comparison study). ECOG study.
	$\overline{43}$	$\overline{7}$	16	Total.

Melanoma

Ref #	# Pts Evaluated	# Pts Responding	% Response	Dose Schedule and Remarks
5	3	1		2-3 mg/kg/day, IV or PO, to response or limiting toxicity. PR.
7	2	1		1 gm/day x 7, IV or PO. PR.
8	1	0		0.8-9.3 mg/kg/day, IV or PO, x 5-35 days. (Majority received total dose in 5 days). Phase I study.
10	5	1		Varied. PR; ECOG study.
13	8	3		(1) ~7.5 mg/kg/day x 6, IV, then 6-20 mg/kg (usually 10 mg/kg)/wk or q 2 wks. (2) 45-100 mg/kg x 1, IV, then 75 to 100% of initial dose "as soon as peripheral blood count began to show a rebound from its lowest point", usually in 19-23 days, and again as tolerated.
16	1	0		100-200 mg/day, IV, to response or limiting toxicity, then PO maintenance as tolerated.
18	5	0		10-20 mg/kg/day, IV, to total of ~40 mg/kg. Then 150-200 mg/day, PO as tolerated.
31	6	2		(1) 100-200 mg/day, PO. (2) 30 mg/kg x 1, IV, then 10-15 mg/kg q 1-2 wks after WBC recovery to $\geq$ 4000. Mean remission duration = 10.3 mo. WCCG study.
	31	8	26	Total.

Lung

Ref #	# Pts Evaluated	# Pts Responding	% Response	Dose Schedule and Remarks
6	3	0		Total dose 20–40 mg/kg, IV or PO – no further details.
8	6	1		0.8–9.3 mg/kg/day x 5–35, IV or PO. (Majority received total dose in 5 days). Phase I study.
9	6	3		Varied; "optimal dose is between 2.5 and 3.0 mg/kg/day." MWCCG study.
10	30	3	10	Varied. ECOG study.
12	4	3		Varied. Two "excellent" responses.
13	9	2		(1) ~7.5 mg/kg/day x 6, then 6–20 (usually 10 mg/kg)/wk or q 2 wks. (2) 45–100 mg/kg x 1, IV, then 75–100% of initial dose "as soon as the peripheral blood count began to show a rebound from its lowest point", usually in 19–23 days, and again as tolerated.
16	7	0		100–200 mg/day, IV, to response or toxicity, then PO maintenance as tolerated.
17	27	8	30	200 mg/day, IV, to WBC of 2000, then 100–200 mg/day, PO. British study. 6 responses >3 mo duration, but all <6 mo.
18	25	5	20	10–20 mg/kg/day, IV to total of 40 mg/kg. Then 150–200 mg/day, PO as tolerated. All classed as "fair" objective responses.

Lung (cont.)

Ref #	# Pts Evaluated	# Pts Responding	% Response	Dose Schedule and Remarks
20	70	11		8 mg/kg/day x 5, IV, repeat in 28 days (CTX), -- vs 0.4 mg/kg over 2 days, IV, repeat in 28 days (HN$_2$). VA CCG study. HN$_2$→6/53 responses (difference not significant).
21	7	1		30-40 mg/kg over 5-10 days, IV; then 150-200 mg/day, PO as tolerated. PR, <2 mo duration.
31	4	0		(1) 100-200 mg/day, PO. (2) 30 mg/kg x 1, IV, followed by 10-15 mg/kg q 1-2 wks after WBC recovery to $\geq$ 4000. WCCG study.
45	157	64	41	Initial IV "loading dose", followed by daily PO maintenance as tolerated. Summed results of several reported British trials.
51	49	25	51	200 mg x 1, IV, then daily PO dosage up to 400 mg/day, to total dose 5 gm if possible (CTX), -- vs 10 mg every other day x 4, IV (HN$_2$). British study; 16/48 responses with HN$_2$ therapy. All patients also received 50 mg nandrolone phenylpropionate weekly and prednisone, 20 mg/day. No increase in survival time demonstrated.
55	13	1		400 mg/day, IV, to WBC 2000, then 100-200 mg/day, PO. British study. Patients with squamous cell carcinoma. Response = 1 mo.
55	6	3		400 mg/day, IV, to WBC 2000, then 100-200 mg/day, PO. Patients with "anaplastic" carcinoma. Mean response = 1 mo.

Lung (cont.)

Ref #	# Pts Evaluated	# Pts Responding	% Response	Dose Schedule and Remarks
55	21	21		400 mg/day, IV, to WBC 2000, then 100-200 mg/day, PO. Patients with "oat cell" carcinoma. Mean response = 6 mo.
70	35	14	40	$1 \rightarrow 2.5$ gm/m², IV, repeated as soon as WBC returns twoard normal (17-21 days; nadir reached between days 9 and 12). 1-1.5 gm/m² = "optimal" dose. MST = 142 days. MST for similar (non-randomized) prior patient group treated with HN_2 = 54 days.
76	-	-		(1) 125 mg/day x 90, PO. (2) 8 mg/kg/day x 5, IV; repeat at 30 and 60 days. (3) 200 mg/day x 5, IV; then 200 mg/day, PO as tolerated. (4) 8 mg/kg/day x 5, IV; then 200 mg/day, PO as tolerated -- vs 0.4 mg/kg/wk x 6, IV (HN_2). (Patients randomized to inert compound for each schedule above). MST = 81 days -- vs 61 for placebo (P = 0.02). See discussion.
78	30	3	10	15 mg/kg/wk, IV (CTX) -- vs 0.15 mg/kg/wk, PO (Uracil mustard) -- vs 0.2 mg/kg/day x 2, IV, off 2 wks; then 0.1 mg/kg/wk, IV (HN_2). Uracil mustard→0/30, HN_2→0/36 in Eastern Cooperative Chemotherapy Group study. Strict response criteria (>50% decrease in <u>all</u> measured lesions).
	509	168	33	Total.

Lung (cont.)

Ref #	# Pts Evaluated	# Pts Responding	% Response	Dose Schedule and Remarks
	236	46	20	Total, American studies.
	273	122	45	Total, British studies.
	114	27	24	Total, intermittent schedule (all American or Canadian). But MST ↑; see discussion.
Hodgkin's Disease				
4	3	2		50–100 mg/day, PO, to total dose 25–70 mg/kg. Both CR.
5	2	2		2–3 mg/kg/day, IV or PO, to response or limiting toxicity. Both PR.
6	3	3		20–40 mg/kg, IV or PO, total dose. No further details. None >6 mo duration.
7	12	7		1 gm/day x 7, IV or PO. 2 CR.
8	6	3		0.8–9.3 mg/kg/day x 5–35, IV or PO. (Majority received total dose in 5 days). All PR. Phase I study.
9	26	12	46	Varied; "optimal dose is 2.5–3.0 mg/kg/day." MWCCG study.
10	11	6		Varied.

Hodgkin's Disease (cont.)

Ref #	# Pts Evaluated	# Pts Responding	% Response	Dose Schedule and Remarks
16	29	14	48	100-200 mg/day, IV, to response or limiting toxicity, then PO maintenance as tolerated. Ten responses >4 mo duration.
17	5	3		200 mg/day, IV, to WBC of 2000, then 100-200 mg/day, PO. Two responses >6 mo duration.
18	41	17	41	5-10 mg/kg/day, IV, to total of ~20 mg/kg. Then 100-250 mg/day, PO as tolerated. 5 CR. SECCG study.
19	20	9	45	15 mg/kg/day x 2, IV; off 2 wks, then 10 mg/kg q 7-14 days, for 3 mo (CTX); -- vs 0.2 mg/kg/day x 2, IV; off 2 wks, then 0.1 mg/kg q 7-14 days, for 3 mo (HN_2). 3 CR. HN_2→3 CR, 10 PR of 17.
20	33	22	67	8 mg/kg/day x 5, IV; repeat in 28 days (CTX) -- vs 0.4 mg/kg over 2 days, IV; repeat in 28 days (HN_2). 0 CR. HN_2→22/31 responses, with 2 CR.
21	4	2		30-40 mg/kg over 5-10 days, IV; then 50-150 mg/day, PO as tolerated. Both responses <2 mo duration.
24	2	2		(1) 150-200 mg/m^2/day, IV or subcutaneously x 7-14 (good marrow reserve); (2) 50-150 mg/m^2/day, IV as tolerated (poor marrow reserve). Daily PO maintenance as tolerated (all patients). 1 CR; children.

Hodgkin's Disease (cont.)

Ref #	# Pts Evaluated	# Pts Responding	% Response	Dose Schedule and Remarks
31	16	6		(1) 100-200 mg/day, PO; (2) 30 mg/kg x 1, IV, then 10-15 mg/kg q 1-2 wks after WBC recovery to $\geq$ 4000. Mean remission duration = 6.8 mo. WCCG study.
34	17	9		30-40 mg/kg x 1; off 2 to 6 wks (to marrow recovery), then 3 mg/kg/day, PO as tolerated. Median response duration = 20 wks for both CTX and HN_2-treated patients. $HN_2 \rightarrow$ 11/18 responses.
40	12	3		15 mg/kg/wk, IV x 4 (as tolerated), then q 2-3 wks. Response durations: 7, 50, and 80+ wks.
41	62	43	69	Varied (? - not stated). British study.
59	14	6		2 mg/kg/day, PO as tolerated (CTX) -- vs Vinblastine. All responses PR. Vinblastine $\rightarrow$ 9 CR, 11 PR of 23.
65	8	5		7.5 mg/kg/day x 6, IV; then maintenance at 2.5 mg/kg/day, PO (CTX) -- vs 0.4 mg/kg x 1, IV (unmaintained) - (HN_2). 2 CR; cross-over comparison study with HN_2, which $\rightarrow$ 2 CR, 7 PR of 12. 5/9 HN_2-resistant patients had CR on CTX as 2nd therapy; 0/2 CTX-resistant patients had response to HN_2 as 2nd therapy. MST of patients initially treated with HN_2= 30.9 mo; of those with CTX, MST = 20.8 mo.

Hodgkin's Disease (cont.)

Ref #	# Pts Evaluated	# Pts Responding	% Response	Dose Schedule and Remarks
70	3	2		$1 \rightarrow 2.5$ gm/m^2 x 1, repeated as soon as WBC counts returned toward normal (17-21 days; nadir reached between days 9 and 12). 1-1.5 gm/m^2 = "optimal" dose.
72	86	46	53.5	15 mg/kg/wk x ~6, IV (induction). Some patients received 3 mg/kg/day, PO maintenance; others placebo. Median duration maintained remission = 32 wks (CTX). Median duration unmaintained remission = 5 wks (CTX). ECOG-ALGB study. Vinblastine $\rightarrow$18 CR, 39 PR of 88. CTX $\rightarrow$12 CR.
73	18	11		40 mg/kg x 1, IV; then daily PO maintenance (CTX) -- vs 0.4 mg/kg x 1, IV (HN$_2$); then daily chlorambucil, PO. HN$_2$-chlorambucil $\rightarrow$ 11/19, with median response = 10 mo. Median CTX response duration = 8 mo.
78	19	10		15 mg/kg/wk, IV as tolerated (CTX) -- vs 0.15 mg/kg/wk, PO as tolerated (UM) -- vs 0.2 mg/kg x 2, IV; off 2 wks, then 0.1 mg/kg/wk, IV (HN$_2$). See discussion. HN$_2$ $\rightarrow$17/26, uracil mustard (UM) $\rightarrow$6/20. MST = 7 mo for CTX-, 20 mo for UM-, and 17 mo for HN$_2$-treated patients. ECOG study.

Hodgkin's Disease (cont.)

Ref #	# Pts Evaluated	# Pts Responding	% Response	Dose Schedule and Remarks
	$\overline{452}$	$\overline{245}$	54	Total. 27 CR of 227 evaluated = 22%.
	173	92	53	Total, intermittent induction. 15 CR of 106 evaluated with weekly or biweekly induction = 14%. 0 CR of 33 evaluated on monthly induction schedule.

Lymphosarcoma

5	1	1		2-3 mg/kg/day to response or limiting toxicity. PR.
6	7	7		Total dose 20-40 mg/kg. No further details. 3/7 responses >6 mo duration.
7	1	1		1 gm/day x 7, IV or PO. CR, 8+ mo duration.
8	4	3		0.8-9.3 mg/kg/day x 5-35, IV or PO. (Majority received total dose in 5 days). All PR.
9	14	6		Varied; "optimal dose is between 2.5 and 3.0 mg/kg/day." MWCCG study.
10	6	3		Varied.
16	21	15		100-200 mg/day, IV to response or limiting toxicity; then PO maintenance as tolerated. All responses >4 mo duration.

Lymphosarcoma (cont.)

Ref #	# Pts Evaluated	# Pts Responding	% Response	Dose Schedule and Remarks
17	4	0		200 mg/day, IV to WBC 2000, then 100-200 mg/day, PO.
18	9	4		5-10 mg/kg/day, IV, to total of ~20 mg/kg. Then 100-250 mg/day, PO as tolerated. 1 CR, 3 PR. SECCG study.
20	17	12		8 mg/kg/day x 5, IV; repeat in 28 days (CTX) -- vs 0.4 mg/kg over 2 days, IV; repeat in 28 days (HN_2). 1 CR.
24	8	8		(1) 150-200 mg/m^2/day, IV or subcutaneously x 7-14 (good marrow reserve); (2) 50-150 mg/m^2/day, IV as tolerated (poor marrow reserve). Daily PO maintenance as tolerated (all patients). 5 CR. Children.
31	6	4		(1) 100-200 mg/day, PO; (2) 30 mg/kg x 1, IV, then 10-15 mg/kg q 1-2 wks after WBC recovery to $\geq$ 4000. Mean remission duration = 5.9 mo. WCCG study.
40	5	4		15 mg/kg/wk x 4, IV (as tolerated), then q 2-3 wks. 3 responses >4 mo duration.
58	65	40	62	1-3, 3-5, or 5-15 mg/kg/day, IV to response or WBC <3000, followed by daily PO maintenance as tolerated. 34 CR, 6 PR. Peruvian study.

Lymphosarcoma (cont.)

Ref #	# Pts Evaluated	# Pts Responding	% Response	Dose Schedule and Remarks
72	56	38	66	15 mg/kg/wk x ~6, IV (induction). Some patients received 3 mg/kg/day, PO maintenance; others placebo. 6 CR, 32 PR. Vincristine →3 CR, 15 PR of 47. ECOG-ALGB study. Median duration maintained remission = 12 wks (CTX). Median duration unmaintained remission = 7 wks (CTX).
73	19	9		40 mg/kg, IV "loading" dose, then daily PO maintenance as tolerated (CTX) -- vs 0.4 mg/kg x 1, IV (HN$_2$), followed by daily PO maintenance with chlorambucil. Median remission duration = 3 mo. HN$_2$-chlorambucil →8/18 responses, with median duration 7.5 mo.
78	17	13		15 mg/kg/wk, IV as tolerated (CTX) -- vs 0.15 mg/kg/wk, PO as tolerated (UM) -- vs 0.2 mg/kg x 2, IV; off 2 wks, then 0.1 mg/kg/wk, IV (HN$_2$). MST = 8 mo. Uracil mustard (UM) →3/13; HN$_2$→12/20 responses. MST with HN$_2$ = 19 mo.
79	16	5	63	1.5 gm/m^2 x 1, IV; repeated q 3 wks as tolerated. 4 CR, 1 PR. Median duration CR = 22 mo.
	$\overline{276}$	$\overline{173}$	65	Total. CR in 52/172 evaluated = 30%. CR in 18/107 evaluated in American studies = 17%.
	111	72		Total, intermittent induction schedules.

Reticulum-cell Sarcoma

Ref #	# Pts Evaluated	# Pts Responding	% Response	Dose Schedule and Remarks
5	1	1		2-3 mg/kg/day to response or limiting toxicity. PR.
6	3	3		Total dose 20-40 mg/kg. No further details. All <6 mo duration.
8	4	4		0.8-9.3 mg/kg/day x 5-35, IV or PO. (Majority received total dose in 5 days). 1 CR. Phase I study.
9	5	3		Varied; "optimal dose is between 2.5 and 3.0 mg/kg/day." 1 CR. MWCCG study.
10	6	2		Varied.
16	8	1		100-200 mg, IV to response or limiting toxicity; then PO maintenance as tolerated.
17	4	3		200 mg/day, IV to WBC 2000, then 100-200 mg/day, PO. 2 responses >3 mo duration.
18	14	11		5-10 mg/kg/day, IV, to total of ~20 mg/kg. Then 100-250 mg/day, PO as tolerated. 2 CR. SECCG study.
21	8	5		30-40 mg/kg over 5-10 days, IV; then 50-150 mg/day, PO as tolerated. 3 responses >2 mo duration.
24	2	2		(1) 150-200 mg/m²/day, IV or subcutaneously x 7-14 (good marrow reserve); (2) 50-150 mg/m²/day, IV as tolerated (poor marrow reserve).

Reticulum-cell Sarcoma (cont.)

Ref #	# Pts Evaluated	# Pts Responding	% Response	Dose Schedule and Remarks
31	9	4		Daily PO maintenance as tolerated (all patients). 0 CR. Children. (1) 100-200 mg/day, PO; (2) 30 mg/kg x 1, IV, then 10-15 mg/kg at 1-2 wk intervals after recovery to ≃ 4000 WBC. Mean remission duration = 4.0 mo. WCCG study.
40	1	0		15 mg/kg/wk x 4, IV, as tolerated, then q 2-3 wks.
58	33	26	79	1-3, 3-5, or 5-15 mg/kg/day, IV, to response or WBC <3000, then daily PO maintenance as tolerated. 19 CR. Peruvian study.
60	66	28	42.5	25-40 mg/kg over 4-5 days, IV; then daily PO maintenance as tolerated. 3 patients had response >14 mo duration. Median response = ~ 5 mo. Patients <13 years of age, with CNS involvement, or in leukemic phase did not respond.
70	3	1		1→→2.5 gm/m^2 x 1, IV, repeated as soon as WBC returned to normal (17-21 days; nadir reached between days 9 and 12). 1 to 1.5 gm/m^2 = "optimal" dose.

Reticulum-cell Sarcoma (cont.)

Ref #	# Pts Evaluated	# Pts Responding	% Response	Dose Schedule and Remarks
72	33	17	51.5	15 mg/kg/wk x ~6, IV (induction). Some patients received 3 mg/kg/day, PO maintenance; others placebo. 4 CR. Vincristine →4 CR, 8 PR of 32. ECOG-ALGB study. Median duration of maintained remission = 12-16 wks (CTX). Median duration of unmaintained remission = 6 wks (CTX).
73	7	5		40 mg/kg x 1, IV; then daily PO maintenance (CTX) -- vs 0.4 mg/kg x 1, IV (HN_2)· then daily PO maintenance (chlorambucil). Median remission duration = 3 mo. HN_2 + chlorambucil →0/5 responses.
78	10	4		15 mg/kg/wk, IV as tolerated (CTX) -- vs 0.15 mg/kg/wk, PO as tolerated (UM) -- vs 0.2 mg/kg/day x 2, IV, off 2 wks; then 0.1 mg/kg/wk, IV (HN_2)· Uracil mustard (UM) →1/6, HN_2 →1/6 responses. MST = 5 mo for CTX-, 5 mo for UM-, and 3 mo for HN_2-treated patients.
79	2	2		1.5 gm/m^2 x 1, IV; repeated q 3 wks as tolerated. 1 CR.
	219	122	56	Total. CR in 28/93 evaluated = 30%. CR in 9/60 evaluated in American studies = 15%.
	49	24	49	Total, intermittent induction schedules.

"Non-Hodgkin's Lymphoma"

Ref #	# Pts Evaluated	# Pts Responding	% Response	Dose Schedule and Remarks
12	7	5		Varied. 3 "excellent" responses, 1 in HN₂-resistant patient.
13	13	9		(1) ~7.5 mg/kg/day x 6, then 6-20 (usually 10) mg/kg/wk or q 2 wks, IV; (2) 45-100 mg/kg x 1, IV, then 75-100% of initial dose as soon as peripheral blood count began to rise (usually 19-23 days), and again as tolerated.
19	11	5		15 mg/kg/day x 2, IV; off 2 wks, then 10 mg/kg q 7-14 days, for 3 mo (CTX) -- vs 0.2 mg/kg x 2, IV; off 2 wks, then 0.1 mg/kg q 7-14 days, for 3 mo (HN₂). All PR. HN₂→2 CR, 6 PR of 14.
34	25	12	48	30-40 mg/kg x 1, IV; then (after 2-6 wks for marrow recovery), 3 mg/kg/day, PO.
59	15	10		2 mg/kg/day, PO as tolerated. 3 CR; vinblastine→1 CR, 5 PR of 17.
65	16	5		7.5 mg/kg/day x 6, IV; then 2.5 mg/kg/day, PO as tolerated (CTX) -- vs 0.4 mg/kg x 1, IV (HN₂) - unmaintained. Children. 1 CR, 4 PR, with median duration 54 days. HN₂→0 CR, 1 PR of 11, with duration 51 days.
77	2	2		10 mg/kg/day, IV or PO, to median WBC of 1500 (usually reached in 9-14 days). Repeat ~ 4 wks later. 1 CR.

"Non-Hodgkin's Lymphoma"

Ref #	# Pts Evaluated	# Pts Responding	% Response	Dose Schedule and Remarks
	89	48	54	Total. CR in 5/44 = 11%.

Burkitt's Lymphoma

Ref #	# Pts Evaluated	# Pts Responding	% Response	Dose Schedule and Remarks
52	63	52		30-40 mg/kg IV, repeat if possible in 10-14 days. 24 CR.

ALL-AUL

Ref #	# Pts Evaluated	# Pts Responding	% Response	Dose Schedule and Remarks
4	1	1 (0 CR)		50-100 mg/day, PO, to total dose 25-70 mg/kg. 1 mo duration.
8	1	1 (0 CR)		0.8-9.3 mg/kg/day x 5-35 days, IV "loading" followed by PO maintenance. (Majority received total dose in 5 days). Phase I study.
11	7	0		4 mg/kg/day, IV or PO, often IV x 14, then PO as tolerated. All received concomitant prednisone or halotestin.
24	16	11 (2 CR)		(1) 150-200 mg/m^2/day, IV or subcutaneously x 7-14 days. Then daily PO maintenance. (2) 50-150 mg/m^2/day, IV (for poor marrow reserve) as tolerated, followed by daily PO maintenance.

ALL-AUL (cont.)

Ref #	# Pts Evaluated	# Pts Responding	% Response	Dose Schedule and Remarks
25	25	10 (5 CR)	40	15 mg/kg/wk, IV, to response or limiting toxicity. All patients unresponsive to 6 MP, MTX, and prednisone. 8 patients received <21 days treatment, classed as inadequate trials. CR = 20% of total, 47% of adequate trials.
26	44	13 (8 CR)	30	(1) "Priming" IV dose, then 2-7.5 mg/kg/day PO maintenance. (2) 5 mg/kg/day, PO; then 2.5 mg/kg/day, PO. (50% of patients received "steroids" concomitantly). Steroid administration did not influence response rate (all patients were unresponsive to steroids, 6 MP, and MTX). No effect on CNS leukemia. 10/44 = 23% had M_1 marrows. SWCCG study.
27	17	1 (0 CR)		2 mg/kg/day, PO, to response or limiting toxicity. ALGB study. All children previously treated. Daily dose less than that in other studies.
27	33	6 (2 CR)	18	10 mg/kg/wk, PO, to response or limiting toxicity. ALGB study. All children previously treated.
27	14	2 (1 CR)		Weekly "sliding scale", starting at 10 mg/kg, PO, and adjusted down as appropriate. ALGB study. All children previously treated.

ALL-AUL (cont.)

Ref #	# Pts Evaluated	# Pts Responding	% Response	Dose Schedule and Remarks
31	2	0		(1) 100-200 mg/day, PO or (2) 30 mg/kg x 1, IV, followed by 10-15 mg/kg at 1 to 2 wk intervals after recovery to $\geq$ 4000 WBC. WCCG study.
61	73	25 (9 CR)	34	3 mg/kg/day, PO as tolerated. CCGA study. Median duration disease prior to CTX = 228 days. 18/73 = 25% had M_1 marrows. 12 patients received <28 days treatment, classed as inadequate trials. CR = 12% of total, 15% of adequate trials.
61	69	11 (1 CR)	16	15 mg/kg/wk, IV as tolerated. CCGA study. Median duration disease prior to CTX = 228 days. 1/69 = 1.4% had M_1 marrow. 11 patients received <4 weekly injections, classed as inadequate trials. CR = 1.4% of total, 1.7% of adequate trials.
62,63	-	-		5 mg/kg/day, PO (CTX) + 2.2 mg/kg/day, PO (Prednisone), -- vs 2.5 mg/kg/day, PO (6 MP) + 2.2 mg/kg/day, PO (Prednisone). See discussion. Previously untreated children, combination study (SWCCG).
64	45	20 (18 CR)	44	5 mg/kg/day, PO as tolerated. SWCCG study. Previously untreated patients. No other antileukemic therapy given. Mean days to CR = 53. 19/45 = 42% had M_1 marrows. CR = 40% of total.

ALL-AUL (cont.)

Ref #	# Pts Evaluated	# Pts Responding	% Response	Dose Schedule and Remarks
	347	$\overline{101}$ (46 CR)	29	Total. CR = 13%.
	45	20 (18 CR)	44	Total, previously untreated patients. CR = 40%.
	302	31 (28 CR)	27	Total, previously treated patients. CR = 9%.
	161	52 (19 CR)	32	Total, previously treated patients - daily schedule. CR = 12%. M_1 marrow reported in 28/117 = 24%.
	141	29 (9 CR)	21	Total, previously treated patients - weekly schedule. CR = 6%.

AML-AMoL

Ref #	# Pts Evaluated	# Pts Responding	% Response	Dose Schedule and Remarks
4	1	1 (0 CR)		50-100 mg/day, PO, to total dose 25-70 mg/kg. Response duration 3 mo.
8	6	0		0.8-9.3 mg/kg/day x 5-35 days, IV "loading" followed by PO maintenance. (Majority received total dose in 5 days). Phase I study.
10	2	0		Varied. ECOG study.

AML-AMoL (cont.)

Ref #	# Pts Evaluated	# Pts Responding	% Response	Dose Schedule and Remarks
11	2	0		4 mg/kg/day, IV or PO, often IV x 14, then PO as tolerated. All received concomitant prednisone or halotestin.
16	15	5 (1 CR)		100-200 mg/day, IV or PO, to response or limiting toxicity.
27	45	2 (0 CR)	4.5	(1) 2 mg/kg/day, PO. (2) 10 mg/kg/wk, PO. (3) "Sliding scale" - weekly - 10 mg/kg initially, PO. ALGB study.
31	4	0		(1) 100-200 mg/day, PO or (2) 30 mg/kg x 1, IV, followed by 10-15 mg/kg at 1 to 2 wk intervals after recovery to ≥ 4000 WBC. WCCG study.
	$\overline{76}$	$\overline{8}$ (1 CR)	10	Total. CR = 1.3%.

Multiple Myeloma

Ref #	# Pts Evaluated	# Pts Responding	% Response	Dose Schedule and Remarks
7	4	3		1 gm/day x 7, IV or PO.

Multiple Myeloma (cont.)

Ref #	# Pts Evaluated	# Pts Responding	% Response	Dose Schedule and Remarks
8	1	0		0.8-9.3 mg/kg/day x 5-35 days, IV "loading" followed by PO maintenance. (Majority received total dose in 5 days). Phase I study.
9	12	0		Varied. MWCCG study. 11 patients had no change in disease status.
10	3	0		Varied.
12	5	0		Varied.
16	16	9		100-200 mg/day, IV or PO, to response or limiting toxicity. None had ↓ in M-protein. "Response" parameters largely subjective.
17	2	0		200 mg/day, IV, to WBC 2000, then PO maintenance at 100-200 mg/day.
30	29	6	21	4 mg/kg/day, PO, as tolerated. 0/25 patients on placebo had objective response. MST = 49 wks for CTX-treated patients, 15 wks for placebo-treated (P <.005). VACCG study.
31	6	1		(1) 100-200 mg/day, PO, or (2) 30 mg/kg x 1, IV, followed by 10-15 mg/kg at 1 to 2 wk intervals after recovery to $\geq$ 4000 WBC. WCCG study.

Multiple Myeloma (cont.)

Ref #	# Pts Evaluated	# Pts Responding	% Response	Dose Schedule and Remarks
35	19	16		1.5 mg/kg/day, PO. (Initial IV "loading dose" sometimes given). 4 "good" and 12 "partial" objective responses.
39	165	~41	25	2 mg/kg/day, PO, as tolerated. 24% of patients received prednisone at some time during study. 165 CTX-treated "adequate trials" had MST = 32 mo. 162 controls had MST 9.5 mo. All patients placed on CTX, including inadequate trials, had MST = 24.5 mo. 20% of "adequately" (60 days or more) CTX-treated patients alive at 56 mo; 12% of controls alive at 50 mo.
40	5	0		15 mg/kg/wk, IV, as tolerated x 4, then q 2-3 wks.
42	62	18	29	2-3 gm over 10-15 days, IV, then 150 mg/day PO as tolerated. Summed results of several Btitish trials.
56	8	2		200 mg/day to WBC ~2000, then 50-100 mg/day, PO maintenance. Response included restoration of normal calcium balance.
69	26	15	58	200 mg/day, IV to <3000 WBC, then PO maintenance at 50-100 mg/day. Median response duration = 15 mo.

Multiple Myeloma (cont.)

Ref #	# Pts Evaluated	# Pts Responding	% Response	Dose Schedule and Remarks
75	50	9	18	4 mg/kg/day, PO as tolerated (CTX) -- vs 0.1 mg/kg/day, PO as tolerated (L-PAM). VACCG-PVACCG study. MST 12.3 mo. Melphalan →8/53, with MST 15.5 mo.
	413	120	29	Total. All studies are with continuous dose schedule.
CLL				
5	6	0		2-3 mg/kg/day, IV or PO, to response or limiting toxicity.
7	3	1		1 gm/day x 7, IV or PO.
9	19	8		Varied. MWCCG study.
10	5	1		Varied. ECOG study.
16	8	4		100-200 mg/day, IV or PO, to response or limiting toxicity.
18	28	11	39	5-10 mg/kg/day, IV, to total of ~20 mg/kg. Then 100-250 mg/day, PO as tolerated. 3 "good", 8 "fair" responses. SECCG study.

CLL (cont.)

Ref #	# Pts Evaluated	# Pts Responding	% Response	Dose Schedule and Remarks
31	25	14	56	100-200 mg/day, PO or (2) 30 mg/kg x 1, IV, followed by 10-15 mg/kg at 1 to 2 wk intervals after recovery to $\geq$ 4000 WBC. WCCG study. Mean remission duration = 8.3 mo.
33	18	2		2 mg/kg/day, PO (CTX), for 8-12 wks -- vs 0.2 mg/kg/day, PO (Chlorambucil), for 8-12 wks. VACCG study. Chlorambucil →6/21 responses.
36	12	5		(1) 20 mg/kg, PO, q 2 wks = high-dose intermittent (CTX). (2) 2 mg/kg/day, PO, as tolerated = daily continuous (CTX). -- vs (1) 0.2 mg/kg, PO, q 2 wks = high-dose intermittent (Uracil mustard). (2) 0.02 mg/kg/day, PO, as tolerated = daily continuous (Uracil mustard).
43	18	14		Not stated. British study.
	142	60	42	Total.

CML

Ref #	# Pts Evaluated	# Pts Responding	% Response	Dose Schedule and Remarks
5	4	4		2-3 mg/kg/day, IV or PO, to response or limiting toxicity. All PR.

CML (cont.)

Ref #	# Pts Evaluated	# Pts Responding	% Response	Dose Schedule and Remarks
11	1	0		4 mg/kg/day, IV or PO, often IV x 14, then PO as tolerated. Patient treated concomitantly with steroid.
31	11	6		100-200 mg/day, PO or (2) 30 mg/kg x 1, IV, followed by 10-15 mg/kg at 1 to 2 wk intervals after recovery to ≥ 4000 WBC. WCCG study. Mean response duration = 4.2 mo.
36	15	4		20 mg/kg q 2 wks, PO (CTX) -- vs 0.2 mg/kg q 2 wks, PO (UM). SECCG study. Uracil mustard (UM) →7/16 responses.
36	16	7		2 mg/kg/day, PO as tolerated (CTX) -- vs 0.02 mg/kg/day, PO as tolerated (UM). SECCG study. Uracil mustard (UM) →14/16 responses.
	47	21	44.5	Total.

Head and Neck

Ref #	# Pts Evaluated	# Pts Responding	% Response	Dose Schedule and Remarks
8	4	1		0.8-9.3 mg/kg/day x 5-35 days, IV "loading" followed by PO maintenance. (Majority received total dose in 5 days). Phase I study.
10	10	0		Varied. ECOG study.

Head and Neck (cont.)

Ref #	# Pts Evaluated	# Pts Responding	% Response	Dose Schedule and Remarks
12	4	4		Varied. 2 "excellent" responses.
31	3	1		100-200 mg/day, PO or (2) 30 mg/kg x 1, IV, followed by 10-15 mg/kg at 1 to 2 wk intervals after recovery to $\geq$ 4000 WBC. Response of 7 mo duration.
44	56	22	39	(1) 40 mg/kg intraarterially, single dose. (2) 4 mg/kg/day, PO, to limiting toxicity. (3) 40-60 mg/kg/day, IV, to limiting toxicity. 2 CR. British study. No breakdown of tumor response by dose schedule used.
	$\overline{77}$	$\overline{28}$	36	Total.

Cervix and Uterus

Ref #	# Pts Evaluated	# Pts Responding	% Response	Dose Schedule and Remarks
8	9	1		0.8-9.3 mg/kg/day x 5-35 days, IV "loading" followed by PO maintenance. (Majority received total dose in 5 days). Phase I study. All cervical carcinoma.
10	28	5	18	Varied. ECOG study. All cervical carcinoma.

Cervix and Uterus (cont.)

Ref #	# Pts Evaluated	# Pts Responding	% Response	Dose Schedule and Remarks
13	3	1		(1) 7.5 mg/kg/day x 6, IV, then 6-20 mg/kg (usually 10 mg/kg)/wk or biweekly. (2) 45 to 100 mg/kg x 1, IV, then 75 to 100% of initial dose "as soon as peripheral blood count began to show a rebound from its lowest point," usually in 19-23 days, and again as tolerated. All cervical carcinoma.
18	7	0		10-20 mg/kg/day, IV, to total of ~40 mg/kg. Then 100-250 mg/day, PO as tolerated. SECCG study. "Cervix and uterus".
21	10	4		30-40 mg/kg over 5-10 days, IV; then PO daily maintenance as tolerated (50-150 mg/day). 3/8 responses, all >2 mo, in uterine; 1/2, <2 mo, in cervical carcinoma.
31	2	0		(1) 100-200 mg/day, PO or (2) 30 mg/kg x 1, IV, followed by 10-15 mg/kg at 1 to 2 wk intervals after recovery to $\geq$ 4000 WBC. WCCG study. Both cervical carcinoma.
57	42	9	21	3-4.5 mg/kg/day, IV, to WBC <3000, then PO maintenance at daily dose to maintain WBC <3000. Peruvian study. All cervical carcinoma. 6 CR, one of 25 mo duration. No response of pelvic or abdominopelvic disease.

Cervix and Uterus (cont.)

Ref #	# Pts Evaluated	# Pts Responding	% Response	Dose Schedule and Remarks
78	10	1		15 mg/kg/wk, IV as tolerated (CTX) -- vs 0.15 mg/kg/wk, PO as tolerated (UM) -- vs 0.2 mg/kg/day x 2, IV, off 2 wks, then 0.1 mg/kg/wk, IV (HN$_2$). ECOG study. Uracil mustard (UM) →1/12, HN$_2$ →0/4 responses.
80	76	15	20	(1) 8 mg/kg/day x 5, IV; repeat q 4-6 wks (78 patients). (2) 2.5 mg/kg/day, PO, as tolerated (6 patients). (3) 8 mg/kg/day x 5, IV; then 2.5 mg/kg/day, PO as tolerated (7 patients). All responses between 3 and 10 mo duration (mean = 5 mo). Melphalan →4/20 responses.
	$\overline{187}$	$\overline{36}$	19	Total.

Ovary

6	3	3		Total dose 20-40 mg/kg, IV or PO, duration not given. No responses >6 mo.
8	3	2		0.8-9.3 mg/kg/day x 5-35 days, IV "loading" followed by PO maintenance. (Majority received total dose in 5 days). Phase I study.

Ovary (cont.)

Ref #	# Pts Evaluated	# Pts Responding	% Response	Dose Schedule and Remarks
10	22	7	32	Varied. ECOG study.
11	2	1		4 mg/kg/day, IV or PO, often IV x 14, then PO as tolerated.
12	1	1		Varied. "Excellent" response.
13	9	6		(1) ~7.5 mg/kg/day x 6, IV, then 6-20 mg/kg (usually 10 mg/kg)/wk or biweekly. (2) 45 to 100 mg/kg x 1, IV, then 75 to 100% of initial dose "as soon as peripheral blood count began to show a rebound from its lowest point," usually in 19-23 days, and again as tolerated.
17	1	0		200 mg/day, IV, to WBC 2000, then PO maintenance at 100-200 mg/day.
18	13	1		10-20 mg/kg/day, IV, to total of ~40 mg/kg. Then 100-250 mg/day, PO as tolerated. CR; no PR. SECCG study.
21	7	6		30-40 mg/kg over 5-10 days, IV; then PO daily maintenance as tolerated (50-150 mg/day). 4 responses >2 mo duration.
31	5	3		(1) 100-200 mg/day, PO or (2) 30 mg/kg x 1, IV, followed by 10-15 mg/kg at 1 to 2 wk intervals after recovery to ≥ 4000 WBC. 2 CR. WCCG study.

Ovary (cont.)

Ref #	# Pts Evaluated	# Pts Responding	% Response	Dose Schedule and Remarks
46	17	12		100 mg/day PO – occasionally preceded by IV "loading dose". British study.
47	6	5		IV "loading dose", then PO maintenance as tolerated. British study.
71	126	62	49	~200 mg/day x 10, IV or ~50–150 mg/day, PO. Canadian study. MST 20 mo. MST of (retrospective) control group treated only with surgery and radiation therapy = 11 mo.
78	7	3		15 mg/kg/wk, IV as tolerated (CTX) –– vs 0.15 mg/kg/wk, PO as tolerated (UM) –– vs 0.2 mg/kg/day x 2, IV, off 2 wks, then 0.1 mg/kg/wk (HN$_2$). Uracil mustard (UM) →1/9, HN$_2$ →4/8 responses.
81	40	3	7.5	400 mg/day x 4, IV; then 50–150 mg/day PO maintenance. Response durations 3, 18, and 22 mo. CTX + radiation therapy →9/22 responses, median duration 16 mo.
	$\overline{262}$	$\overline{115}$	44	Total. Intermittent schedules →9/16 responses.

Prostate

| 10 | 8 | 2 | | Varied. ECOG study. |

Prostate (cont.)

Ref #	# Pts Evaluated	# Pts Responding	% Response	Dose Schedule and Remarks
13	1	0		(1) ~7.5 mg/kg/day x 6, IV, then 6-20 mg/kg (usually 10 mg/kg)/wk or biweekly. (2) 45 to 100 mg/kg x 1, IV, then 75 to 100% of initial dose "as soon as peripheral blood count began to show a rebound from its lowest point," usually in 19-23 days, and again as tolerated.
31	1	0		(1) 100-200 mg/day, PO or (2) 30 mg/kg x 1, IV, followed by 10-15 mg/kg at 1 to 2 wk intervals after recovery to $\geq$ 4000 WBC. WCCG study.
50	3	1		(1) 400-500 mg/day, IV, to WBC of ~1000; then PO maintenance as tolerated after marrow recovery. (2) 200-800 mg/day, IV, over 6 days; then PO maintenance as tolerated after marrow recovery. British study. Duration response = 35 wks.
$\overline{13}$		$\overline{3}$	23	Total.

Kidney

8	1	1		0.8-9.3 mg/kg/day x 5-35 days, IV "loading" followed by PO maintenance. (Majority received total dose in 5 days). PR. Phase I study.

Kidney (cont.)

Ref #	# Pts Evaluated	# Pts Responding	% Response	Dose Schedule and Remarks
10	6	0		Varied. ECOG study.
13	1	0		(1) ~7.5 mg/kg/day x 6, IV, then 6–20 mg/kg (usually 10 mg/kg)/wk or biweekly. (2) 45 to 100 mg/kg x 1, IV, then 75 to 100% of initial dose "as soon as peripheral blood count began to show a rebound from its lowest point," usually in 19–23 days, and again as tolerated.
21	5	1		30–40 mg/kg over 5–10 days, IV; then PO daily maintenance as tolerated (50–150 mg/day). Response >2 mo duration.
31	1	0		100–200 mg/day, PO or (2) 30 mg/kg x 1, IV, followed by 10–15 mg/kg at 1 to 2 wk intervals after recovery to ≥ 4000 WBC. WCCG study.
50	7	2		(1) 400–500 mg/day, IV, to WBC of ~1000; then PO maintenance as tolerated after marrow recovery. (2) 200–800 mg/day, IV, over 6 days; then PO maintenance as tolerated after marrow recovery. Response durations 5 and 42 wks.
	$\overline{21}$	$\overline{4}$	19	Total.

Bladder

Ref #	# Pts Evaluated	# Pts Responding	% Response	Dose Schedule and Remarks
10	2	0		Varied. ECOG study.
50	8	2		(1) 400-500 mg/day, IV, to WBC of ~1000; then PO maintenance as tolerated after marrow recovery. (2) 200-800 mg/day, IV, over 6 days; then PO maintenance as tolerated after marrow recovery. British study. Response durations <1 mo.
	$\overline{10}$	$\overline{2}$	20	Total.

Brain Tumors – Primary

Ref #	# Pts Evaluated	# Pts Responding	% Response	Dose Schedule and Remarks
32	2	0		5 mg/kg/day, IV or PO.
39	12	0		400 mg/day, IV, to WBC <2000, then ~100 mg/day PO.
	$\overline{14}$	$\overline{0}$		

Pancreas

Ref #	# Pts Evaluated	# Pts Responding	% Response	Dose Schedule and Remarks
8	1	0		0.8-9.3 mg/kg/day x 5-35 days, IV "loading" followed by PO maintenance. (Majority received total dose in 5 days). Phase I study.

Pancreas (cont.)

Ref #	# Pts Evaluated	# Pts Responding	% Response	Dose Schedule and Remarks
17	2	0		200 mg/day, IV, to WBC of 2000, then 100–200 mg/day, PO.
31	2	1		(1) 100–200 mg/day, PO or (2) 30 mg/kg x 1, IV, followed by 10–15 mg/kg at 1 to 2 wk intervals after recovery to $\geq$ 4000 WBC. Remission duration = 8 mo. WCCG study.
	$\overline{5}$	$\overline{1}$	20	Total.

Rhabdomyosarcoma

4	1	1		50–100 mg/day, PO, to total dose 25–70 mg/kg. CR, 3 mo duration.
7	1	0		1 gm/day x 7, IV or PO.
8	2	1		0.8–9.3 mg/kg/day x 5–35 days, IV "loading" followed by PO maintenance. (Majority received total dose in 5 days). PR. Phase I study.
24	1	1		(1) 150–200 mg/m^2/day, IV or subcutaneously x 7–14 days. Then daily PO maintenance. (2) 50–150 mg/m^2/day, IV (for poor marrow reserve) as tolerated, followed by daily PO maintenance. PR.

Rhabdomyosarcoma (cont.)

Ref #	# Pts Evaluated	# Pts Responding	% Response	Dose Schedule and Remarks
28	7	3		Low-dose daily treatment, PO (most patients) – a few received 600 mg/m^2/wk, IV. All PR; duration 42, 56, and 105 days.
29	4	0		5-5.5 mg/kg/day x 10-13, IV, then PO maintenance as tolerated.
68	11	3		5 mg/kg/day x 10, IV. Then 2.5-5 mg/kg/day, PO. All PR.
68	14	11		30 mg/kg/wk x $\geq$ 4, IV or PO. 7 "good" (>50%), 4 <50% regressions. SWCCG study.
77	5	4		10 mg/kg/day, IV or PO, to median WBC of >1500 (usually reached in 9-14 days). Repeat – 4 wks later. 3 CR, all PR's >50%. CCGA study.
82	10	9		30 mg/kg/wk, PO or IV. 5 "good" responses. SWCCG study.
	56	33	59	Total.
	29	24	83	Total, intermittent schedules.
	27	9	33	Total, daily schedules.

Neuroblastoma

Ref #	# Pts Evaluated	# Pts Responding	% Response	Dose Schedule and Remarks
11	1	1		4 mg/kg/day, IV or PO, often IV x 14, then PO as tolerated.
15	9	5		5-10 mg/kg/day x 7-10, IV. All PR.
24	5	4		(1) 150-200 mg/m^2/day, IV or subcutaneously x 7-14 days. Then daily PO maintenance. (2) 50-150 mg/m^2/day, IV (for poor marrow reserve) as tolerated, followed by daily PO maintenance. 3 CR.
28	8	3		Low-dose daily treatment (most patients) - a few received 600 mg/m^2/wk, IV. Transient PR.
38	24	19	79	5 mg/kg/day x 10, IV; then 2.5 mg/kg/day, PO, as tolerated. SWCCG study. 10 "good" responses.
68	21	11	52	30 mg/kg/wk, PO or IV x $\geq$ 4 wks. SWCCG study. 4 "good" responses. 7 patients had received CTX in initial daily-dose study (Ref #38), of whom 3 obtained PR with high-dose intermittent therapy.
77	10	9		10 mg/kg/day, IV or PO, to median WBC of >1500 (usually reached in 9-14 days). Repeat - 4 wks later. CCGA study. 4 CR; all PR >50% regression.
	78	52	67	Total.

Wilms' Tumor

Ref #	# Pts Evaluated	# Pts Responding	% Response	Dose Schedule and Remarks
4	2	0		50-100 mg/day, PO, to total dose 25-70 gm.
23	11	2		5-5.5 mg/kg/day x 10-13, IV, then PO maintenance as tolerated. Both PR. SWCCG study.
68	22	7		5 mg/kg/day x 10, IV, then 2.5-5 mg/kg/day, PO. All PR. SWCCG study.
68	5	1		30 mg/kg/wk x $\geq$ 4, IV or PO. PR. SWCCG study.
77	3	2		10 mg/kg/day, IV or PO, to median WBC of $>$1500 (usually reached in 9-14 days). Repeat ~ 4 wks later. Both PR. CCGA study.
	$\overline{45}$	$\overline{12}$	27	Total.

Ewing's Sarcoma

7	1	1		1 gm/day x 7, IV or PO. PR.
11	1	1		4 mg/kg/day, IV or PO, often IV x 14, then PO as tolerated. PR.
24	2	1		(1) 150-200 mg/m^2/day, IV or subcutaneously x 7-14 days. Then daily PO maintenance. (2) 50-150 mg/m^2/day, IV (for poor marrow reserve) as tolerated, followed by daily PO maintenance. CR.

Ewing's Sarcoma (cont.)

Ref #	# Pts Evaluated	# Pts Responding	% Response	Dose Schedule and Remarks
28	2	1		Low-dose daily treatment (most patients) – a few received 600 mg/m²/wk, IV. CR.
66	13	7		Varied; often 5 mg/kg/day, PO as tolerated. SWCCG study. (Includes data in Ref #22).
77	2	2		10 mg/kg/day, IV or PO, to median WBC of >1500 (usually reached in 9-14 days). Repeat ~ 4 wks later. CCGA study. 1 CR. 1 patient responded to high dose regimen after lesser dosages had failed.
	$\overline{21}$	$\overline{13}$	62	Total.

Retinoblastoma

Ref #	# Pts Evaluated	# Pts Responding	% Response	Dose Schedule and Remarks
21	16	2		30-40 mg/kg over 5-10 days, IV; then PO daily maintenance as tolerated (50-150 mg/day). Both >2 mo response.
66	9	5		Varied; often 5 mg/kg/day, PO as tolerated. SWCCG study.
	$\overline{25}$	$\overline{7}$	28	Total.

Osteogenic Sarcoma

Ref #	# Pts Evaluated	# Pts Responding	% Response	Dose Schedule and Remarks
28	3	1		Low-dose daily treatment (most patients) - a few received 600 mg/m² /wk, IV. PR of pulmonary metastases.
66	11	0		Varied; often 5 mg/kg/day, PO as tolerated. SWCCG study.
77	2	1		10 mg/kg/day, IV or PO, to median WBC of 1500 (usually reached in 9-14 days). Repeat ≥ 4 wks later. CCGA study. PR in patient who responded to high dose regimen after lesser dosages had failed.
	$\overline{16}$	$\overline{2}$	12.5	Total.

References

(1)   Arnold, H., Bourseaux, F., and Brock, N. Chemotherapeutic
        action of a cyclic nitrogen mustard phosphamide ester
        (B-518-ASTA) in experimental tumors of the rat. Nature 181:
        931, 1958.

(2)   Foley, G., Friedman, O., and Drolet, B. Studies on the
        mechanism of action of Cytoxan. Evidence of activation
        in vivo and in vitro. Cancer Res 21: 57, 1961.

(3)   Santos, G., Owens, A., and Sensenbrenner, L. Effects of
        selected cytotoxic agents on antibody production in man:
        a preliminary report. Ann NY Acad Sci 114: 404, 1964.

(4)   Cramblett, H. Experience with cyclophosphamide in treatment
        of childhood tumors. In "Antibiotics Annual, 1959-1960",
        Antibiotica, Inc., New York; pp 966-969, 1960.

(5)   Haar, H., Marshall, J., Bierman, H., et al. The influence
        of cyclophosphamide upon neoplastic diseases in man.
        Cancer Chemother Rep 6: 41, 1960.

(6)   Papac, R., Petrakis, N., Amini, F., et al. Comparative
        clinical evaluation of two alkylating agents - mannitol
        mustard and cyclophosphamide (Cytoxan). JAMA 172: 1387,
        1960.

(7)   Korst, D., Johnson, F., Frenkel, E., et al. Preliminary
        evaluation of the effect of cyclophosphamide on the course
        of human neoplasms. Cancer Chemother Rep 7: 1, 1960.

(8)   Bergsagel, D., and Levin, W. A prelusive clinical trial
        of cyclophosphamide. Cancer Chemother Rep 8: 120, 1960.

(9)   Bethell, F., Louis, J., Robbins, A., et al. Phase II
        evaluation of cyclophosphamide. A study by the Midwest
        Cooperative Chemotherapy Group. Cancer Chemother Rep 8:
        112, 1960.

(10)   Shnider, B., Gold, G., Hall, T., et al. Preliminary
        studies with cyclophosphamide. Cancer Chemother Rep 8:
        106, 1960.

(11)   Spurr, C., and Hayes, D. Clinical observations on newer
        chemotherapeutic agents. South Med J 53: 1005, 1960.

(12) Foye, L., Chapman, C., Willett, F., et al. Cyclophosphamide.
      A preliminary study of a new alkylating agent. Arch Intern
      Med 106: 365, 1960.

(13) Coggins, P., Ravdin, R., and Eisman, S. Clinical evaluation
      of a new alkylating agent: Cytoxan (cyclophosphamide).
      Cancer 13: 1254, 1960.

(14) Hurley, J., Ellison, E., and Carey, L. Treatment of
      advanced cancer of the gastrointestinal tract with antitumor
      agents. Gastroenterology 41: 557, 1961.

(15) Kontras, S., and Newton, W. Cyclophosphamide (Cytoxan)
      therapy of childhood neuroblastoma. Preliminary report.
      Cancer Chemother Rep 12: 39, 1961.

(16) Wall, R., and Conrad, F. Cyclophosphamide therapy. Its
      use in leukemia, lymphoma and solid tumors. Arch Intern
      Med 108: 456, 1961.

(17) Anders, C., and Kemp, N. Cyclophosphamide in treatment
      of disseminated malignant disease. Brit Med J 2: 1516, 1961.

(18) Rundles, R., Laszlo, J., Garrison, F., et al. The antitumor
      spectrum of cyclophosphamide. Cancer Chemother Rep 16: 407,
      1962.

(19) Laszlo, J., Grizzle, J., Jonsson, U., et al. Comparative
      study of mannitol mustard, cyclophosphamide, and nitrogen
      mustard in malignant lymphomas. Cancer Chemother Rep 16:
      247, 1962.

(20) Spear, P., and Patno, M. A comparative study of the
      effectiveness of HN_2 and cyclophosphamide in bronchogenic
      carcinoma, Hodgkin's disease, and lymphosarcoma. Cancer
      Chemother Rep 16: 413, 1962.

(21) Atkins, H., Gregg, H., and Hyman, G. Clinical appraisal
      of cyclophosphamide in malignant neoplasms. Cancer 15:
      1076, 1962.

(22) Sutow, W., and Sullivan, M. Cyclophosphamide therapy in
      children with Ewing's sarcoma. Cancer Chemother Rep 23:
      55, 1962.

(23) Haddy, T., Whitaker, J., Vietti, T., et al. Clinical
      trials with cyclophosphamide (Cytoxan) in children with
      Wilms' tumor - preliminary report. Cancer Chemother
      Rep 25: 81, 1962.

(24) Sweeney, M., Tuttle, A., Etteldorf, J., et al.
      Cyclophosphamide in the treatment of common neoplastic
      diseases of childhood. J Pediat 61: 702, 1962.

(25) Brubaker, C., Sonley, K., Hyman, C., et al. Cyclophosphamide
      therapy of acute leukemia in children. Clin Res 10: 107, 1962.

(26) Fernbach, D., Sutow, W., Thurman, W., et al. Clinical
      evaluation of cyclophosphamide. A new agent for the
      treatment of children with acute leukemia. JAMA 182: 30,
      1962.

(27) Hoogstratten, B. Cyclophosphamide in acute leukemia.
      Cancer Chemother Rep 16: 167, 1962.

(28) Pinkel, D. Cyclophosphamide in children with cancer. Cancer
      15: 42, 1962.

(29) Steinberg, J., Haddy, T., Porter, F., et al. Clinical
      trials with cyclophosphamide in children with soft tissue
      sarcoma. Cancer Chemother Rep 28: 39, 1963.

(30) Rivers, S., Whittington, R., and Patno, M. Comparison of
      effect of cyclophosphamide and a placebo in treatment of
      multiple myeloma. Cancer Chemother Rep 29: 115, 1963.

(31) Solomon, J., Alexander, M., and Steinfeld, J. Cyclophosphamide.
      A clinical study. JAMA 183: 165, 1963.

(32) Holcomb, T., Haggard, M., and Windmiller, J. Cyclophosphamide
      (NSC 26271) in uncommon malignant neoplasms in children.
      Cancer Chemother Rep 36: 73, 1964.

(33) Kaung, D., Whittington, R., and Patno, M. Treatment of chronic
      lymphocytic leukemia with chlorambucil and cyclophosphamide.
      Cancer Chemother Rep 39: 41, 1964.

(34) Papac, R., and Wood, D. Long term results achieved with
      the use of alkylating agents in malignant lymphoma and
      Hodgkin's disease. Acta Un Int Contra Cancer 20: 377, 1964.

(35) Korst, D., Frenkel, E., and Nixon, J. Multiple myeloma.
      Studies of mouse plasma cell tumor and human myeloma
      responsiveness to cyclophosphamide (Cytoxan). Ann Intern
      Med 60: 217, 1964.

(36) Frommeyer, W. Comparison of cyclophosphamide (Cytoxan) and
      uracil mustard (U-8344) in chronic granulocytic leukemia.
      Cancer 17: 288, 1964.

(37) Korst, D., Clifford, G., Fowler, W., et al. Multiple myeloma - II. Analysis of cyclophosphamide therapy in 165 patients. JAMA 189: 758, 1964.

(38) Thurman, W., Fernbach, D., and Sullivan, M. Cyclophosphamide therapy in childhood neuroblastoma. New Eng J Med 270: 1336, 1964.

(39) Rose, F., Meikle, R., and Lord, P. Endoxana (cyclophosphamide) in the treatment of intracerebral malignancy. J Neurol Neurosurg Psychiat 27: 470, 1964.

(40) Foley, J., and Kennedy, B. Effect of cyclophosphamide on far-advanced neoplasia. Cancer Chemother Rep 34: 55, 1964.

(41) Fairley, G., and Healy, J. Hodgkin's disease. In "Cyclophosphamide" (Fairley, G., and Simister, J., eds.), Williams and Wilkins Co., Baltimore; pp 1-4, 1965.

(42) Matthias, J., Newall, J., Pugh, D., et al. Myeloma. In "Cyclophosphamide" (Fairley, G., and Simister, J., eds.), Williams and Wilkins Co., Baltimore; pp 7-15, 1965.

(43) Fairley, G., and Hall, R. Leukemia. In "Cyclophosphamide" (Fairley, G., and Simister, J., eds.), Williams and Wilkins Co., Baltimore; pp 16-18, 1965.

(44) Harrison, D., Espiner, H., and Glazebrook, G. Cyclophosphamide in head and neck cancer. In "Cyclophosphamide" (Fairley, G., and Simister, J., eds.), Williams and Wilkins Co., Baltimore; pp 48-55, 1965.

(45) Ross, W., Jack, G., Helm, W., et al. Carcinoma of the lung. In "Cyclophosphamide" (Fairley, G., and Simister, J., eds.), Williams and Wilkins Co., Baltimore; pp 55-82, 1965.

(46) Anderson, T. Carcinoma of the ovary. In "Cyclophosphamide" (Fairley, G., and Simister, J., eds.), Williams and Wilkins Co., Baltimore; pp 92-97, 1965.

(47) Eton, B. Carcinoma of the ovary and uterus. In "Cyclophosphamide" (Fairley, G., and Simister, J., eds.), Williams and Wilkins Co., Baltimore; pp 98-100, 1965.

(48) Mengel, C., Kelly, M., Carbone, P., et al. Clinical and biochemical effects of cyclophosphamide in patients with malignant carcinoid. Amer J Med 38: 396, 1965.

(49) Wilson, W., and de la Garza, J. Systemic chemotherapy
      for CNS metastases of solid tumors. Arch Intern Med 115:
      710, 1965.

(50) Fox, M. The effect of cyclophosphamide on some urinary
      tract tumors. Brit J Urol 37: 399, 1965.

(51) Barran, K., Helm, W., King, D. Bronchial carcinoma treated
      with nitrogen mustard and cyclophosphamide. Brit Med J
      5463: 685, 1965.

(52) Burkitt, D., Hutt, M., and Wright, D. The African lymphoma.
      Preliminary observations on response to therapy. Cancer 18:
      399, 1965.

(53) Gordon, I., and McArthur, J. Thiotepa and cyclophosphamide
      in the treatment of advanced mammary cancer. Scot Med J
      10: 27, 1965.

(54) Talley, R., Vaitkevicius, V., and Leighton, G. Comparison
      of cyclophosphamide and 5-fluorouracil in the treatment
      of patients with metastatic breast cancer. Clin Pharm Ther
      6: 740, 1965.

(55) McLean, R. Cyclophosphamide in the management of advanced
      bronchial carcinoma. Thorax 20: 555, 1965.

(56) Skoog, W., and Adams, W. Clinical and metabolic investigations
      of eight cases of multiple myeloma during prolonged
      cyclophosphamide administration. Amer J Med 41: 76, 1966.

(57) Solidoro, A., Esteves, L., Castellano, C., et al. Chemotherapy
      of advanced cancer of the cervix. Experience in 55 cases
      treated with cyclophosphamide. Amer J Obstet Gyn 94: 208,
      1966.

(58) Solidoro, A., and Saenz, R. Effects of cyclophosphamide on
      127 patients with malignant lymphoma. Cancer Chemother Rep
      50: 265, 1966.

(59) Stutzman, L., and Ezdinli, E. Vinblastine sulfate vs
      cyclophosphamide in the therapy for lymphoma. JAMA 195: 173,
      1966.

(60) Hyman, G., and Cassileth, P. Efficacy of cyclophosphamide
      in the management of reticulum-cell sarcoma. Cancer 19:
      1386, 1966.

(61) Pierce, M., Shore, N., Sitarz, A., et al. Cyclophosphamide
      therapy in acute leukemia of childhood. Cancer 19: 1551, 1966.

(62) Fernbach, D., Griffith, K., Haggard, M., et al. Chemotherapy
      of acute leukemia in childhood. New Eng J Med 275: 451, 1966.

(63) Fernbach, D. Chemotherapy for acute leukemia in children:
      comparison of cyclophosphamide (NSC 26271) and 6-mercaptopurine
      (NSC 755). Cancer Chemother Rep 51: 381, 1967.

(64) Holcomb, T. Cyclophosphamide (NSC 26271) in the treatment of
      acute leukemia in children. Cancer Chemother Rep 51: 389,
      1967.

(65) Sullivan, M. Cyclophosphamide therapy for children with
      generalized lymphoma and Hodgkin's disease. Cancer Chemother
      Rep 51: 393, 1967.

(66) Haggard, M. Cyclophosphamide in the treatment of children with
      malignant neoplasms. Cancer Chemother Rep 51: 403, 1967.

(67) Thurman, W., and Donaldson, M. Cyclophosphamide therapy for
      children with neuroblastoma. Cancer Chemother Rep 51: 399,
      1967.

(68) Sutow, W. Cyclophosphamide in Wilms' tumor and rhabdomyosarcoma.
      Cancer Chemother Rep 51: 407, 1967.

(69) Choi, O., English, A., Hilton, J., et al. Cyclophosphamide in
      the treatment of myelomatosis. Canad Med Assoc J 97: 1133,
      1967.

(70) Bergsagel, D., Robertson, G., and Hasselback, R. Effect of
      cyclophosphamide on advanced lung cancer and the hematological
      toxicity of large, intermittent intravenous doses. Canad Med
      Assoc J 98: 532, 1968.

(71) Beck, R., and Boyes, D. Treatment of 126 cases of advanced
      ovarian carcinoma with cyclophosphamide. Canad Med Assoc J
      98: 539, 1968.

(72) Carbone, P., and Spurr, C. Management of patients with
      malignant lymphoma: a comparative study with cyclophosphamide
      and vinca alkaloids. Cancer Res 28: 811, 1968.

(73) Jacobs, E., Peters, F., Luce, J., et al. Mechlorethamine
      HCl and cyclophosphamide in the treatment of Hodgkin's
      disease and the lymphomas. JAMA 203: 392, 1968.

(74) Firat, D., and Olshin, S. Treatment of metastatic carcinoma
      of the female breast with combination of hormones and other
      chemotherapy. Cancer Chemother Rep 52: 743, 1968.

(75) Rivers, S., and Patno, M. Cyclophosphamide vs melphalan in
      treatment of plasma cell myeloma. JAMA 207: 1328, 1969.

(76) Green, R., Humphrey, E., Close, H., et al. Alkylating agents
      in bronchogenic carcinoma. Amer J Med 46: 516, 1969.

(77) Finklestein, J., Hittle, R., and Hammond, D. Evaluation of a
      high dose cyclophosphamide regimen in childhood tumors. Cancer
      23: 1239, 1969.

(78) Gold, G., Shnider, B., Salvin, L., et al. The use of
      mechlorethamine, cyclophosphamide, and uracil mustard in
      neoplastic disease: a cooperative study. J Clin Pharmacol
      New Drugs 10: 110, 1970.

(79) Mendelson, D., Block, J., and Serpick, A. Effect of large
      intermittent doses of cyclophosphamide in lymphoma. Cancer
      25: 715, 1970.

(80) Smith, J., Ruttedge, F., Burns, B., et al. Systemic
      chemotherapy for carcinoma of the cervix. Amer J Obstet
      Gynec 97: 800, 1967.

(81) Decker, D., Malkasian, G., Mussey, E., et al. Cyclophosphamide.
      Evaluation in recurrent and progressive ovarian cancer. Amer
      J Obstet Gynec 97: 656, 1967.

(82) Haddy, T., Nora, H., Sutow, W., et al. Cyclophosphamide
      treatment for metastatic soft tissue sarcoma. Amer J Dis
      Child 114: 301, 1967.

Chlorambucil

Synonyms: Leukeran, CB-1348.

Structure:

$$ClCH_2CH_2-N(C_6H_4)-CH_2CH_2CH_2COOH \quad / \quad ClCH_2CH_2$$

Dosage: 0.1-0.2 mg/kg/day x 3-6 wks, PO. Maintenance therapy
               may be given at a lower dose, depending on toxicity
               and response.

Toxicity: I.   Hematological - usually dose-limiting
                    A.   Leukopenia
                    B.   Thrombocytopenia
                    C.   Anemia

               II. Gastrointestinal
                    A.   Nausea, vomiting, anorexia - usually minimal
                         or absent at standard doses

               III. Dermatitis - unusual

               IV. Hepatotoxicity - unusual

Mechanism of Action: Chlorambucil is an alkylating agent. Like
               other nitrogen mustards, it reacts with (alkylates)
               nucleophilic substances within the cell, including a
               number of biologically important groups, e.g.,
               phosphate, amino, sulfhydryl, hydroxyl, imidazole, and
               carboxyl. This takes place through formation of the
               highly reactive, electrophilic ethylenimonium
               derivative from the tertiary amine in neutral or
               alkaline aqueous solution, according to the following
               general reaction:

$$
\begin{array}{ccc}
R-N\begin{cases} CH_2CH_2Cl \\ CH_2CH_2Cl \end{cases} & \rightarrow & R-\overset{+}{N}\begin{cases} \overset{CH_2}{\underset{CH_2}{|}} \\ CH_2CH_2Cl \end{cases} \qquad +Cl-
\end{array}
$$

               Internal cyclization of a bis (β-chloroethyl) grouping
               is necessary to the biological activity of the mustard
               derivatives.

                              Role in Cancer Therapy

     Chlorambucil is an agent which has been used primarily in CLL,
ovarian carcinoma, and lymphomas. It appears to be the most
effective single chemotherapeutic agent yet introduced for the
treatment of CLL, with a 61% overall recorded response rate, as
opposed to 34% for CTX. A randomized comparison study of these
two compounds was carried out by Kaung et al,[21] who found
chlorambucil effective in about twice as many patients, although
the numbers involved were too small to demonstrate significance at
the .05 level.

In ovarian cancer, chlorambucil has produced an objective
response rate of 52.6% in 422 reported cases, which represents
activity at least as great as that of the other two alkylating
agents often used in this disease, CTX and melphalan. Chlorambucil
possesses the advantage of causing little or no cystitis or
alopecia, and many clinicians feel that its use carries the least
risk of irreversible myelosuppression. For these reasons, it may
be the alkylating agent of choice against this tumor type.

Chlorambucil is an effective agent used alone in the
treatment of Hodgkin's disease, with a 61% overall reported response
rate. It has also successfully been used, because of its slower
onset of action at the dose schedule routinely employed, for
maintenance of remissions induced with HN_2. Chlorambucil appears
to be equally effective in the treatment of lymphosarcoma, and
somewhat less so against reticulum-cell sarcoma, in which the
results obtained may be inferior to those obtained with CTX.

Chlorambucil is also an effective agent for the treatment
of CML. Rundles et al compared it directly with busulfan in a
randomized study[14] and found that the latter agent produced a
higher proportion of "good" responses (100% vs 50%). Busulfan
also caused more severe myelosuppression, however, and the authors
made the following comment: "Large doses of chlorambucil than
those administered could have been given. This or a longer period
of treatment might have made the final results of therapy more
nearly equal."

The treatment of Waldenstrom's macroglobulinemia with this
agent has been notably successful.[19,27] It may have activity
against multiple myeloma equivalent to that of CTX or melphalan,
the more commonly used alkylating agents, but the number of
reported cases treated with chlorambucil is too small to
accurately assess this.

Other tumor types against which chlorambucil has been
reported to exert significant effects are carcinoma of the cervix,
pancreas, breast, Kaposi's sarcoma, and connective tissue
sarcomas in general. Its activity against colorectal carcinoma
and malignant melanoma, like that of other alkylating agents,
appears to be minimal when used alone. A small number of cases of
bronchogenic carcinoma treated with chlorambucil indicates that it
may be less effective here than HN_2 or CTX.

Chlorambucil has received an insufficient trial against
either ALL-AUL or AML-AMoL to judge its effectiveness, although
it is of interest that responses, including one CR, have been
reported in the latter disease.[11]

Practically without exception, chlorambucil has been given on a chronic oral, low-dose daily regimen. The statement is frequently made that chlorambucil is an agent with slow, gradual onset of effect, suitable for use in relatively indolent or subacute disease, but inferior to HN_2 or CTX for use in more acute situations. In fact, however, chlorambucil has not been used on a high-dose intermittent schedule, which is the usual way of administering HN_2, and the manner in which CTX is often given to achieve "quick" results.

Finally, Moore et al[28] have raised the possibility that chlorambucil could be given in a more optimal manner, even on a chronic daily dose schedule. Their study of the drug, carried out by the Eastern Clinical Drug Evaluation Program in 374 patients with advanced cancer, provides some provocative data. In this report, the median number of days to the beginning of a clinically evident response was 28, and 80% of patients who responded had developed evidence of tumor regression by day 37. The median number of days to the onset of thrombocytopenia was 45, and 51 days to the onset of leukopenia. Thus, 4 of 5 clinical responses were evident more than a week before half the patients had first manifested marrow toxicity. Furthermore, in those patients who demonstrated a tumor response, the median number of days to onset of hematologic depression was even greater: 45 for thrombocytopenia and 55 for leukopenia. This group's experience **appears** to indicate that it is most often not necessary to give a dose of chlorambucil causing appreciable myelosuppression, at least by this dose schedule, in order to achieve clinical response.

Tumor Type or Site

Breast

Ref #	# Pts Evaluated	# Pts Responding	% Response	Dose Schedule (always PO) and Remarks
8	2	1		Varying daily dose. PR.
28	52	10		0.2 mg/kg/day x 42, as tolerated (see discussion). 2 CR, 8 PR. PR defined as $\geq$ 50% regression.
	$\overline{54}$	$\overline{11}$	20.4	Total.

Colon and Rectum

| 28 | 55 | 5 | 9.1 | 0.2 mg/kg/day x 42, as tolerated (see discussion). 1 CR, 4 PR. PR defined as $\geq$ 50% regression. |

Melanoma

| 28 | 22 | 2 | 9.0 | 0.2 mg/kg/day x 42, as tolerated (see discussion). 1 CR, 1 PR. PR defined as $>$ 50% regression. |

Lung

8	2	1		Varying daily dose. PR.
28	21	1		0.2 mg/kg/day x 42 as tolerated (see discussion). PR defined as $\geq$ 50% regression.
	$\overline{23}$	$\overline{2}$	8.8	Total.

ALL-AUL

Ref #	# Pts Evaluated	# Pts Responding	% Response	Dose Schedule (always PO) and Remarks
11	1	0		0.3 mg/kg/day x 21-28, as tolerated.

AML-AMoL

Ref #	# Pts Evaluated	# Pts Responding	% Response	Dose Schedule (always PO) and Remarks
5	-	-		Varying daily dose. "Distinct improvement" in some patients with AMoL.
11	16	1		0.3 mg/kg/day x 21-28, as tolerated. Response was CR of 20 mo duration in patient with AMoL.
12	2	2		0.1-0.2 mg/kg/day x 4 to 8 wks per course. Both PR.
	$\overline{18}$	$\overline{3}$	16.7	Total.

Hodgkin's Disease

Ref #	# Pts Evaluated	# Pts Responding	% Response	Dose Schedule (always PO) and Remarks
1	23	18		Usually 0.1-0.2 mg/kg/day x 3-6 wks. Only 4 were felt to have achieved significant clinical benefit.
3	52	32		0.2-0.25 mg/kg/day. 17 "definite and prolonged", 15 "moderate" remissions. Some patients received steroids.

Hodgkin's Disease (cont.)

Ref #	# Pts Evaluated	# Pts Responding	% Response	Dose Schedule (always PO) and Remarks
6	22	17		0.1-0.9 mg/kg/day. 5 CR, 12 PR.
8	3	3		Varying daily dose. 2 "good" and 1 PR.
9	7	5		0.2 mg/kg/day x 21. All were transient PR. All had received prior HN_2 and x-ray therapy.
10	8	2		Varying daily dose, average = 10 mg. Both PR.
11	47	22		0.3 mg/kg/day x 21-28. 22 responses were all $\geq$ 4 mo duration. 5 patients had remissions >1 year duration.
12	35	25		0.1-0.2 mg/kg/day x 4 to 8 wks per course. 4 "CR" of $\geq$ 6 mo duration.
15	38	19		0.1-0.2 mg/kg/day, as tolerated. 11 "marked", 8 "moderate" responses. Mean remission duration >12 wks.
17	4	3		Varying daily dose to total of 100-400 mg/m^2. All PR.
24	43	26		6-12 mg/day x 4-8 wks. A few patients also received steroids. Mean response duration 5.7 mo.
	282	172	61.0	Total.

Lymphosarcoma

Ref #	# Pts Evaluated	# Pts Responding	% Response	Dose Schedule (always PO) and Remarks
1	12	10		Usually 0.1-0.2 mg/kg/day x 3-6 wks. 7/12 had significant "benefit".
3	13	10		0.2-0.25 mg/kg/day. 7 "good", 3 "moderate" responses. Some patients received steroids.
8	5	5		Varying daily dose. 1 "good", 4 PR.
10	14	7		Varying daily dose, average = 10 mg. 1 CR, 6 PR.
12	20	12		0.1-0.2 mg/kg/day x 4 to 8 wks per course. 7 responses $\geq$ 6 mo duration.
15	6	6		0.1-0.2 mg/kg/day, as tolerated. All were "marked" responses. Mean response duration = 19 wks.
24	20	11		6-12 mg/day x 4-8 wks. A few patients also received steroids. Mean response duration = 16.5 mo.
	90	61	67.8	Total.

Reticulum-cell Sarcoma

Ref #	# Pts Evaluated	# Pts Responding	% Response	Dose Schedule (always PO) and Remarks
1	11	6		Usually 0.1-0.2 mg/kg/day x 3-6 wks. None had "benefit".

Reticulum-cell Sarcoma

Ref #	# Pts Evaluated	# Pts Responding	% Response	Dose Schedule (always PO) and Remarks
11	5	1		0.3 mg/kg/day x 21-28. 6 mo duration.
12	13	8		0.1-0.2 mg/kg/day x 4-8 wks per course. All PR.
15	5	2		0.1-0.2 mg/kg/day, as tolerated. Both responses "marked". Mean duration 5 wks.
24	12	1		6-12 mg/kg/day x 4-8 wks. A few patients also received steroids.
	46	18	39.1	Total.
			"Lymphoma"	
28	23	16		0.2 mg/kg/day x 42. 1 CR.
			CLL	
1	8	5		Usually 0.1-0.2 mg/kg/day x 3-6 wks. 4 had "benefit".
3	40	23		0.2-0.25 mg/kg/day. Some patients received steroids. All had "marked and prolonged" response.
4	8	5		0.1 mg/kg/day as tolerated.

CLL (cont.)

Ref #	# Pts Evaluated	# Pts Responding	% Response	Dose Schedule (always PO) and Remarks
7	15	4		Usually 6 mg/day for "first few wks", then 2–4 mg/day as tolerated. Response defined as significant improvement for >3 mo.
8	2	2		Varying daily dose. 1 "good", 1 PR.
9	2	1		0.2 mg/kg/day x 21. PR in patient who had previous total-body x-ray.
10	32	21		Varied daily dose, average = 10 mg. 4 CR, 17 PR.
11	18	12		0.15–0.2 mg/kg/day x 21. 5 of the 12 had previously failed to respond to P^{32} or x-ray.
12	27	21		0.1–0.2 mg/kg/day x 4–8 wks. 12 responses $\geq$ 6 mo duration.
14	23	17		12 mg/day as tolerated (chlorambucil) -- vs 6 mg/day as tolerated (busulfan). 3 excellent, 12 good, 2 fair. Myleran→3 PR of 17.
15	19	12		0.1–0.2 mg/kg/day as tolerated. 6 "marked", 6 "moderate". Mean duration = 11 wks.
18	43	33		0.1–0.2 mg/kg/day x 4–8 wks. 24 had "benefit". Further treatment required "usually" within 1 year.

CLL (cont.)

Ref #	# Pts Evaluated	# Pts Responding	% Response	Dose Schedule (always PO) and Remarks
20	34	12		0.1-0.2 mg/kg/day to WBC <12,000 or to 6 mo (chlorambucil) -- vs 0.015-0.066 mg/kg/wk to WBC <12,000 or to 6 mo (TEM). 11 good, 1 fair response. TEM→14/40 responses, with 1 CR. See discussion.
21	21	14		0.2 mg/kg/day as tolerated (chlorambucil) -- vs 2 mg/kg/day as tolerated (CTX). CTX→6/18 responses. No CR in either group.
24	51	26		6-12 mg/day x 4-8 wks. A few patients also received steroids. Mean response duration 13.2 mo.
29	24	18		0.2 mg/kg/day, chlorambucil -- vs .004 mg/kg/day, streptonigrin, each for 6 wks. Streptonigrin →21/25.
	367	226	61	Total.

CML

Ref #	# Pts Evaluated	# Pts Responding	% Response	Dose Schedule (always PO) and Remarks
8	1	1		Varying daily dose.
13	2	2		8 mg/day, PO.
14	21	20		12 mg/day as tolerated (chlorambucil) -- vs 6 mg/day as tolerated (CTX). 2 CR, 18 PR. 10 "good" responses. Myleran→8 CR, 13 PR of 21 (all "good" responses). See discussion.

CML (cont.)

Ref #	# Pts Evaluated	# Pts Responding	% Response	Dose Schedule (always PO) and Remarks
15	6	6	97	0.1-0.2 mg/kg/day as tolerated. 5 "marked", 1 "moderate". Mean duration = 6 wks.
	30	29		Total.
			Ovary	
8	2	2		Varying daily dose. Both had "marked benefit".
16	30	20		0.2-0.4 mg/kg/day x 28. Repeat courses as tolerated. 6 CR.
22	62	38	61	0.3 mg/kg/day →leukopenia, then 0.2 mg/kg/day. 16 CR. 27/65 had "worthwhile" responses. Median remission = 7.5 mo.
23	280	140	50	0.2 mg/kg/day x 4-6 wks. (Maintenance: repeated 2-4 wk courses with intervening 1-3 wk "rest" periods). 40 patients, on maintenance treatment, in remission ≥ 2 years = 14.3%.
25	28	11	40	Not stated.
28	20	11		0.2 mg/kg/day x 42, as tolerated. 1 CR.
	422	222	52.6	Total.

Pancreas

Ref #	# Pts Evaluated	# Pts Responding	% Response	Dose Schedule (always PO) and Remarks
28	6	4	66.7	0.2 mg/kg/day x 42, as tolerated. All responses PR.

Kidney

Ref #	# Pts Evaluated	# Pts Responding	% Response	Dose Schedule (always PO) and Remarks
28	14	2	14.3	0.2 mg/kg/day x 42, as tolerated. Both PR.

Bladder

Ref #	# Pts Evaluated	# Pts Responding	% Response	Dose Schedule (always PO) and Remarks
8	2	0		Varying daily dose.
28	8	0		0.2 mg/kg/day x 42, as tolerated.
	$\overline{10}$	$\overline{0}$		Total.

Multiple Myeloma

Ref #	# Pts Evaluated	# Pts Responding	% Response	Dose Schedule (always PO) and Remarks
5	6	4		Varying daily dose. Patients who responded had weight gain, ↓bone pain. ? objective response.
9	2	1		0.2 mg/kg/day x 21. PR, 8 mo duration.
10	6	0		Varying daily dose, average = 10 mg.
11	1	0		0.15-0.2 mg/kg/day x 21, PO.
	$\overline{15}$	$\overline{5}$	33.3	Total.

Waldenstrom's Macroglobulinemia

Ref #	# Pts Evaluated	# Pts Responding	% Response	Dose Schedule (always PO) and Remarks
19	2	2		Varying daily dose.
27	13	11		6-12 mg/day to leukopenia, then 2-8 mg/day as tolerated. Patients had prolonged, "good to excellent" response as long as they were kept on therapy.
	$\overline{15}$	$\overline{13}$	86.7	Total.

Cervix

Ref #	# Pts Evaluated	# Pts Responding	% Response	Dose Schedule (always PO) and Remarks
23	18	4	22.2	0.2 mg/kg/day x 4-6 wks. (Maintenance: repeated 2-4 wk courses with intervening 1-3 wk "rest" periods. 5-FU→2/11.
28	26	7		0.2 mg/kg/day x 42 as tolerated. 1 CR, 6 PR.
	$\overline{44}$	$\overline{11}$	25.0	Total.

Uterus

Ref #	# Pts Evaluated	# Pts Responding	% Response	Dose Schedule (always PO) and Remarks
23	5	0		0.2 mg/kg/day x 4-6 wks. (Maintenance: repeated 2-4 wk courses with intervening 1-3 wk "rest" periods. Hydroxyprogesterone→7/38.
28	6	0		0.2 mg/kg/day x 42 as tolerated.
	$\overline{11}$	$\overline{0}$		Total.

Head and Neck

Ref #	# Pts Evaluated	# Pts Responding	% Response	Dose Schedule (always PO) and Remarks
28	34	5	14.7	0.2 mg/kg/day x 42 as tolerated. 1 CR, 4 PR.

"Connective Tissue Sarcomas"

| 28 | 28 | 7 | 25 | 0.2 mg/kg/day x 42 as tolerated. 1 CR, 6 PR. |

Stomach

| 28 | 18 | 3 | 16.7 | 0.2 mg/kg/day x 42 as tolerated. |

Salivary Gland

| 28 | 7 | 2 | 28.6 | 0.2 mg/kg/day x 42 as tolerated. Both PR. |

Neuroblastoma

| 17 | 10 | 2 | 20.0 | Varying daily dose to total of 100-400 mg/m^2. Both PR. |

Kaposi's Disease

| 26 | 6 | 5 | 83.3 | Varying daily dose. 1 CR of 18 mo. |

References

(1)   Galton, D., Israels, L., Nabarro, J., and Till, M.   Clinical
       trials of p-(di-2-chloroethyl-amino)-phenylbutyric acid (CB
       1348) in malignant lymphoma.   Brit Med J 2: 1172, 1955.

(2)   Bouroncle, B., Doan, C., Wiseman, B., and Frajola, W.
       Evaluation of CB 1348 in Hodgkin's disease and allied
       disorders.   Arch Intern Med 97: 703, 1956.

(3)   Bernard, J., Mathe, G., and Weil, M.   Therapeutic trial with
       para-(di-2-chloroethylamino)-phenylbutyric acid in Hodgkin's
       disease, chronic lymphoid leukemia and various sarcomas of
       the lymphoid tissue.   (Study on 100 patients).   Rev Franc
       Et Clin Biol 1: 1121, 1956.

(4)   Altman, S., Haut, A., Cartwright, G., and Wintrobe, M.   Early
       experience with p-(N, N-di-2-chloroethyl)-aminophenylbutyric
       acid (CB 1348), a new chemotherapeutic agent effective in the
       treatment of chronic lymphocytic leukemia.   Cancer 9: 512,
       1956.

(5)   Shanbrom, E., Knudson, A., and Rapaport, S.   Clinical
       evaluation of chlorambucil.   Clin Res Proc 5: 31, 1957.

(6)   Rottino, A.   Therapeutic results in treatment of Hodgkin's
       disease with CB 1348 and R-48.   Blood 12: 755, 1957.

(7)   Hansen, P.   Clinical experience with CB 1348 in the treatment
       of chronic lymphatic leukaemia.   Acta Radiol 47: 210, 1957.

(8)   Gumport, S., Golomb, F., and Wright, J.   Summary of results
       obtained with CB 1348.   Ann N Y Acad Sci 68: 1024, 1958.

(9)   Olson, K.   P-(di-2-chloroethyl) aminophenylbutyric acid
       (CB 1348) in the treatment of cancer.   Ann N Y Acad Sci
       68: 1017, 1958.

(10)   Ultmann, J., Hyman, G., and Collhorn, A.   Chlorambucil and
       triethylene thiophosphoramide in the treatment of neoplastic
       disease.   Ann N Y Acad Sci 68: 1007, 1958.

(11)   Doan, C., Wiseman, B., and Bouroncle, B.   Clinical evaluation
       of CB 1348 in leukemias and lymphomas.   Ann N Y Acad Sci 68:
       979, 1958.

(12)   Israels, L., Galton, D., Till, M., and Wiltshaw, E.   Clinical
       evaluation of CB 1348 in malignant lymphoma and related diseases.
       Ann N Y Acad Sci 68: 915, 1958.

(13) Krakoff, I., Karnofsky, D., and Burchenal, J. Remissions
      induced by chlorambucil in chronic granulocytic leukemia.
      JAMA 166: 629, 1958.

(14) Rundles, R., Grizzle, J., Bell, W., et al. Comparison of
      chlorambucil and Myleran in chronic lymphocytic and
      granulocytic leukemia. Amer J Med 27: 424, 1959.

(15) Miller, D., Diamond, H., and Craver, L. The clinical use of
      chlorambucil. A critical study. New Eng J Med 261: 525,
      1959.

(16) Masterson, J., Calame, R., and Nelson, J. A clinical study
      on the use of chlorambucil in the treatment of cancer of the
      ovary. Amer J Obstet Gyn 79: 1002, 1960.

(17) Pinkel, D. Chlorambucil in childhood cancer. Cancer 14:
      36, 1961.

(18) Galton, D., Wiltshaw, E., Szur, L., and Dacie, J. The use of
      chlorambucil and steroids in the treatment of chronic
      lymphocytic leukaemia. Brit J Haemat 7: 73, 1961.

(19) Clatanoff, D., and Meyer, O. Response to chlorambucil in
      macroglobulinemia. JAMA 183: 40, 1963.

(20) Bigley, R. Treatment of chronic lymphocytic leukemia with
      triethylene melamine (TEM) and chlorambucil (CB 1348).
      Cancer Chemother Rep 30: 27, 1963.

(21) Kaung, D., Whittington, R., and Patno, M. Treatment of chronic
      lymphocytic leukemia with chlorambucil (NSC 3088) and
      cyclophosphamide (NSC 26271). Cancer Chemother Rep 39: 41,
      1964.

(22) Wiltshaw, E. Chlorambucil in the treatment of primary
      adenocarcinoma of the ovary. J Obstet Gynaec Brit Cmwlth
      72: 586, 1964.

(23) Masterson, J., and Nelson, J. The role of chemotherapy in
      the treatment of gynecologic malignancy. Amer J Obstet Gynec
      93: 1102, 1965.

(24) Ezdinli, E., and Stutzman, L. Chlorambucil therapy for
      lymphomas and chronic lymphocytic leukemia. JAMA 191: 444,
      1965.

(25) Keettel, W. The treatment of ovarian cancer. Ca 16:
      245, 1966.

(26) Degos, R., et al. Treatment of Kaposi's disease with
      chlorambucil (chloraminophene). Dermatologica 135: 345, 1967.

(27) McCallister, B., Bayrd, E., Harrison, E., and McGuckin, W.
      Primary macroglobulinemia. Review with a report on thirty-
      one cases and notes on the value of continuous chlorambucil
      therapy. Amer J Med 43: 394, 1967.

(28) Moore, G., Bross, I., Ausman, R., et al. Effects of
      chlorambucil (NSC 3088) in 374 patients with advanced cancer.
      Cancer Chemother Rep 52: 661, 1968.

(29) Kaung, D., Whittington, R., Spencer, H., and Patno, M.
      Comparison of chlorambucil and streptonigrin in the
      treatment of chronic lymphocytic leukemia. Cancer 23:
      597, 1969.

Melphalan

Synonyms: phenylalanine mustard, Alkeran, L-PAM, L-sarcolysin

Structure:

$$Cl-CH_2CH_2 \diagdown \atop Cl-CH_2CH_2 \diagup N \!-\! \bigcirc \!-\! CH_2-\underset{\underset{NH_2}{|}}{CH}-COOH$$

HCl

Dosage: 1. 0.25 mg/kg/day x 4, PO, q 6 wks or
                2. 0.15 mg/kg/day x 7, PO, followed by rest period for
                    bone marrow recovery; then up to 0.05 mg/kg/day, PO,
                    maintenance as tolerated or
                3. 0.05-0.1 mg/kg/day, PO, continuously as tolerated.

Toxicity: I. Hematological - usually dose-limiting
                    A. Leukopenia
                    B. Thrombocytopenia
                    C. Anemia

               II. Gastrointestinal
                    A. Nausea, vomiting, anorexia

Mechanism of Action: L-PAM is an alkylating agent. Like other
                nitrogen mustards, it reacts with (alkylates)
                nucleophilic substances within the cell, including
                a number of biologically important groups, e.g.,
                phosphate, amino, sulfhydryl, hydroxyl, imidazole, and
                carboxyl. This takes place through formation of the
                highly reactive, electrophilic ethylenimonium
                derivative from the tertiary amine in neutral or
                alkaline aqueous solution, according to the following
                general reaction:

$$R-N\begin{array}{c} CH_2CH_2Cl \\ \\ CH_2CH_2Cl \end{array} \rightarrow R-^+N\begin{array}{c} CH_2 \\ | \diagdown CH_2 \\ CH_2CH_2Cl \end{array} + Cl^-$$

Internal cyclization of a bis (β-chloroethyl) grouping
is necessary to the biological activity of the mustard
derivatives.

The initial rationale in synthesizing L-PAM was that
addition of the amino acid group might allow for more
selective cytotoxic action against cancer cells,
especially against melanoma cells, which utilize
phenylalanine in melanin synthesis. Unfortunately, this
theoretical advantage has not been substantiated by
results obtained clinically.

Role in Cancer Therapy

    Multiple myeloma is the one tumor type in which L-PAM is
widely considered to be the drug of choice. Superficially, this
conclusion appears to be supported by the recorded overall objective

response rate of 42%, as opposed to 29% for CTX, its closest rival.
However, the reliability of attempts to measure objective response
as a parameter of therapeutic effect is particularly questionable
in this tumor type. The range in recorded objective responses from
15% to 78% for melphalan used alone, as cited here in two large
series carried out by reputable investigators (and on a similar
dose schedule),[19,24] points up this fact. The single published
study comparing the two drugs in a randomized, prospective trial
in fact found no difference in either median survival time or
response rate between patients receiving CTX and those receiving
L-PAM.[24] To quote the authors of this study, "The only significant
difference between the two study drugs in this dose regimen was an
increased incidence of thrombocytopenia in the melphalan-treated
patients." On the other hand, CTX consistently induces alopecia,
and melphalan rarely does. An ongoing study in Britian under
auspices of the Medical Research Council, when completed, may offer
more definitive information as to the relative merits of these two
drugs in this disease.

It is probable that either L-PAM or CTX is capable of prolonging
the survival of patients who respond. Every study which has
measured survival time has shown a significant increase in the
lifespan of melphalan-treated patients with multiple myeloma who
respond to therapy, vs those who do not. In a recently completed
study of the PVACCG, Brook[26] found the mean survival to be 40 months
for responders and 6.8 months for non-responders. Patients with
only subjective improvement had a mean survival of 19.0 months, an
increase in the mean survival time over that for non-responders,
but not as good as the groups with one or more objective parameters
of response. Brook, whose patients received daily therapy, does
not feel that intermittent therapy offers any therapeutic advantage.
This viewpoint is shared by Hoogstraten, who has reported the results
of Acute Leukemia Group B studies utilizing both continuous and
intermittent maintenance regimens.[19,25] In fact, in patients on
intermittent maintenance, recurrence of pain in the third and fourth
week of the five-week interval between courses was appreciable:
"a normal performance status was obtained in only 10% (5) of the
patients [on intermittent maintenance] as compared to more than one
half of those in the previous study [continuous maintenance]."
Median survival and response rates were not markedly different,
although the latter were also somewhat superior for continuous
therapy.

The findings of Acute Leukemia Group B are in definite and
unexpalined opposition to those of the Southwest Cancer Chemotherapy
Study Group, as summarized by **Alexanian**.[27] These investigators
found the response rate more than twice as high for intermittent
as for continuous maintenance therapy, with no increase in toxicity.

In the treatment of ovarian carcinoma, L-PAM appears to be the equal of CTX, with 47% of 367 patients showing a significant objective response. Here, the results of a daily schedule seem inferior to those for an intermittent schedule; according to Burns and Rutledge[6], the attempt to use continuous oral therapy resulted in much more myelosuppression and in "tumor escape", although there seemed to be no difference[23] between the results of intermittent oral and intermittent intravenous thearpy.

L-PAM has activity equivalent to that of other alkylating agents in the treatment of breast cancer. Against malignant melanoma, its systemic use has proved a disappointment; if anything, it may be inferior to CTX as an alkylating agent in the treatment of this disease, and it appears definitely inferior to either hydroxyurea or imidazole carboxamide as single-agent therapy. Studies are under way currently to evaluabe the benefit of L-PAM administered by regional perfusion as an adjuvant to surgery in melanoma; the results of these are not yet available.

The activity of L-PAM appears to be substantially less than that of CTX in lung cancer, lymphomas, acute leukemia, and Ewing's sarcoma. There has been no published trial of the agent against colorectal carcinoma.

Tumor Type or Site

Breast

Ref #	# Pts Evaluated	# Pts Responding	% Response	Dose Schedule and Remarks
2	1	0		Varied, PO and IV (intermittent).
15	9	1		0.1 mg/kg/day, PO, to limiting toxicity. Independent study.
15	25	4	16	1 mg/kg over 3 or 8 hr, IV, q 3 wks or longer as tolerated. Independent study.
15	40	12	30	0.2–0.3 mg/kg/day, PO, x 4–6 days; repeat q 3–6 wks as tolerated. Two complete responses. Median remission duration 4 mo, 52 treated, only 40 evaluable ($\geq$ 2 courses). SWCCG study.
	$\overline{75}$	$\overline{17}$	23	Total.

Colorectal

No published data.

Melanoma

Ref #	# Pts Evaluated	# Pts Responding	% Response	Dose Schedule and Remarks
1	16	2		.089–0.37 mg/kg/day, PO, to median total dose 1.41 mg/kg. Repeat course after median of 3 wks (in those patients who received a second course). One remission of 10 months' duration.

Melanoma (cont.)

Ref #	# Pts Evaluated	# Pts Responding	% Response	Dose Schedule and Remarks
1	6	0		~25 mg/day, IV, x 4 to total dose 100 mg.
2	1	0		Varied, PO and IV (intermittent).
3	12	2		8-16 mg/day x 21-28, PO, or to toxicity. Remission durations of 4 mo and 9 mo.
5	2	1		2-3 mg/kg in 4-5 days, PO. Repeat as tolerated.
	37	5	13.5	Total.

Lung

Ref #	# Pts Evaluated	# Pts Responding	% Response	Dose Schedule and Remarks
2	2	0		Varied, PO and IV (intermittent).
	2	0		Total.

Lymphoma

Ref #	# Pts Evaluated	# Pts Responding	% Response	Dose Schedule and Remarks
2	14	7		Varied, PO and IV (intermittent). Hodgkin's; responses transient.
2	6	0		Varied, PO and IV (intermittent). Reticulum-cell sarcoma.
5	5	1		2-3 mg/kg in 4-5 days, PO. Repeat as tolerated. 0/3 reticulum-cell sarcoma, 1/2 Hodgkin's - PR.

Lymphoma (cont.)

Ref #	# Pts Evaluated	# Pts Responding	% Response	Dose Schedule and Remarks
5	14	4		2-3 mg/kg in 4-5 days, PO. Repeat as tolerated. Burkitt's - all PR.
	39	12	31	Total.

ALL-AUL

Ref #	# Pts Evaluated	# Pts Responding	% Response	Dose Schedule and Remarks
13	27	0		0.2 mg/kg/day, PO or IV. IV treatment not to exceed 5 days consecutively. 11 daily IV, 16 daily PO treatment. All patients far-advanced; had received at least 3 agents previous to melphalan therapy. SWCCG study.

AML-AMoL

No published data.

Multiple Myeloma

Ref #	# Pts Evaluated	# Pts Responding	% Response	Dose Schedule and Remarks
4	24	14	58	0.2 mg/kg/day, PO to total dose of 1.8-9.4 mg/kg. Daily schedule; 8/24 "significantly improved".
7	25	13	52	10 mg/day x 7-10 days, PO. At recovery (4-8 wks), 2-4 mg/day, PO maintenance as tolerated. Daily schedule.

Multiple Myeloma (cont.)

Ref #	# Pts Evaluated	# Pts Responding	% Response	Dose Schedule and Remarks
9	36	13	36	.05-0.1 mg/kg/day x >3 wks. Pacific VACCG study. 8/36 "significantly improved".
10	42	14	33	5-6 mg/day x 10 days, PO; then 5-6 mg eod x 20 days, PO; then 5-6 mg weekly or biw, PO. Range of remission, 2 wks to 30 mo. Mean remission duration = 12.8 mo. Swedish study.
11	70	?		5 mg/day x 16-25 days, PO as tolerated; then 2 mg/day maintenance after recovery of bone marrow function. See cited reference.
12	20	8	40	10 mg/day x 5-7, PO; repeated q 4-8 wks (usually at 6 wk intervals). British study. Intermittent schedule.
19	64	50	78	0.15 mg/kg/day x 7, PO, followed by rest period for bone marrow recovery; then up to .05 mg/kg/day, PO, maintenance as tolerated. 35/64 had response as defined in study. ALGB study.
24	53	8	15	4 mg/kg/day, PO (CTX); 0.1 mg/kg/day, PO (L-PAM). Comparative study with CTX, which gave 9/50 - all PR; 15.5 mo MST -- vs 13 mo for CTX. Daily schedule. VACCG study.
25	27	48	31	0.15 mg/kg/day x 7, PO; repeat course q 5 wks as tolerated. ALGB study. 19/48 responses as defined in study. Intermittent schedule.

Multiple Myeloma (cont.)

Ref #	# Pts Evaluated	# Pts Responding	% Response	Dose Schedule and Remarks
27	35	6	17	0.025 mg/kg/day, PO as tolerated. SWCCG; 6/30 evaluable had objective response.
27	152	55	36	0.25 mg/kg/day x 4, PO q 6 wks. SWCCG; 55/115 evaluable had objective response.
	499	212	42	Total.
	237	104	44	Total, daily schedule.
	262	108	42	Total, intermittent schedule.

Ovary

Ref #	# Pts Evaluated	# Pts Responding	% Response	Dose Schedule and Remarks
2	1	0		Varied, PO and IV (intermittent).
21	28	6	21	"Loading dose" 60-100 mg over 16-30 days, PO; then PO maintenance as tolerated, daily or eod.
23	239	118	50	1 mg/kg over 8 hr IV q 4 wks.
23	99	49	50	1 mg/kg over 5 days, PO q 4 wks.
	367	173	47	Total.

Cervix

Ref #	# Pts Evaluated	# Pts Responding	% Response	Dose Schedule and Remarks
17	20	4	20	(1) 1 mg/kg over 8 hr, IV; repeat q 3 wks. (2) 0.2 mg/kg/day x 5, repeat q 4 wks.
	$\overline{20}$	$\overline{4}$	20	Total.

Osteogenic Sarcoma

Ref #	# Pts Evaluated	# Pts Responding	% Response	Dose Schedule and Remarks
8	7	2		(Modified to) 0.2 mg/kg/day x 5, IV q 4 wks. SWCCG study.
	$\overline{7}$	$\overline{2}$	29	Total.

Ewing's Sarcoma

Ref #	# Pts Evaluated	# Pts Responding	% Response	Dose Schedule and Remarks
18	5	0		(1) 1 mg/kg/day x 2-4 days, monthly x 3 (3 patients). (2) 1.5 mg/kg IV, q 4-6 wks (2 patients). 7/11 treated with CTX responded, including 2 melphalan failures.

Neuroblastoma

Ref #	# Pts Evaluated	# Pts Responding	% Response	Dose Schedule and Remarks
20	13	0		(1) 0.2 mg/kg/day x 28, PO or (2) 0.2 mg/kg/day x 5, IV; off 21 days, then (may) repeat. All patients CTX-resistant or unresponsive. SWCCG study.

Polycythemia Vera

Ref #	# Pts Evaluated	# Pts Responding	% Response	Dose Schedule and Remarks
22	25	25	100	6-10 mg/day x 7, then 2-4 mg/day to response; then 2 mg eod maintenance (all PO). No marrow aplasia seen. All responses "good" or "excellent".

References

(1)   Holland, J., and Regelson, W.   Studies of phenylalanine
        nitrogen mustard (CB 3025) in metastatic malignant
        melanoma of man.   Ann N Y Acad Sci 68: 1122, 1958.

(2)   Papac, R., Galton, D., Till, M., et al.   Preliminary
        clinical trial of p-di-2-chloroethyl-amino-1-phenylalanine
        (CB 3025, melphalan) and of di-2-chloroethyl methanesulfonate
        (CB 1506).   Ann N Y Acad Sci 68: 1126, 1958.

(3)   Hall, B., Willett, F., and Hales, D.   Observations on the
        effects of alkylating agents in human neoplastic disease.
        Ann Intern Med 52: 602, 1960.

(4)   Bergsagel, D., Sprague, C., Austin, C., et al.   Evaluation
        of new chemotherapeutic agents in the treatment of multiple
        myeloma.   IV.   L-phenylalanine mustard (NSC 8806).   Cancer
        Chemother Rep 21: 87, 1962.

(5)   Clifford, P., Clift, R., and Gillmore, J.   Oral melphalan
        therapy in advanced malignant disease.   Brit J Cancer 17:
        381, 1963.

(6)   Burns, B., Rutledge, F., and Gallager, H.   Phenylalanine
        mustard in the palliative management of carcinoma of the
        ovary.   Obstet Gyn 22: 30, 1963.

(7)   Osserman, E.   Therapy of plasma cell myeloma with melphalan.
        Proc Amer Assoc Cancer Res 4: 50 (#197), 1963.

(8)   Sullivan, M., Sutow, W., and Taylor, G.   L-phenylalanine
        mustard as a treatment for metastatic osteogenic sarcoma in
        children.   J Pediat 63: 227, 1963.

(9)   Brook, J., Bateman, J., and Steinfeld, J.   Evaluation of
        melphalan in treatment of multiple myeloma.   Cancer Chemother
        Rep 36: 25, 1964.

(10)   Norin, T.   Melphalan (phenylalanine nitrogen mustard) -
        treatment in myelomatosis.   Acta Un Int Cancer 20: 382, 1964.

(11)   Waldenstrom, J.   Melphalan therapy in myelomatosis.   Brit Med
        J 5387: 859, 1964.

(12)   Speed, D., Galton, D., and Swan, A.   Melphalan in the
        treatment of myelomatosis.   Brit Med J 5399: 1664, 1964.

(13)   Holcomb, T., Berry, D., Haggard, M., et al. L-sarcolysin
       therapy for acute leukemia in children. Cancer Chemother
       Rep 48: 45, 1965.

(14)   Sullivan, M., Fernbach, D., Haggard, M., et al. L-
       phenylalanine mustard in uncommon malignant disease in
       children. Cancer Chemother Rep 45: 63, 1965.

(15)   Sears, M., Haut, A., and Eckles, N. Melphalan in advanced
       breast cancer. Cancer Chemother Rep 50: 271, 1966.

(16)   Rutledge, F., and Burns, B. Chemotherapy for advanced
       ovarian cancer. Amer J Obstet Gyn 96: 761, 1966.

(17)   Smith, J., Rutledge, F., Burns, B., et al. Systemic
       chemotherapy for carcinoma of the cervix. Amer J Obstet
       Gyn 97: 800, 1966.

(18)   Samuels, M., and Howe, C. Cyclophosphamide in the
       management of Ewing's sarcoma. Cancer 20: 961, 1967.

(19)   Hoogstraten, B., Sheehe, P., Cuttner, J., et al. Melphalan
       in multiple myeloma. Blood 30: 74, 1967.

(20)   Fernbach, D., Haddy, T., Holcomb, T., et al. L-sarcolysin
       therapy for children with metastatic neuroblastoma. Cancer
       Chemother Rep 52: 293, 1968.

(21)   Frick, H., Tretter, P., Tretter, W., et al. Disseminated
       carcinoma of the ovary treated by 1-phenylalanine mustard.
       Cancer 21: 508, 1968.

(22)   Laszlo, J. Effective treatment of polycythemia vera with
       phenylalanine mustard. Blood 32: 506, 1968.

(23)   Rutledge, F. Chemotherapy of ovarian cancer with melphalan.
       Clin Obstet Gyn 11: 354, 1968.

(24)   Rivers, S., and Patno, M. Cyclophosphamide vs melphalan in
       treatment of plasma cell myeloma. JAMA 207: 1328, 1969.

(25)   Hoogstraten, B., and Costa, J. Intermittent melphalan therapy
       in multiple myeloma. JAMA 209: 251, 1969.

(26)   Brook, J. (Personal communication). Unpublished data,
       PVACCG, 1969.

(27)   Alexanian, R., (Personal communication) Chemotherapy of
       multiple myeloma by the Southwest Cancer Chemotherapy Study
       Group. Unpublished data, 1969, and Alexanian, R., Bergsagel,
       D., Migliore, P., et al. Melphalan therapy for plasma cell
       myeloma. Blood 31: 1, 1968.

Busulfan

Synonyms: Myleran, GT-41, 1, 4-dimethanesulfonyl-oxybutane

Structure:

$$CH_3-SO_2-O-CH_2-(CH_2)_2-CH_2-O-SO_2-CH_3$$

Dosage: 1.   4-6 mg/day to WBC $\overset{<}{-}$10,000; then no treatment
                  until WBC↑ to $\geq$50,000, and resume as before.
                  (Chronic, interrupted therapy), or
             2.   4-6 mg/day to WBC of 10-20,000, then daily
                  maintenance at reduced dose as necessary to
                  maintain this level of WBC. (Chronic,
                  continuous therapy).

Toxicity: I.   Hematological - common, dose-limiting, and
                    occasionally irreversible
                    A.   Thrombocytopenia
                    B.   Leukopenia
                    C.   Anemia

              II.   "Endocrinological" - poorly understood
                    A.   Amenorrhea - occasional
                    B.   Skin hyperpigmentation - occasional
                    C.   Wasting syndrome with features of Addison's
                         disease - rare, and not usually accompanied
                         by objective evidence of adrenal hypofunction.

             III.   Pulmonary - rare
                    A.   "Busulfan lung"
                         1.   Syndrome of persistent cough and
                              progressive dyspnea
                         2.   Due to intra-alveolar exudation of fibrin
                              with subsequent organization

             Note: Both the "wasting syndrome" and the syndrome of
                    "Busulfan lung" typically appear in patients on
                    long-term busulfan therapy, although their
                    appearance has been reported after only a few
                    months.

Mechanism of Action: Busulfan is an alkylating agent. It acts
                  analogously to the nitrogen mustards, but the property
                  of biological alkylation here is conferred on the
                  ethyl groups of a diethylarylamine by the introduction
                  of aromatic sulfonic acid ester groups.[2] In the
                  nitrogen mustards this property is associated with the
                  bis-β-chloroethyl grouping. "Stripping" of the sulfur
                  from organic sulfhydryl groups may represent an important
                  molecular site of alkylation for this compound.[3]

                         Role in Cancer Therapy

     Busulfan is the most commonly used chemotherapeutic agent for
the treatment of chronic myelogenous leukemia (CML). It produces
remission of the clinical evidence of this disease in almost all

patients who receive the drug as primary therapy, and a recently
reported study by a Medical Research Council Working Party[39]
indicated that busulfan is superior to splenic radiation for CML:
30/48 busulfan-treated patients were alive at 3 years, as opposed
to only 18/54 in the radiation therapy group (P <0.01). The MST
of the busulfan-treated patients was 170 wks (about 40 mo) and was
120 wks (less than 30 mo) for the radiation therapy group (P <0.03).
These results are even more impressive when one considers that many
of the patients who received primary radiation subsequently were
treated with busulfan and other drugs, having become unfit for
further radiation treatment, and the survival of this group was
still significantly shorter than that for the group treated with
drug only.

However, evidence is lacking that busulfan treatment
definitely alters life expectancy for patients with CML. A study
by Minot et al[4] in 1924 yielded a median survival of 31 mo for
patients receiving only supportive care, and, with the advent of
blood transfusions and antibiotics, such a group today might well
survive as long as a group treated with the drug. What busulfan
does convincingly do for the patient with CML is to improve the
quality of life; most patients have few or no symptoms related to
its use, and, when in remission, are able to carry on relatively
normal, productive lives.

In about 90% of patients with CML, the erythroblasts,
megakaryocytes, and granulocytes demonstrate deletion of part of
the long arm of one member in one pair of small acrocentric (G
group) chromosomes. This is usually called the "Philadelphia" or
"Ph[1]" chromosome, and acts as a marker for the presence of the
malignant cell line. It has been shown by Carbone et al[35] that,
even in the presence of complete bone marrow remission (including
reduction in the myeloid: erythroid ratio to <4:1) induced by
busulfan or other drugs, there is no change in the incidence of
the Ph[1] chromosome in the marrow. Thus, it is not surprising
that therapy to date has failed to lengthen appreciably the time
before patients with CML develop "blast crisis" and die of their
disease.

Other drugs are also effective in CML, including 6 MP,
hydroxyurea, dibromomannitol (DBM), and chlorambucil. Studies
comparing busulfan with chlorambucil[27] and with 6 MP[33,34] against
the disease have concluded that busulfan, at the schedules used,
provides smoother and more reliable control of the disease. No
comparative studies have yet been reported with hydroxyurea and
DBM.

The other disorder in which busulfan has been widely used is
polycythemia vera. Gilbert,[41] in the largest reported series of

patients treated with this agent, found that unmaintained remissions after busulfan treatment were considerably longer than those obtained after similar treatment with CTX or chlorambucil. However, with the use of cyclic maintenance therapy employing either of the latter two drugs (not feasible with busulfan because of its severe myelosuppressive potential), prolonged remissions could be obtained. Furthermore, an initial response to chlorambucil occurred in a slightly higher percentage of patients, and chlorambucil was the most effective of the three in reducing splenomegaly. Busulfan-induced leukopenia and thrombocytopenia were more frequent and longer in duration than those seen with chlorambucil or CTX. Probably the only indication for preferring busulfan over chlorambucil in the treatment of polycythemia vera is in the situation cited by Killman and Cronkite:[32] "...it is a major advantage of Myleran that it can safely be given in the presence of a normal hematocrit in order to bring an existing thrombocytosis under control..." There are, of course, a number of other effective drugs in polycythemia vera, such as 6 MP and hydroxyurea, with which busulfan has not been directly compared. A comparison study with procarbazine[40] showed essentially equivalent results.

In general, busulfan has proved inferior to other alkylating agents for the treatment of CLL. The small series of Bean[36] is, however, worth noting: using the drug in single, very high doses, he reported objective remissions in 4 patients with CLL refractory to the use of nitrogen mustards. This is a potentially important observation, with obvious implications, both relative to the optimal dose schedule for busulfan and to its widely presumed cross-resistance with other alkylating agents. A test of this observation remains to be reported by others.

In a related vein, Sullivan[22], using an unorthodox, high-dose "bolus" regimen, reported objective responses to busulfan in 6/17 patients with bronchogenic carcinoma over ten years ago. This observation, too, remains provocative and untested by others. It is notable, on the minus side, that two of the four patients who received two such high-dose courses developed persistent pancytopenia as a result.

Tumor Type or Site

Ref #	# Pts Evaluated	# Pts Responding	% Response	Dose Schedule (always PO) and Remarks
Breast				
10	8	0		10 mg/day to WBC = 25% of baseline level. Maintenance, if necessary, at 2–4 mg/day.
Colorectal				
10	1	0		10 mg/day to WBC = 25% of baseline level. Maintenance, if necessary, at 2–4 mg/day.
Lung				
10	2	0		10 mg/day to WBC = 25% of baseline level. Maintenance, if necessary, at 2–4 mg/day.
22	17	6		Majority of patients received a single course of 1.0 mg/kg/day x 4. Four patients received 2 such courses, 2 of whom had resulting persistent pancytopenia. Onset of leukopenia between 11 and 30 days after onset of therapy, with improvement by day 24–54. Response duration of 2 wk–3+ mo.
	$\overline{19}$	$\overline{6}$	32	Total.

Melanoma

Ref #	# Pts Evaluated	# Pts Responding	% Response	Dose Schedule (always PO) and Remarks
10	1	0		10 mg/day to WBC = 25% of baseline level. Maintenance, if necessary, at 2-4 mg/day.

"Lymphoma"

Ref #	# Pts Evaluated	# Pts Responding	% Response	Dose Schedule (always PO) and Remarks
6	3	0	0	6 mg/day x 4-6 wks, then lower dose daily maintenance.
21	21	6	29	Often, 25 mg/day x 2 or 4, off 2 wks, then "dosage was continued, based on the blood picture and the therapeutic response". 1 CR and 2 PR were in patients with CLL. Overall, 2 CR, 4 PR.
	24	6	25	Total.

ALL-AUL

Ref #	# Pts Evaluated	# Pts Responding	% Response	Dose Schedule (always PO) and Remarks
5	1	0	0	(1) 200-500 mg total dose in 4-16 wks; (2) 100-150 mg in 1-6 days.

AML-AMoL

Ref #	# Pts Evaluated	# Pts Responding	% Response	Dose Schedule (always PO) and Remarks
5	6	0	0	(1) 200-500 mg total dose in 4-16 wks; (2) 100-150 mg in 1-6 days.

AML-AMoL (cont.)

Ref #	# Pts Evaluated	# Pts Responding	% Response	Dose Schedule (always PO) and Remarks
6	11	0		6 mg/day x 4-6 wks, then maintenance at lower daily dose. Patients had "subacute" AML.
7	6	1		(1) 100-150 mg total dose in 4-6 days; (2) 50-100 mg in 10-14 days; weekly maintenance at 6-20 mg/dose. One of 4 patients with AMoL had "excellent" response to busulfan, but "required cortisone for CR", duration 6 mo.
8	2	0		Varied daily doses.
12	4	0		Varied, usually 4-6 mg/day until Hb ~normal, then maintenance at 1-4 mg/day. Patients had "adult acute leukemia."
17	3	0		.06 mg/kg/day for induction, maintenance as needed. "Subacute" leukemia.
	$\overline{32}$	$\overline{1}$	3	Total.
			CLL	
6	3	0		6 mg/day x 4-6 wks, then maintenance at lower daily dose.
21	—	—		See under "Lymphoma" - no denominator for response given.

CLL (cont.)

Ref #	# Pts Evaluated	# Pts Responding	% Response	Dose Schedule (always PO) and Remarks
27	17	3		6 mg/day for 2-4 wks (busulfan) -- vs 12 mg/day for 2-4 wks (chlorambucil); dose then adjusted and continued for at least 3 mo. Responses to busulfan only "fair"; chlorambucil →3 "excellent", 12 "good", and 2 "fair" responses in 23 patients treated. SECCG study.
36	4	4		200 mg as single dose, repeated at irregular intervals as required. All 4 patients were "refractory" to nitrogen mustards and obtained "worthwhile" remissions with the use of busulfan. See discussion.
	24̄	7̄	29	Total.
			CML	
6	33	26	79	6 mg/day x 4-6 wks, then maintenance at lower daily dose. 13/18 previously untreated, 13/15 previously treated patients responded.
7	11	8		(1) 100-150 mg total dose in 4-6 days; (2) 50-100 mg in 10-14 days; weekly maintenance at 6-20 mg/dose.
8	7	6		Varied daily doses. Mean remission duration = 5 mo.

CML (cont.)

Ref #	# Pts Evaluated	# Pts Responding	% Response	Dose Schedule (always PO) and Remarks
9	24	22	92	Induction: 4-14 mg/day (mean daily dose, 7 mg). Maintenance: varied. "In no instances were normal bone marrows (i.e., without some degree of granulocytic hyperplasia) found during remission."
10	21	17	81	Induction: 10 mg/day to WBC = 25% of baseline level. Maintenance, if necessary, at 2-4 mg/day.
11	11	10		Usually 6 mg/day for induction, 2 mg/day for maintenance.
12	19	15		Varied, usually 4-6 mg/day until Hb ~normal, then maintenance at 1-4 mg/day. 10/19 had "excellent", 4/19 patients had "fair" or "good" responses.
13	22	19	86	Induction: 4 mg/day until "no further improvement in blood count"; maintenance (in some patients): 1-2 mg/day.
14	10	10		Induction: 2-6 mg/day. Maintenance: varied (or none).
15	12	7		Induction: 4-12 mg/day (to WBC ~10,000). No maintenance. Responses "good" or "excellent".

CML (cont.)

Ref #	# Pts Evaluated	# Pts Responding	% Response	Dose Schedule (always PO) and Remarks
16	35	29	83	Induction: 8-16 mg/day (usually for 1-2 wks); then daily dose adjusted downward as appropriate. 11/17 patients with prior radiation therapy or alkylating agent had "excellent" response; 18/18 previously untreated patients had "excellent" response.
17	36	28	78	Induction: .06 mg/kg/day; maintenance as needed. 0/5 patients with "advanced" disease (all previously treated), 12/15 "other" previously treated, and 16/16 new patients had "good" responses.
18	31	26	84	Busulfan, 6 mg/day (most patients) for induction, and varied dose for maintenance. -- vs TEM, 5 mg eod (most patients) for induction, and varied dose for maintenance. Busulfan→ 8 "excellent", 18 "good" responses; TEM→ 2 "excellent", 15 "good" of 41 (41%). "In cases becoming refractory to either of these agents, it has not been possible to obtain significant benefit by substituting the other."
19	42	41	98	Induction: ~4 mg/day; maintenance varied (in 25 patients treated continuously). MST in 25 patients treated with continuous busulfan = 37 mo.

CML (cont.)

Ref #	# Pts Evaluated	# Pts Responding	% Response	Dose Schedule (always PO) and Remarks
25	53	48	91	Induction: 4-6 mg/day (10-20 days); lowered dose for maintenance. Mean duration of remission = 17.9 mo.
26	17	13		6-10 mg/day. Responses characterized as "good".
27	21	21	100	6 mg/day for 2-4 wks (busulfan) -- vs 12 mg/day for 2-4 wks (chlorambucil); dose then adjusted and continued for at least 3 mo. Busulfan→ 8 "excellent", 13 "good" responses; chlorambucil →2 "excellent", 10 "good" of 21. SECCG study.
28	46	38	83	Usually 8-12 mg/day to WBC of 40-60,000, then 2-4 mg/day to WBC of 10,000. Therapy then interrupted until WBC ↑ to 50,000. Mean duration (unmaintained) remission = 6.5 mo. Indian study.
29	–	–		See discussion.
30	30	29	97	4-6 mg/day to WBC ≤10,000; treatment then interrupted until WBC ↑ to ≥50,000, and resumed as before. MST = 42 mo. See discussion.
31	25	18	72	4-6 mg/day (induction). Maintenance varied, aimed at maintaining WBC of 10-20,000. 0/4 responses in patients resistant to prior radiation, 2/2 in patients with prior radiation who were not resistant to it. 1/2 responses in patients with prior 6 MP, 1/1 in patient with prior TEM.

CML (cont.)

Ref #	# Pts Evaluated	# Pts Responding	% Response	Dose Schedule (always PO) and Remarks
33	-	-		See discussion.
34	47	42	89	Busulfan, 6 mg/day for 2 wks -- vs 6 MP, 3 mg/kg/day for 2 wks; dose then adjusted and effects evaluated at 12 wks. Busulfan→12 "excellent", 30 "good". 6 MP→5 "good" of 15 (33%).
35	14	13		1-8 mg/day. 9 CR, 4 PR of 14 trials (number of patients not given). See discussion.
39	-	-		Busulfan, 4 mg or .065 mg/kg/day, to WBC of 15-20,000. "Treatment resumed when necessary to stabilize total leukocyte count at ~ 10,000." See discussion.
	567	486	86	Total.

Polycythemia Vera

Ref #	# Pts Evaluated	# Pts Responding	% Response	Dose Schedule (always PO) and Remarks
6	2	1		6 mg/day x 4-6 wks, then maintenance at lower daily dose.
23	5	5		Varied daily dose. 3 CR, 2 PR.
24	18	18		Induction: 2-10 mg/day. Maintenance: 2 mg/wk to 8 mg/day. Two patients developed pancytopenia after therapy, one still persisting and severe at 20 wks.

Polycythemia Vera (cont.)

Ref #	# Pts Evaluated	# Pts Responding	% Response	Dose Schedule (always PO) and Remarks
32	12	12		Induction: usually 4-6 mg/day. Maintenance: usually 2-4 mg/day. See discussion.
37	8	8		Varied daily administration. All "CR". One case of pancytopenia. Three of 3 patients with hemorrhagic thrombocythemia had less complete responses.
40	19	19		Busulfan, 4-6 mg/day for induction, reduced dose for maintenance -- vs Procarbazine, 250 mg/day for induction, reduced dose for maintenance. All responses CR. Procarbazine→ 9/9 CR. Nine of 19 busulfan-treated and 3/9 procarbazine-treated patients had "toxic leuko- and/or thrombopenias".
41	32	27	84	Busulfan, 4-6 mg/day, induction. No maintenance, repeated courses as necessary; -- vs Chlorambucil, 6-8 mg/day, induction. Often maintenance at 3 mg/day x 3-4 wks, off 3-4 wks, and repeat; -- vs CTX, 100-150 mg/day, induction. Often maintenance at 50 mg/day x 3-4 wks, off 3-4 wks, and repeat. Chlorambucil→40/44 (91%) satisfactory Hct response, CTX→33/38 (87%). See discussion.
42	15	15		4 mg/day, induction. 2 mg/day, maintenance. Busulfan stopped when platelets reached 300,000. Greater effect on WBC and platelet count than on Hb noted. Mean remission duration, 6-12 mo.

Polycythemia Vera (cont.)

Ref #	# Pts Evaluated	# Pts Responding	% Response	Dose Schedule (always PO) and Remarks
	$\overline{111}$	$\overline{105}$	95	Total.
			Prostate	
38	16	1		4 mg/day to early toxicity (15 patients) - no responses. Escalating dose schedule (1 patient) →response, then death from aplasia.

References

(1)   Galton, D. Chemotherapy of chronic myelocytic leukemia.
       Seminars Hemat 6: 333, 1969.

(2)   Haddow, A., and Timmis, G. Myleran in chronic myeloid
       leukemia. Chemical constitution and biological action.
       Lancet 1: 207, 1953.

(3)   Calabresi, P., and Welch, A. In "The Pharmacological Basis
       of Therapeutics" (Goodman, L., and Gilman, A., eds.), 3rd
       edition, Macmillan Co., New York; pp. 1345-1360, 1965.

(4)   Minot, G., Buckman, T., and Isaacs, R. Chronic myelogenous
       leukemia: age incidence, duration and benefit derived from
       irradiation. JAMA 82: 1489, 1924.

(5)   Galton, D. Myleran in chronic myeloid leukemia. Results
       of treatment. Lancet 264: 208, 1953.

(6)   Hansen, P. Clinical experience with Myleran therapy,
       especially in myeloid leukaemia. In "Ciba Foundation
       Symposium on Leukemia Research", pp. 205-215, 1954.

(7)   Petrakis, N., Bierman, H., Kelly, K., et al. The effect of
       1,4-dimethanesulfonyloxybutane (GT-41 or Myleran) upon
       leukemia. Cancer 7: 383, 1954.

(8)   Videbaek, A. Myleran (GT 41) in the treatment of leukemia.
       Acta Med Scand 151: 295, 1955.

(9)   Louis, J., Limarzi, L., and Best, W. Treatment of chronic
       granulocytic leukemia with Myleran. Arch Intern Med 97:
       299, 1956.

(10)   Hyman, G., and Gellhorn, A. Myleran therapy in malignant
       neoplastic disease. JAMA 161: 844, 1956.

(11)   Spurr, C., Wilson, W., and McDonald, J. Myleran in the
       treatment of chronic myeloid leukemia: results of treatment.
       Southern Med J 49: 847, 1956.

(12)   Schilling, R., and Meyer, O. Treatment of chronic
       granulocytic leukemia with 1,4-dimethanesulfonyloxybutane
       (Myleran). New Eng J Med 254: 986, 1956.

(13)   Greig, H. Myleran in the treatment of chronic myeloid
       leukaemia. Acta Haemat 16: 171, 1956.

(14)   Frost, J., and Jackson, C. Myleran in the treatment of
       chronic granulocytic leukemia. JAMA 161: 54, 1956.

(15)   Early, I., and Prichard, R. The treatment of chronic
       granulocytic leukemia with Myleran. N Carolina Med J 17:
       315, 1956.

(16)   Unugur, A., Schulman, E., and Dameshek, W. Treatment of
       chronic granulocytic leukemia with Myleran. New Eng J Med
       256: 727, 1957.

(17)   Turesson, D. Myleran treatment in chronic granulocytic
       leukemia. Brit J Haemat 3: 220, 1957.

(18)   Bethell, F. Myleran and triethylene melamine in the
       treatment of chronic granulocytic leukemia. Ann N Y
       Acad Sci 68: 996, 1958.

(19)   Galton, D., Till, M., and Wiltshaw, E. Busulfan (1,4-
       dimethanesulfonyloxybutane, Myleran): summary of clinical
       results. Ann N Y Acad Sci 68: 967, 1958.

(20)   Dameshek, W., Granville, N., and Rubio, F. Therapy of the
       myeloproliferative disorders with Myleran. Ann N Y Acad Sci
       68: 1001, 1958.

(21)   Sykes, M. Myleran in the treatment of lymphomas. Ann N Y
       Acad Sci 68: 1035, 1958.

(22)   Sullivan, R. Myleran therapy in bronchogenic carcinoma.
       Ann N Y Acad Sci 68: 1038, 1958.

(23)   Wald, N., Hoshino, T., and Sears, M. Therapy of polycythemia
       vera with Myleran. Blood 13: 757, 1958.

(24)   Louis, J. Treatment of polycythemia vera with busulfan
       (Myleran). JAMA 168: 1882, 1958.

(25)   Wilkinson, J., and Turner, R. Chemotherapy of chronic myeloid
       leukemia, with special reference to Myleran. In "Progress in
       Hematology", (Tocantins, L., ed.), Grune and Stratton, New
       York and London, Volume 2, pp. 227-238, 1959.

(26)   Desai, R. Treatment of chronic granulocytic and lymphocytic
       leukemia and allied disorders with Myleran and Leukeran in
       Indian subjects. Acta Haemat Jap 22: 160, 1959.

(27)   Rundles, R., Grizzle, J., Bell, W., et al. Comparison of
       chlorambucil and Myleran in chronic lymphocytic and
       granulocytic leukemia. Amer J Med 27: 424, 1959.

(28)   Ghose, S., and Chatterjea, J.   Chronic myeloid leukemia: a
       study of 116 cases.   J Indian Med Assoc 34: 381, 1960.

(29)   Xefteris, E., Mitus, W., Mednicoff, I., et al.   Leukocytic
       alkaline phosphatase in busulfan induced remissions of chronic
       granulocytic leukemia.   Blood 18: 202, 1961.

(30)   Haut, A., Abbott, W., Wintrobe, M., et al.   Busulfan in the
       treatment of chronic myelocytic leukemia.   The effect of long
       term intermittent therapy.   Blood 17: 1, 1961.

(31)   Bridges, J., Hayes, D., and Nelson, M.   Busulfan in the
       treatment of chronic granulocytic leukemia.   Brit J Cancer
       15: 468, 1961.

(32)   Killmann, S., and Cronkite, E.   Treatment of polycythemia
       vera with Myleran.   Amer J Med Sci 241: 218, 1961.

(33)   Shullenberger, C.   Evaluation of the comparative
       effectiveness of Myleran and 6 MP in the management of
       patients with chronic myelocytic leukemia.   Cancer Chemother
       Rep 16: 203, 1962.

(34)   Huguley, C., Grizzle, J., Rundles, R., et al.   Comparison of
       6-mercaptopurine and busulfan in chronic granulocytic
       leukemia.   Blood 21: 89, 1963.

(35)   Carbone, P., Tjio, J., Whang, J., et al.   The effect of
       treatment in patients with chronic myelogenous leukemia.
       Hematologic and cytogenetic studies.   Ann Intern Med 59:
       622, 1963.

(36)   Bean, R.   Myleran in the treatment of chronic lymphatic
       leukemia.   Israel J Med Sci 1: 801, 1965.

(37)   Epstein, I.   The treatment of polycythemia vera and
       thrombocythemia with Myleran (busulphan).   Israel J Med Sci
       1: 797, 1965.

(38)   Arduino, L., and Mellinger, G.   Clinical trial of busulfan
       (NSC 750) in advanced carcinoma of prostate.   Cancer Chemother
       Rep 51: 295, 1967.

(39)   Witts, L.   (Medical Research Council Working Party).   Chronic
       granulocytic leukemia: comparison of radiotherapy and
       busulfan therapy.   Brit Med J 1: 201, 1968.

(40)   Penttila, O., and Ikkala, E.   Procarbazine (Natulan) and
       busulfan in the treatment of polycythemia vera.   Ann Med Int
       Fenn 57: 99, 1968.

(41) Gilbert, H. Problems relating to control of polycythemia
       vera: the use of alkylating agents. Blood 32: 500, 1968.

(42) Brodsky, I., Kahn, S., and Brady, L. Polycythaemia vera:
       differential diagnosis by ferrokinetic studies and
       treatment with busulphan (Myleran). Brit J Haemat 14:
       351, 1968.

Methotrexate

Synonyms: amethopterin, MTX.

Structure:

Dosage: Varied. See discussion under "Role in Cancer Therapy"
               and tables.

Toxicity: I.   Hematological
                    A. Leukopenia
                    B. Thrombocytopenia

               II. Gastrointestinal
                    A. Stomatitis – common; an indication for
                        interruption of therapy
                    B. Diarrhea – an indication for interruption of
                        therapy
                        1. Hemorrhagic enteritis and intestinal
                            perforation can occur if therapy is
                            continued after the appearance of
                            diarrhea

               III. Hepatic dysfunction – usually reversible and
                    subclinical. Not ordinarily an indication for
                    discontinuation of therapy

               IV. Dermatological
                    A. Alopecia – uncommon
                    B. Dermatitis – uncommon

               V.   Osteoporosis – seen occasionally in children
                    on long-term MTX maintenance. May result in
                    pathologic fractures.[1]

Mechanism of Action: Folic acid serves as the precursor for a
               coenzyme, tetrahydrofolic acid (THF), and a group of
               structurally related derivatives. The formation of
               dihydrofolate and THF from folate is accomplished by
               the dihydrofolate reductase enzyme system. The THF
               so formed is of critical importance in the metabolic
               transfer of one-carbon units in a variety of bio-
               chemical reactions. Those reactions which are of
               special importance in cellular reproduction are the
               biosynthesis of thymidylic acid from deoxyuridine 5'-
               monophosphate (thymidylic acid is the nucleotide
               specific to DNA), and the biosynthesis of inosinic
               acid, the precursor of adenine and guanine nucleotides
               in de novo purine biosynthesis.

               MTX competitively inhibits dihydrofolate reductase, thus
               restricting the availability of THF to cells.[2,3] In
               human leukocytes, the synthesis of DNA appears to be
               more sensitive than that of RNA to inhibition by MTX,[4,5]
               suggesting that the most important effect of the drug

is on thymidylate synthesis. It has been shown in
mouse leukemias that MTX can block the in vivo incorporation of deoxyuridine into DNA in a sensitive cell
line, without causing a significant change in deoxyuridine incorporation into drug-induced resistant or
innately insensitive lines.[6]

A common mechanism of resistance to MTX occurs through
the development of increased dihydrofolate reductase
activity,[7,8] and it appears that in resistant cells
the rate of enzyme synthesis may exceed the rate of
MTX uptake.[9] The rate of MTX uptake by cells has been,
in itself, shown to correlate with the drug's ability
to prolong the life of tumor-bearing mouse hosts.[10]

Role in Cancer Therapy

MTX has been used clinically for more than 20 years, first
against acute childhood leukemia, and more recently in a wide variety
of malignancies. It is one of the most useful anticancer agents so
far developed, and one of the most commonly employed. Yet there
remain a number of incompletely answered questions about how best
to use MTX. One of the most critical is to what extent modification
of the dose schedule influences therapeutic effectiveness.

This issue was first raised by Goldin and Venditti,[11] who
demonstrated experimentally that administration of MTX every 4
days was superior to daily administration of the drug in two
situations: (1) against early transplanted L1210 mouse leukemia
(one or two days after tumor inoculation), and (2) against advanced
L1210 leukemia, after other chemotherapeutic agents had been used
to markedly reduce the leukemic cell load. On the other hand, they
found that daily administration of the drug was necessary for
optimal therapeutic effect against "advanced" disease (in which
treatment was not started until 7 or 8 days after tumor inoculation,
at a time when the mice had an enormous leukemic cell load). It
has since been demonstrated that intermittent (twice weekly) MTX
is superior to daily MTX for remission maintenance in ALL-AUL.[68,73]
In a group of patients with disease refractory to other agents in
whom both induction and maintenance therapy were given with MTX
alone, Selawry et al[73] found the median duration of CR to be 4.5
months for patients who received semi-weekly MTX, as opposed to 2
months for those who received it daily. Subsequently,[68] they
demonstrated an even more striking superiority for intermittent MTX
maintenance in previously untreated patients who were induced with
vincristine and prednisone, then randomized to either 30 mg/m^2 x 2/
week or 3 mg/m^2/day of MTX. The median duration of CR was 11.5
months for the former and two months for the latter group, and the

median survival time of the intermittently maintained children is
in excess of 25 months. Acute Leukemia Group B has now demonstrated
that orally administered twice-weekly MTX is just as effective as
parenteral drug for remission maintenance.[109]

The greater effectiveness of MTX on an intermittent schedule
for maintenance (i.e., in the presence of a much-reduced leukemic
cell load) correlates well with the prediction of Goldin and
Venditti, based on L1210 data. On the basis of their data, one
would predict that chronic, daily administration of the drug might
be superior to an intermittent schedule for remission induction in
ALL-AUL. An early study of Frei et al[17] appeared to lend some
support to this contention: children induced and maintained with
daily MTX + daily 6 MP had a median remission duration of 4.5
months, as opposed to 2.2 months for children who received MTX
every third day (equivalent total dose) + daily 6 MP during
induction and maintenance. These results, however, were only
"marginally" significant ($P = 0.05$-0.10). There was no
difference in the rate of induction of remission between the two
groups: about one-sixth obtained CR and one-sixth PR in each group.

By contrast, the data tabulated in this review show an 80%
overall response rate for MTX given alone in high, single doses every
two weeks, as against a 35% overall response rate with daily treatment. Unfortunately, the numbers are too small in the "intermittent"
group to draw conclusions; however, it is especially impressive that
most of the remissions so obtained were in patients "resistant" or
"refractory" to previously administered daily MTX.[22,44]

Freireich[68] reportedly obtained remissions in 15 of 18
children with ALL who were induced with MTX on a q 4 day schedule
at doses up to 40 mg/m^2 (in most cases also with intrathecal MTX).

Selawry and James,[73] administering MTX for induction according
to a twice-weekly vs a daily schedule, found no difference between
the two in the remission rate obtained (31% CR vs 28%, respectively).

A substantial body of data which compares intermittent with
daily MTX for induction in ALL-AUL is contained in studies by
Children's Cancer Group A. In each of these, MTX was given in
conjunction with prednisone; the dose and schedule of prednisone
was, however, essentially identical for each study, so that
variations observed probably relate to differences in MTX administration. In the first, Krivit et al[79] compared daily 6 MP +
prednisone with daily MTX + prednisone in previously untreated
patients. There was no significant difference between the two as
to rate of induction, with MTX + prednisone yielding 80% M_1
marrows in ALL-AUL (113 patients were evaluated, most of whom were
in this disease category). Alteration of the dose or discontinuance

of MTX was required in 27% of the patients treated, due to bone
marrow or GI toxicity. At the Children's Hospital of Los Angeles,
one of the institutions participating in that study, 5 of 14
patients with ALL attained an M_1 marrow in 28 days, and 7 of the
14 after 42 days of induction treatment. Subsequently at the same
hospital, Brubaker et al[99] used MTX, 3 mg/kg IV on days 1 and 14,
together with prednisone in 14 consecutive untreated patients,
and obtained M_1 marrows in all by day 28 of therapy. "No instances
of nausea, vomiting, diarrhea, skin rash, or bone marrow depression
were observed. One patient developed buccal ulceration following
the second dose of methotrexate." Because of this encouraging
initial experience, Children's Group A has instituted two group-
wide protocols examining prednisone + intermittent MTX as an
induction regimen. The results of these latter studies should,
when published, provide more definite answers to the question of
whether daily or intermittent MTX is preferable for induction.

A discussion of MTX scheduling in ALL-AUL must include the
work of Djerassi;[88] although he uses a number of other drugs, both
for induction and maintenance, intermittent MTX given by prolonged
IV infusion is central to his program. With it, he has successfully and repeatedly reinduced children who have relapsed on
"conventional" MTX therapy. The toxicity associated with this
program has been quite marked, and this, coupled with the individ-
ualization of dose and drug schedule required, has made it difficult
for others to attempt to apply Djerassi's methods. Nevertheless,
he has shown that "resistance" to MTX, at least in ALL, is relative
rather than absolute, and may be overcome by revising the schedule
of drug administration.

Intrathecal MTX is extremely effective therapy for central
nervous system leukemia, even in cases where the hematologic
disease is "resistant". Most series have reported rather short
remission durations, which may have been related to inadequate
treatment. Selawry first proposed treatment beyond the period of
clearing of the cerebrospinal fluid of leukemic blast cells, with
encouraging preliminary results.[102] Sullivan et al[110] from the
SWCCG have now reported a study in 102 children with meningeal
leukemia which offers powerful confirmation of this concept. All
of the patients received twice weekly intrathecal MTX until the
cerebrospinal fluid WBC count fell below $10/mm^3$, and remission was
induced in 83. These were then randomly assigned to one of
three maintenance regimens: (1) intrathecal MTX, 12 mg/m^2 every
8 weeks; (2) BCNU (bis-chloroethyl nitrosourea), 100 mg/m^2 IV
every 8 weeks; or (3) no therapy. Because of a high relapse
rate at the time of the first follow-up lumbar puncture, the
treatment interval in the MTX and BCNU-treated patients was
subsequently shortened to 6 weeks. Remission maintenance was
evaluated in 46 children (MTX-19; BCNU-14; no therapy-13). The

median duration of remission in each maintenance group was as
follows: MTX, 488 days; BCNU, 94 days; and no therapy, 116
days. The differences among these median values were highly
significant in favor of MTX (P <0.01). Severe toxicity on the
maintenance program which required discontinuation of the drug
occurred in one of the patients treated with MTX, and two of
those who received BCNU. Sullivan et al concluded: "The
superiority of the MTX regimen is of such degree that it should
be considered for all children with CNS leukemia after CNS
remission is achieved."

In summary, MTX, the first agent shown to have activity
against ALL-AUL, remains the treatment of choice, used alone,
for meningeal leukemia. As a single agent, MTX appears less active
in systemic disease than vincristine or prednisone for induction,
and about equivalent to 6 MP or CTX. Its future role, if any,
for induction of remission in this disease will lie in
combination with other drugs, an area which continues to be
extensively explored. A third role for MTX in ALL-AUL lies in its
usefulness as a maintenance agent, either alone or in combination
therapy. The optimal way to use it for maintenance appears to be
twice weekly, and the oral route is just as effective as the
parenteral.

MTX has been much less effective against AML-AMoL. The most
successful dose schedule has been that of Vogler, Huguley et al[54,87]
(5-day courses of divided-daily-dose, oral administration), which
produced an overall reported response rate of 25%, 7/40 (17.5%)
obtaining CR. At all dose schedules combined, in 140 patients,
a 16% response rate is obtained, with 9/83 (11%) obtaining CR.
The overall response rate is thus lower than that reported for
6 MP, but the CR rate is essentially equivalent. Neither agent
appears as potent, at the schedules employed, for remission induction
as Ara-C or daunorubicin.

MTX has been employed extensively in the treatment of
epithelial malignancies involving the head and neck. The results
have been tabulated separately for patients who received the
drug by intra-arterial infusion and those who received it intravenously or by mouth ("systemically"). The overall response
rates are not markedly different for the two forms of therapy,
(53% of 340 vs 43% of 232), in spite of the fact that patients
selected for intra-arterial therapy undoubtedly were a group with
more localized disease. If one looks only at the results of weekly
and semiweekly MTX administration by the systemic route, the
response rate is 56%, actually slightly higher than that for
intra-arterial MTX. There thus appears to be no justification for
the use of intra-arterial MTX on the basis of response, and there
is every reason not to use it on the basis of toxicity. The "best"
series in terms of toxicity is probably that of Watkins and

Sullivan,[61] summarized in 1964: of 68 patients catheterized, 8
died of hemorrhage and 4 had "major" embolization related to the
treatment (17.5%), while 6 obtained CR of $\geq$ 6 months' duration.
The experience of others has been, on the whole, even worse,
as in the series of Tindel,[91] who reported 4 patient deaths and
serious complications in 10 others out of a total group of 24.
Creech, best known himself as a "regional perfusion" chemotherapist,
has summarized the arguments against this approach to therapy
(JAMA 200: 983, 1967): "To be sure, immediate results of intra-
arterial infusion may be impressive and, in fact, some remissions
have been protracted. But general results do not differ remarkably
from those of systemic chemotherapy, which is safer. Tindel's
report is timely because it shows the slight therapeutic value of
an extremely dangerous method of using cancericidal drugs."

The usefulness of MTX in trophoblastic malignancy is well-
known. Eighty-eight of 176 reported patients = 50% have obtained
a sustained CR and are apparently "cured" with MTX alone. It
should be noted that actinomycin D appears to be just as active
in a smaller series of patients, and may be effective in patients
who no longer respond to MTX.

Intra-arterial and "systemic" MTX have been tabulated separately
with respect to results obtained in cervical cancer. The same
considerations probably apply here as in treatment of head and
neck tumors. Although the response rate seems much better for intra-
arterial therapy, the toxicity is again a major drawback, and
systemic MTX has not received an adequate trial: 19 of the 25
reported patients are from a series in India, treated with "loading
dose" daily oral therapy in 5-day courses.

MTX deserves further evaluation in brain tumors. The reported
results, especially of administration by the intrathecal route,
are impressive, with medulloblastoma apparently the most responsive
tumor.

MTX has usually been used in combination with actinomycin D
and chlorambucil against testicular cancer. It may be equally
effective when used alone.[93]

MTX is a drug with significant activity against two of the
most common types of lethal tumor in man: breast and lung cancer.
The overall reported response rate of 33.6% for MTX against
breast cancer is slightly superior to that reported for CTX or
for 5-FU. "Loading-dose" monthly treatment appears clearly
inferior to other dose schedules, and if the results of such
therapy are excluded, the response rate exceeds 40%.

The dose-schedule effect does not seem so marked for MTX against lung cancer, at least in terms of response rate, although it should be noted that none of the reported trials employed low-dose, chronic treatment. Selawry and Ross[71] found twice-weekly MTX to be less toxic than either intermittent "loading-dose" or high single-dose, widely spaced administration, with therapeutic results which appeared to be at least as good. The VA Lung Group, in an unpublished study,[111] found monthly "loading-dose" MTX to be inferior to CTX, as measured by per cent survival, at up to 150 days on study; however, 11.7% of MTX-treated patients in their "extensive disease" category were alive at the end of a year, compared to 8.1% for CTX and 7.1% for a placebo-treated group.

MTX appears to have inferior activity, relative to CTX, BCNU, or imidazole carboxamide, against malignant melanoma. This judgment must be modified by the very small numbers reported, and the dose schedules employed.

Besides the question of what represents the best dose schedule for MTX, at least two other major issues remain, regarding its optimal clinical use: (1) is there an advantage in giving very large doses of MTX, and subsequently administering citrovorum factor; and (2) is MTX best used in combination with other drugs? With reference to the first, Goldin, Venditti et al[112] noted improved survival in mice with leukemia L1210 who received MTX followed by citrovorum factor (leukovorin) at an interval of 12 hours, over a group which received the same doses of MTX alone, or a group which received MTX + simultaneous citrovorum factor. Apparently, the implication of this finding was that the tumor cells had been irreversibly damaged by MTX at a time when toxicity to normal cells could still be largely reversed. Selawry[113] has reported preliminary studies in man which indicate that "rescue" of normal cells by citrovorum factor from increased toxicity due to MTX is possible at intervals as long as 72 hours after MTX administration. It remains to be seen whether the therapeutic index of MTX in man will be increased by the use of delayed citrovorum factor, but the feasibility of such an approach is now demonstrated.

MTX is clearly more effective for induction of remission in ALL-AUL when used in combination with prednisone than is either drug alone.[79] Whether it will prove more useful against solid tumors when used in concert with other agents remains to be determined.

* aminopterin data included

Tumor Type or Site

Breast

Ref #	# Pts Evaluated	# Pts Responding	% Response	Dose Schedule and Remarks
15	11	3		Varied, IM and PO, daily. Usually 2.5-5 mg/day in children, 5-10 mg/day in adults, as single daily dose. Transient PR.
16	9	4		5-20 mg/day, PO (MTX), 0.5-2 mg/day PO, (Aminopterin).
19	36	10	28	2.5-7.5 mg/day, PO, to toxicity or response.
33	37	20	54	~5 mg/day, PO as tolerated. British study.
36	9	2		2.5-10.0 mg/kg IV q 2 wk, as tolerated; "tolerated dose": 5 mg/kg q 2 wk.
65	13	7		.05 mg/kg (50 mcg/kg) daily, PO as tolerated [2-5 mg/day].
66	9	6		(1) 1.25-5.0 mg q 6 hr = 5-20 mg/day x 5, PO, repeated as tolerated (q 2-3 wks, generally). (2) 25 mg/day, IM x 5 (single daily injection). (3) 2, 4, or 6 mg/kg, IV q 2 wk. 3 "good" PR.
84	35	5	14	MTX, 0.4 mg/kg/day x 4, then 0.2 mg/kg eod x 4. Repeat in 4 wks (IV) -- vs 5-FU, 15 mg/kg/day x 4, then 7.5 mg/kg eod x 4. Repeat in 4 wks (IV) -- vs FUDR, 30 mg/kg/day x 4, then 15 mg/kg eod x 4. Repeat in 4 wks

Breast (cont.)

Ref #	# Pts Evaluated	# Pts Responding	% Response	Dose Schedule and Remarks
				(IV) -- ECOG study. 5-FU→8/30, FUDR→9/31 responses.
90	28	14	50	(1) 1.25 mg, PO, qid = 5 mg/day x 5-10 days; repeat when toxicity allows. (2) 5 mg/24 hr, continuous IV infusion, x 5-10 days; repeat when toxicity allows. All responders had ≥ 50% regression. Divided daily dose or continuous IV infusion for 5-10 days per course.
96	19	2	11	0.2 mg/kg/day x 4, then 0.1 mg/kg eod x 4, PO. Repeat one mo later (starting on day 42). COG study. 1 CR, 1 PR. "Loading-dose" monthly treatment.
103	20	5	25	MTX, 0.2 mg/kg/day x 4, IV or PO, then 0.1 mg/kg/day eod x 4 -- vs Testosterone propionate, 100 mg x 3/wk, IM. "Loading-dose" treatment. All patients without previous chemotherapy.
104	21	7	33	1.25-2.5 mg q 6 hr = 5-10 mg/day, PO x 5 days -- repeated q 2-4 wk, depending on toxicity (MTX) -- given alone in 21 patients. SECCG study. 4/21 had ≥ 50% objective regression.

Breast (cont.)

Ref #	# Pts Evaluated	# Pts Responding	% Response	Dose Schedule and Remarks
104	12	2		1.25-2.5 mg q 6 hr = 5-10 mg/day, PO x 5 days -- repeated q 2-4 wk, depending on toxicity (MTX) + fluoxymesterone, 15-30 mg/day, PO, or estrogen (dose not stated), and/or prednisone, 30 mg/day, PO, in 12 patients. SECCG study. Steroids added to treatment, but all patients already steroid-"resistant".
	$\overline{259}$	$\overline{87}$	33.6	Total.
	106	44	41.5	Total, single-dose daily treatment. Criteria of objective response not clearly defined.
	74	12	16.2	Total, loading-dose monthly treatment. Criteria of response clearly defined.
	70	29	41.5	Total, divided dose schedule or infusion. Criteria of response clearly defined.

Colorectal

Ref #	# Pts Evaluated	# Pts Responding	% Response	Dose Schedule and Remarks
16	1	0		5-20 mg/day, PO (MTX). 0.5-2 mg/day, PO (Aminopterin).
36	12	3		2.5-10.0 mg/kg IV q 2 wk, as tolerated; "tolerated dose": 5 mg/kg q 2 wk.

Colorectal (cont.)

Ref #	# Pts Evaluated	# Pts Responding	% Response	Dose Schedule and Remarks
65	6	2		.05 mg/kg (50 mcg/kg) daily, PO as tolerated [2-5 mg/day].
84	40	4	10	MTX, 0.4 mg/kg/day x 4, then 0.2 mg/kg eod x 4. Repeat in 4 wks (IV) -- vs 5-FU, 15 mg/kg/day x 4, then 7.5 mg/kg eod x 4. Repeat in 4 wks (IV) -- vs FUDR, 30 mg/kg/day x 4, then 15 mg/kg eod x 4. Repeat in 4 wks (IV). Median response duration = 22 wks. 5-FU →13/48, FUDR→2/46. ECOG study.
90	17	7		(1) 1.25 mg, PO, qid = 5 mg/day x 5-10 days; repeat when toxicity allows. (2) 5 mg/24 hr, continuous IV infusion, x 5-10 days; repeat when toxicity allows. All responders had regression of ≥ 2 mo duration.
96	14	1		0.2 mg/kg/day x 4, then 0.1 mg/kg eod x 4, PO. Repeat one mo later (starting on day 42). PR of 3 wk duration. COG study.
114	38	2	5	50 mcg/kg/day, PO as tolerated or 1.5 mg q 6 hr, PO in daily courses up to 8 days, with treatment repeated 4 wks after onset of the preceding course. 3 drug-related deaths among 51 patients treated. (All at 50 mcg/kg/day).
	$\overline{128}$	$\overline{19}$	15	Total.

Lung

Ref #	# Pts Evaluated	# Pts Responding	% Response	Dose Schedule and Remarks
36	7	1		2.5-10.0 mg/kg IV q 2 wk, as tolerated; "tolerated dose": 5 mg/kg q 2 wk.
66	3	0		(1) 1.25-5.0 mg q 6 hr = 5-20 mg/day x 5, PO, repeated as tolerated (q 2-3 wks, generally). (2) 25 mg/day, IM x 5 (single daily injection). (3) 2, 4, or 6 mg/kg, IV q 2 wk.
71	14	6		0.4 mg/kg/day, IV x 4; repeat q 3 wk. All PR.
71	12	5		0.8 mg/kg x 2/wk, IV to progression or limiting toxicity. 3 CR. "Least toxic" schedule.
71	13	4		10 mg/kg x 1, IV; repeat q 3 wk. All PR.
90	16	5		(1) 1.25 mg, PO, qid = 5 mg/day x 5-10 days; repeat when toxicity allows. (2) 5 mg/24 hr, continuous IV infusion, x 5-10 days; repeat when toxicity allows. All responders had regression of $\geq$ 2 mo duration.
95	21	3	14	0.6 mg/kg, IM, "semiweekly" as tolerated. Transient PR's. Only 1 patient in this series classed as "oat cell" carcinoma.
96	15	1		0.2 mg/kg/day x 4, then 0.1 mg/kg eod x 4, PO. Repeat one mo later (starting on day 42). Transient PR. COG study.

Lung (cont.)

Ref #	# Pts Evaluated	# Pts Responding	% Response	Dose Schedule and Remarks
111	—	—		10 mg/day x 5, IV; repeated monthly as tolerated. See discussion. VA Lung Group study.
	$\overline{101}$	$\overline{25}$	25	Total.

Malignant Melanoma

Ref #	# Pts Evaluated	# Pts Responding	% Response	Dose Schedule and Remarks
15	3	0		Varied, IM and PO, daily. Usually 2.5-5 mg/day in children, 5-10 mg/day in adults, as single daily dose.
38	1	1		50 mg/day x 5, by continuous (common carotid) intra-arterial infusion. CF given simultaneously, 6 mg q 6 hr, IM. CR; intra-arterial treatment of orbital tumors.
66	2	0		(1) 1.25-5.0 mg q 6 hour = 5-20 mg/day x 5, PO, repeated as tolerated (q 2-3 wks, generally). (2) 25 mg/day, IM x 5 (single daily injection). (3) 2, 4, or 6 mg/kg, IV q 2 wks.
90	12	2		(1) 1.25 mg, PO, qid = 5 mg/day x 5-10 days; repeat when toxicity allows. (2) 5 mg/24 hr, continuous IV infusion, x 5-10 days; repeat> when toxicity allows. Both responses were l- 50% regression.

Malignant Melanoma (cont.)

Ref #	# Pts Evaluated	# Pts Responding	% Response	Dose Schedule and Remarks
96	9	0		0.2 mg/kg/day x 4, then 0.1 mg/kg eod x 4, PO. Repeat one mo later (starting on day 42). Monthly loading-dose. COG study.
	27	3	11.1	Total. 2/26 = 7.7% by systemic treatment.

Lymphoma (not mycosis fungoides)

Ref #	# Pts Evaluated	# Pts Responding	% Response	Dose Schedule and Remarks
15	16	1		*Varied, IM and PO, daily. Usually 2.5-5 mg/day in children, 5-10 mg/day in adults, as single daily dose. Most patients received aminopterin. All adults.
15	7	3		*Varied, IM and PO, daily. Usually 2.5-5 mg/day in children, 5-10 mg/day in adults, as single daily dose. Children; all had lymphosarcoma, responders showed "significant improvement".
66	1	0		(1) 1.25-5.0 mg q 6 hr = 5-20 mg/day x 5, PO, repeated as tolerated (q 2-3 wks, generally). (2) 25 mg/day, IM x 5 (single daily injection). (3) 2, 4, or 6 mg/kg, IV q 2 wk.

Lymphoma (cont.)

Ref #	# Pts Evaluated	# Pts Responding	% Response	Dose Schedule and Remarks
63	14	8	57	0.15 mg/kg/day, PO. 3/10 CR in lymphosarcoma, 1/4 CR in Hodgkin's disease (34 wk duration).
63	7	1		.075 mg/kg/day, PO. 1/4 PR in lymphosarcoma, 0/3 in Hodgkin's disease.
	$\overline{45}$	$\overline{13}$	29	Total, non-Burkitt's lymphoma.

Burkitt's Lymphoma

Ref #	# Pts Evaluated	# Pts Responding	% Response	Dose Schedule and Remarks
69	19	10		MTX, 1 mg/kg/day x 5-8, PO -- vs CTX, 30-40 mg/kg x 1, IV; repeat at 10-14 days. 6 CR, 4 PR. CTX→52/63 with 24 CR, 28 PR.

ALL-AUL (systemic) MTX alone

Ref #	# Pts Evaluated	# Pts Responding	% Response	Dose Schedule and Remarks
12	14	6		*Varied, daily (various antifols used).
13	7	2		*MTX, 2-4 mg/day, IM to toxicity or response. Aminopterin, 0.5-2.0 mg/day, IM. 1 CR.
15	60	23	38	*Varied, IM and PO, daily. Usually 2.5-5 mg/day in children, 5-10 mg/day in adults, as single daily dose. 19 "good", 4 PR.
16	8	5		*5-20 mg/day, PO (MTX). 0.5-2 mg/day, PO (Aminopterin). 3 CR, 2 PR.

ALL—AUL (cont.)

Ref #	# Pts Evaluated	# Pts Responding	% Response	Dose Schedule and Remarks
22	3	2		1-5 mg/kg q 2-4 wk, IV. 2 CR; one in patient with previous daily MTX treatment.
32	55	15	27	(1) MTX, 1.25 mg/day for patients <1 year; 2.5 mg/day for patients 2-10 years old; 5 mg/day for patients >10 (Phase I) - PO as tolerated; followed by (Phase II) - 6 MP, 3 mg/kg/day, PO as tolerated. (2) (Phase I) 6 MP, followed by (Phase II) MTX (same doses). (3) 6 MP + MTX (same doses). [Prednisone used for "serious clinical situations" but not electively]. 12 CR, 3 PR. 6 MP→22/54, with 12 CR, 12 PR. MTX + 6 MP→23/40, with 17 CR. ALGB study.
44	12	10		3 mg/kg q 2 wk, IV push. All 12 had relapsed after previous exposure to both 6 MP and daily MTX. Mean duration remission = 4.4 mo; MST = 19.5 mo for this group.
109	-	-		Vincristine + prednisone induction, followed by maintenance with 30 mg/m^2 MTX twice weekly, IM vs PO. See discussion. ALGB study.
88	-	-		Varied -- see original paper and discussion.

ALL-AUL (cont.)

Ref #	# Pts Evaluated	# Pts Responding	% Response	Dose Schedule and Remarks
73	–	–		(1) MTX, 30 mg/m^2, IM, x 2/wk, for induction and maintenance -- vs (2) MTX, 3 mg/m^2/day, PO, for induction and maintenance. See discussion.
	159	69	40	Total. 18/73 CR = 24.6%.
	15	12	80	Total, high single-dose intermittent treatment.
	144	51	35.4	Total, daily treatment. 16/70 CR = 23%.

ALL-AUL (CNS disease)

Ref #	# Pts Evaluated	# Pts Responding	% Response	Dose Schedule and Remarks
18	5	5		0.1-0.5 mg/kg, intrathecally x 1, repeated as indicated. Duration remission ~6 wks.
20	14	12		0.25-0.5 mg/kg, q 2-5 days to clearing of CSF, given intrathecally. Mean remission duration = 5 mo. All patients presented with ↑ CSF pressure.
20	9	0		0.25-0.5 mg/kg, q 2-5 days to clearing of CSF, given intrathecally. All patients presented with lower extremity weakness.
25	2	2		0.5 mg/kg q 3-4 days x 3.

ALL-AUL (cont.)

Ref #	# Pts Evaluated	# Pts Responding	% Response	Dose Schedule and Remarks
31	2	2		5-10 mg intrathecally, repeat to clearing of CSF.
55	-	-		MTX, 0.5 mg/kg x 1, intrathecally or 400 r (radiation) to brain. 44/50 episodes responded to MTX→3.7 mo mean symptom-free interval. 49/50 responded to radiation therapy→2.8 mo mean symptom-free interval.
83	29	29		5 to 10 mg q 2-3 days, intrathecally, until CSF cell count fell below 10 cells/mm^3.
102	-	-		12 mg/m^2 once or twice weekly, intrathecally. Some patients received 2-3 doses of MTX after normalization of CSF; others received a median of 5.5 semiweekly doses after onset of CNS remission. See discussion.
110	102	83	81	MTX, 12 mg/m^2 x 2/wk, intrathecally, to CSF WBC count <10/mm^3. Patients then received: (1) MTX, 12 mg/m^2, intrathecally, q 8 wks or (2) BCNU, 100 mg/m^2 IV q 8 wks or (3) no prophylactic therapy. All patients responsive to MTX; lack of remission due to toxicity (4 cases), early death (6), or "other causes" (9). SWCCG study. See discussion.
	$\overline{162}$	$\overline{133}$	82	Total.

AML-AMoL

Ref #	# Pts Evaluated	# Pts Responding	% Response	Dose Schedule and Remarks
13	7	1		*MTX, 2-4 mg/day, IM to toxicity or response. Aminopterin, 0.5-2.0 mg/day, IM. CR.
14	21	3	14	*MTX, 2-5 mg/day, PO. (See original for doses of other antifols used).
15	28	5	18	*Varied, IM and PO, daily. Usually 2.5-5 mg/day in children, 5-10 mg/day in adults, as single daily dose. 1 "good", 4 "partial".
22	1	0		1-5 mg/kg q 2-4 wks, IV. Patient with AMoL.
32	43	4	9	(1) MTX, 1.25 mg/day for patients <1 year; 2.5 mg/day for patients 2-10 years old; 5 mg/day for patients >10 (Phase I) - PO as tolerated, followed by (Phase II) - 6 MP, 3 mg/kg/day, PO as tolerated. (2) (Phase I) 6 MP, followed by (Phase II) MTX (same doses) (3) 6 MP + MTX (same doses). [Prednisone used for "serious clinical situations" but not electively]. 2 CR, 2 PR. 6 MP→8/42, with 4 CR; 6 MP + MTX→6/46, 5 CR. ALGB study.
54	18	7	39	1.25-2.5 mg q 6 hr, daily x 5, PO. (Total dose 5-10 mg/day x 5), repeat courses at 10-14 day intervals. 6 CR. Median remission duration ~3 mo.

AML–AMoL (cont.)

Ref #	# Pts Evaluated	# Pts Responding	% Response	Dose Schedule and Remarks
87	22	3	14	(1) MTX, 1.25–2.5 mg q 6 hr = 5–10 mg/day, PO x 5 days. Repeat as soon as toxicity subsides (usually 10–14 days after initiation of treatment). (2) Prednisone, 15 mg tid, PO + 6 MP, 3 mg/kg/day as tolerated, PO. Both regimens continued for ~ 6 wks, if possible. 1 CR, 2 PR. 6 MP + Prednisone →7/26, 1 CR and 6 PR. SECCG study.
	$\overline{140}$	$\overline{23}$	16	Total. 9/83 CR = 11%.
	40	10	25	Total, divided daily dose treatment. 7/40 CR = 17.5%.
Head and Neck				
41	13	3		MTX, 50 mg/day by continuous intra-arterial infusion, with intermittent, concomitant CF administration. "Moderate" or "definite" objective regressions.
50	30	8	27	MTX, 50 mg/day by continuous intra-arterial infusion, with concomitant CF, 5 mg q 4 hr, IM. Only 1 response >3 mo duration.

Head and Neck (cont.)

Ref #	# Pts Evaluated	# Pts Responding	% Response	Dose Schedule and Remarks
51	13	7		40-50 mg MTX/day by continuous intra-arterial infusion, with concomitant CF at .085-0.125 mg/kg/day, IM in divided daily doses.
52	16	5		~50 mg/day MTX by continuous intra-arterial infusion, with CF, 20 mg/day, given concomitantly in divided daily doses, IM. 3-6 mo duration. Responses classed as "good results".
59	74	56	76	MTX, 50 mg/day by continuous intra-arterial infusion to local or systemic limiting toxicity (usually 5-6 days). CF given simultaneously, 18 mg/day, IM. 11 CR, one of 14+ mo duration. 74 patients considered evaluable.
61	68	42	62	50 mg/24 hr by continuous intra-arterial infusion, with CF, 6 mg q 6 hr, IM, for duration of the MTX infusion. Infusion continued until drug toxicity obtained in the region of infusion (7-30 days), repeated as tolerated for up to 3 mo. 15 CR, 27 PR of 53 "evaluable" patients. Summary report. 6 patients had CR of >6 mo duration; 8 patients died of hemorrhage, 4 had "major" embolization related to treatment.

Head and Neck (cont.)

Ref #	# Pts Evaluated	# Pts Responding	% Response	Dose Schedule and Remarks
62	7	0		MTX, 340–610 mg total dose over 10–14 days by continuous intra-arterial infusion, with administration of "intermittent" CF.
64	21	7	33	MTX, 50 mg/day by continuous intra-arterial infusion, with concomitant intermittent CF -- vs 5-FU, 1 gm/day by continuous intra-arterial infusion, for average duration of 6 days. 5-FU→2/18 responses.
72	45	25	56	MTX, 50 mg/day by continuous intra-arterial infusion, with concomitant CF, 6 mg q 6 hr IM -- as tolerated. 4 CR.
77	11	7		Continuous intra-arterial infusion of varying daily doses MTX, up to 25 mg/day, with 3 mg CF q 6 hr.
91	14	4		MTX, 25–50 mg/day by continuous intra-arterial infusion for varying intervals together with CF, 9 mg tid, IM. All ≥ 50% regressions. Four patients died as result of treatment, of 25 treated.
100	28	17	61	MTX, 50 mg/day by continuous intra-arterial infusion, with concomitant CF (dose not stated) -- administered for 5 days to 3 wks. 1 CR. All patients had oral cancer.

Head and Neck (cont.)

Ref #	# Pts Evaluated	Responding	Response	Dose Schedule and Remarks
	340	181	53.2	Total, intra-arterial infusion. All of above series utilized intra-arterial mode of MTX administration.
36	9	4		2.5-10.0 mg/kg IV q 2 wks, as tolerated; "tolerated dose": 5 mg/kg q 2 wks.
40	8	3		25 mg total dose over 5 days, PO -- repeat at one-month intervals if possible.
45	23	12	52	25 mg/day x 5, IV (23 patients); repeated q 4 wks as tolerated. Only 4 had >50% regression. Median remission = 4 wks.
45	24	9	37.5	15-20 mg/day x 5, PO (24 patients); repeated q 4 wks as tolerated. 4 had >50% regression. Median remission = 4 wks.
58	20	7	35	(1) 1.3-23 mg/kg, IV (occasionally intra-arterial), at varying intervals. Usual dose 3-5 mg/kg. (2) MTX as above + short, intensive courses of radiation therapy. (3) MTX + protracted radiation therapy. 1 CR, 5 mo duration. MTX + radiation therapy→6/11, with 4 CR.
60	10	2		0.2 mg/kg/day, IV x 5; repeat q 4-6 wks as tolerated. Both >50% regression.

Head and Neck (cont.)

Ref #	# Pts Evaluated	# Pts Responding	% Response	Dose Schedule and Remarks
66	8	2		(1) 1.25-5.0 mg q 6 hr = 5-20 mg/day x 5, PO, repeated as tolerated (q 2-3 wks, generally). (2) 25 mg/day, IM x 5 (single daily injection). (3) 2, 4, or 6 mg/kg, IV q 2 wks. 1 "good" PR.
74	11	5		0.2 mg/kg/day x 5, IV (MTX) followed by radiation therapy beginning on day 15. Response apparently seen prior to radiation therapy (sequential study).
90	13	7		(1) 1.25 mg, PO, qid = 5 mg/day x 5-10 days; repeat when toxicity allows. (2) 5 mg/24 hr, continuous IV infusion, x 5-10 days; repeat when toxicity allows.
92	18	4		1 to 3 mg/kg over 24 hour by continuous IV infusion, followed in some cases by CF, 6 mg q 12 hr x 6, IM. All patients received CF, 6 mg, IM, before MTX infusion. Infusions repeated (at higher dose, if possible) after 2-3 wk interval. All PR. 3 were >75% regression.
94	15	9		0.8 mg/kg q 4 days, IV to toxicity. 8 responses >50%. Median remission duration = 2 mo.

Head and Neck (con't)

Ref #	# Pts Evaluated	# Pts Responding	% Response	Dose Schedule and Remarks
96	11	3		0.2 mg/kg/day x 4, then 0.1 mg/kg eod x 4, PO. Repeat one mo later (starting on day 42). Transient PR. COG study.
101	27	14	52	25 mg (poor-risk) or 50 mg (good risk) q 4-7 days, IV. SWCCG study. 4 CR, 2 >300 days. Median response duration = 3 mo. 23 patients previously irradiated.
105	35	20	57	60 mg/m^2/wk, IV (30 patients) or 40 mg/m^2 x 2/wk, IV (5 patients). "Same dose administered at 3-4 wk intervals served to maintain remission." 11 CR, mean duration 5+ mo. 2 patients had remissions >300 days. Weekly MTX in most patients, semiweekly "too toxic."
	232	101	43.5	Total, systemic MTX administration (non-arterial).
	77	43	55.8	Total, weekly and semiweekly MTX.
			Cervix	
26	8	–		MTX, 50 mg/day by continuous intra-arterial infusion with concomitant CF, 24 mg/day in divided doses, IM. 3 deaths associated with treatment; intra-arterial.

Cervix (con't)

Ref #	# Pts Evaluated	# Pts Responding	% Response	Dose Schedule and Remarks
28	3	1		MTX, 50 mg/day by continuous intra-arterial infusion into hypogastric arteries, + CF 6 mg q 4 hr, IM. Infusion continued to toxicity. 25% PR for 3 mo.
61	20	11		50 mg/24 hr by continuous intra-arterial infusion, with CF, 6 mg q 6 hr, IM for duration of the MTX infusion. Infusion continued until drug toxicity obtained in the region of infusion (7-30 days), repeated as tolerated for up to 3 mo. 1 CR, 10 PR. 15 considered evaluable. Summary report. Intra-arterial.
70	16	4		50 mg/24 hr to 200-1700 mg MTX total dose over 4-48 days of continuous intra-arterial perfusion of the internal iliac (hypogastric) arteries, with intermittent administration of CF, IM, at 36 mg q 6-8 hr. 2 "considerable" responses. One patient had CR >18 mo. 3 died of drug-related sepsis.
80	4	2		MTX, 50 mg/24 hr x 5 days, if tolerated. CF, 6 mg q 6 hr, given concurrently, IM. 1/4 died of drug toxicity.

Cervix (con't)

Ref #	# Pts Evaluated	# Pts Responding	% Response	Dose Schedule and Remarks
81	12	7		5 mg/24 hr by continuous intra-arterial (internal iliac) infusion, given to appearance of toxicity. CF given (amount not stated) bid into vagina and rectum; no systemically administered CF given. All PR.
91	2	0		MTX, 25-50 mg/day by continuous intra-arterial infusion for varying intervals together with CF, 9 mg tid, IM.
	$\overline{71}$	$\overline{33}$	46.5	Total, intra-arterial MTX.
36	5	1		2.5-10.0 mg/kg IV q 2 wk, as tolerated; "tolerated dose": 5 mg/kg q 2 wk.
67	1	0		10-30 mg/day x 5, IM (MTX), repeated as tolerated. 7-12 mcg/kg/day x 5, IV (Actinomycin D), repeated as tolerated.
82	19	4		MTX, daily x 5, PO (dose not stated) -- repeat courses q 7-10 days as tolerated.
	$\overline{25}$	$\overline{5}$	20	Total, systemic MTX.

Brain Tumors

Ref #	# Pts Evaluated	# Pts Responding	% Response	Dose Schedule and Remarks
34	6	2		MTX, 12–14 mg/day by continuous intra-arterial infusion, with concomitant (delayed) intermittent CF. 12 and 16+ mo regression of neurologic deficits in glioblastoma patients.
47	5	2		MTX, 100 mg over 6 or 7 days, intra-arterially, or during the course of several wks; concomitant CF given IM.
76	–	–		MTX, 50 mg/day by continuous intra-arterial infusion, with 6 mg CF given q 6 hr IM. "Caused marked regressive changes in gliomatous tissue".
	11	4	36.4	Total, intra-arterial MTX.
75	7	2		MTX, varying doses by intraventricular perfusion, 5–7 hr once or twice weekly. "Definite" improvement – 3 mo. Glioblastoma.
98	18	15		0.2 mg/kg/day x 5–7, intrathecally. 9 patients had medulloblastoma. Remissions of 1.5–5 mo duration in most patients.

Brain Tumors (cont.)

Ref #	# Pts Evaluated	# Pts Responding	% Response	Dose Schedule and Remarks
108	11	6		0.25 mg/kg intrathecally, eod during initial hospitalization then q 1-2 wks (dose varied somewhat according to response). Medulloblastomas showed best response.
	$\overline{36}$	$\overline{23}$	64	Total, intrathecal MTX.

Trophoblastic Malignancies

Ref #	# Pts Evaluated	# Pts Responding	% Response	Dose Schedule and Remarks
27	7	3		(Usual) total dose 1.5 mg/kg over 4 days, PO. Repeat q 2 wks as tolerated.
29	12	9		15-30 mg/day chronically, after surgical removal of primary tumor. (Route and duration not given). 3 drug deaths. 5 CR, living and well beyond 3 years.
30	63	57	90	(1) 10-30 mg/day, IM, for 5 days (MTX). (2) 3-6 mg bid, IV, for 3 days consecutively (vinblastine). 28 sustained CR and apparent cure = 44.5%, with MTX alone.
43	-	-		3-5 days of 6 MP + MTX -- MTX total dose 75-125 mg, PO; 6 MP total dose 300-3000 mg, PO.

Trophoblastic Malignancies (cont.)

Ref #	# Pts Evaluated	# Pts Responding	% Response	Dose Schedule and Remarks
46	22	22	100	MTX alone (14 patients) according to "previous schedule" or MTX followed by Actinomycin D (2 patients). 20 CR. All patients had localized disease, received MTX as primary therapy.
49	5	4		MTX, 15-50 mg/day by continuous intra-arterial infusion, with CF concomitantly in divided daily doses; in addition, 50-100 mg 6 MP bid, PO. Intra-arterial infusion for localized tumor. One patient required systemic MTX to obtain CR.
53	-	-		15-30 mg/day x 5, IM, repeated as tolerated. 45/87 who received MTX as primary chemotherapy had sustained CR, apparent cures = 52%. Actinomycin D→7/13 sustained CR as primary chemotherapy.
56	28	20	71	(1) 0.5 mg/kg/day x 5, PO (MTX) or (2) 10 mcg/kg/day x 5, IV (Actinomycin D) or (3) 5 mg MTX, PO + 10 mg chlorambucil PO + 0.5 mg Actinomycin D -- daily x 5. 7 patients relapsed, all within 6 mo; overall sustained CR with MTX alone = 13/28.

Trophoblastic Malignancies (cont.)

Ref #	# Pts Evaluated	# Pts Responding	% Response	Dose Schedule and Remarks
57	11	7		5 mg four times daily, PO, for 5 or more days, repeated as tolerated. 3 patients relapsed at 3, 12, and 18 mo. 4 had CR, were disease-free at 11, 41, 45, and 48 mo.
67	–	–		10-30 mg/day x 5, IM (MTX), repeated as tolerated. 7-12 mcg/kg/day x 5, IV (Actinomycin D), repeated as tolerated. 17/36 = 47% had sustained CR with MTX alone. Actinomycin D→8/14 sustained CR.
78	2	2		25 mg/day x 5, divided daily doses, PO. Sustained CR, localized disease.
85	12	8		20 mg/day x 5, PO, repeated as tolerated. All CR, all >1 year duration.
86	58	54	93	15-25 mg/day, IM x 5, repeated as tolerated. 4 patients relapsed on MTX; all patients in this series had localized disease.
97	10	10		20-25 mg/day x 5, IV; repeated courses given in varying dosages at 2-4 wk intervals. 7/10 CR, free of disease. 1 patient died of cerebral hemorrhage, 2 relapsed on MTX.

Trophoblastic Malignancies (cont.)

Ref #	# Pts Evaluated	# Pts Responding	% Response	Dose Schedule and Remarks
107	—	—		Hysterectomy + MTX, 10–25 mg/day, PO x 5. Repeated at intervals of 1–4 wks as tolerated — vs hysterectomy without MTX. (These patients also apparently received radiation and/or alkylating agents). 2/8 2-year survivors with MTX + hysterectomy.
	$\overline{230}$	$\overline{196}$	85	Total.
			Testicular Cancer	
93	10	4	40	2.5–5.0 mg/day, PO, as tolerated. Each responder survived >5 years. Mean survival time for non-responders = 4 mo.

References

(1)   Ragab, A., Frech, R., and Vietti, T.   Osteoporotic fractures
      secondary to methotrexate therapy of acute leukemia in
      remission.   Cancer 25: 580, 1970.

(2)   Bertino, J.   The mechanism of action of the folate antagonists
      in man.   Cancer Res 23: 1286, 1963.

(3)   Werkheiser, W.   The biochemical, cellular, and pharmacological
      action and effects of the folic acid antagonists.   Cancer Res
      23: 1277, 1963.

(4)   Wells, W., and Winzler, R.   Metabolism of human leukocytes
      in vitro.   III.   Incorporation of formate-C^{14} into cellular
      components of leukemic human leukocytes.   Cancer Res 19:
      1086, 1959.

(5)   Winzler, R., Williams, A., and Best, W.   Metabolism of human
      leukocytes in vitro.   I.   Effects of a-methopterin on
      formate-C^{14} incorporation.   Cancer Res 17: 108, 1957.

(6)   Roberts, D., and Wodinsky, I.   On the poor correlation
      between the inhibition by methotrexate of dihydrofolate
      reductase and of deoxynucleoside incorporation into DNA.
      Cancer Res 28: 1955, 1968.

(7)   Fischer, G.   Increased levels of folic acid reductase as
      a mechanism of resistance to amethopterin in leukemic cells.
      Biochem Pharmacol 7: 75, 1961.

(8)   Hakala, M., Lakrzewski, S., and Nichol, C.   Relation of folic
      acid reductase to amethopterin resistance in cultured
      mammalian cells.   J Biol Chem 236: 952, 1961.

(9)   Hakala, M.   On the role of drug penetration in amethopterin
      resistance of sarcoma-180 cells in vitro.   Biochim Biophys
      Acta 102: 198, 1965.

(10) Kessel, D., Hall, T., Roberts, D., et al.   Uptake as a
      determinant of methotrexate response in mouse leukemias.
      Science 150: 752, 1965.

(11) Goldin, A., Venditti, J., Humphreys, S., et al.   Modification
      of treatment schedules in the management of advanced mouse
      leukemia with amethopterin.   J Nat Cancer Inst 17: 203,
      1956.

(12) Dameshek, W. The use of folic acid antagonists in the treatment of acute and subacute leukemia. Blood 4: 168, 1949.

(13) Sacks, M., Bradford, G., and Schoenbach, E. The response of acute leukemia to the administration of the folic acid antagonists, aminopterin and a-methopterin: report of 14 cases. Ann Intern Med 32: 80, 1950.

(14) Dameshek, W., Freedman, M., and Steinberg, L. Folic acid antagonists in the treatment of acute and subacute leukemia. Blood 5: 898, 1950.

(15) Burchenal, J., Karnofsky, D., Kingsley-Pillers, E., et al. The effects of the folic acid antagonists and 2, 6-diaminopurine on neoplastic disease. Cancer 4: 549, 1951.

(16) Schoenbach, E., Colsky, J., and Greenspan, E. Observations on the effects of the folic acid antagonists, aminopterin and amethopterin, in patients with advanced neoplasms. Cancer 5: 1201, 1952.

(17) Frei, E., Holland, J., Schneiderman, M., et al. A comparative study of two regimens of combination chemotherapy in acute leukemia. Blood 13: 1126, 1958.

(18) Whiteside, J., Philips, F., Dargeon, H., and Burchenal, J. Intrathecal amethopterin in neurological manifestations of leukemia. Arch Intern Med 101: 279, 1958.

(19) Wright, J., Cobb, J., Golomb, F., Gumport, S., Lyall, D., and Safadi, D. Chemotherapy of disseminated carcinoma of the breast. Ann Surg 150: 221, 1959.

(20) Murphy, M. Leukemia and lymphoma in children. Pediat Clin N Amer 6: 611, 1959.

(21) Wright, J., Gumport, S., and Golomb, F. Remissions produced with the use of methotrexate in patients with mycosis fungoides. Cancer Chemother Rep 9: 11, 1960.

(22) Condit, P., and Eliel, L. Effects of large infrequent doses of a-methopterin on acute leukemia in children. JAMA 172: 451, 1960.

(23) Sullivan, R., Miller, E., Wood, A., Clifford, P., Duff, J., Trussell, R., and Burchenal, J. Continuous infusion cancer chemotherapy in humans--effects of therapy with intra-arterial methotrexate plus intermittent intramuscular

citrovorum factor.   Cancer Chemother Rep 10: 39, 1960.

(24)   Sullivan, R., Wood, A., Clifford, P., Duff, J., Trussell, R.,
       Nary, D., and Burchenal, J.   Continuous intra-arterial
       methotrexate with simultaneous, intermittent, intramuscular
       citrovorum factor therapy in carcinoma of the cervix.   Cancer
       Chemother Rep 8: 1, 1960.

(25)   Laurance, B.   Intracranial complications of leukemia treated
       with intrathecal amethopterin.   Arch Dis Childh 36: 107, 1961.

(26)   Trussell, R., and Mitford-Barberton, G.   Carcinoma of the
       cervix treated with continuous intra-arterial methotrexate
       and intermittent intramuscular leucovorin.   Lancet 1: 971,
       1961.

(27)   Hreshchyshyn, M., Graham, J., and Holland, J.   Treatment
       of malignant trophoblastic growth in women, with special
       reference to amethopterin.   Amer J Obstet Gyn 81:
       688, 1961.

(28)   Cahill, J., and Zeit, P.   Intra-arterial infusions of pelvic
       tumors with amethopterin.   Amer J Obstet Gyn 81: 970, 1961.

(29)   Manahan, C., Benitez, I., and Estrella, F.   Amethopterin in
       the treatment of trophoblastic tumors.   Amer J Obstet Gyn
       82: 641, 1961.

(30)   Hertz, R., Lewis, J., and Lipsett, M.   Five years'
       experience with the chemotherapy of metastatic chorio-
       carcinoma and related trophoblastic tumors in women.   Amer
       J Obstet Gyn 82: 631, 1961.

(31)   Shanbrom, E., Miller, S., and Fairbanks, V.   Intrathecal
       administration of amethopterin in leukemic encephalopathy
       of young adults.   New Eng J Med 265: 169, 1961.

(32)   Frei, E., et al.   Studies of sequential and combination
       antimetabolite therapy in acute leukemia: 6-mercaptopurine
       and methotrexate.   Blood 18: 431, 1961.

(33)   Greening, W.   Methotrexate in the treatment of advanced
       cancer of the breast.   In "Methotrexate in the Treatment
       of Cancer," (Porter and Wiltshaw, eds.), pp 29-33, 1962.

(34)   Perese, D., Day, C., and Chardack, W.   Chemotherapy of
       brain tumors by intra-arterial infusion.   J Neurosurg 19:
       215, 1962.

(35) Balla, G., Mallams, J., Hutton, S., et al. The treatment
      of head and neck malignancies by continuous intra-arterial
      infusion of methotrexate. Amer J Surg 104: 699, 1962.

(36) Condit, P., Shnider, B., and Owens, A. Studies on the folic
      acid vitamins VII. The effect of large doses of amethopterin
      in patients with cancer. Cancer Res 22: 706, 1962.

(37) Perrin, J., and Mauer, A. Evaluation of intravenous
      amethopterin therapy in acute leukemia. J Pediat 61:
      283, 1962.

(38) Levick, S., Belmont, O., Cohen, E., and Steinmetz, C.
      Treatment of malignant melanoma of the orbit with intra-
      arterial methotrexate. JAMA 182: 300, 1962.

(39) Elliot, J. Treatment of bladder cancer with amethopterin.
      Cancer Chemother Rep 20: 147, 1962.

(40) Huseby, R., and Downing, V. The use of methotrexate orally
      in treatment of squamous cancers of the head and neck. Cancer
      Chemother Rep 16: 511, 1962.

(41) Yollick, B., and Corgill, D. Regional chemotherapy of head
      and neck tumors by intra-arterial infusion techniques. Texas
      State J Med 59: 423, 1963.

(42) Benson, J., Kiehn, C., and Holden, W. Cancer chemotherapy
      by arterial infusion. Arch Surg 87: 125, 1963.

(43) Bagshawe, K. Trophoblastic tumors. Chemotherapy and
      developments. Brit Med J 5368: 1303, 1963.

(44) Perrin, J., Mauer, A., and Sterling, T. Intravenous
      methotrexate (amethopterin) therapy in the treatment of
      acute leukemia. Pediatrics 31: 833, 1963.

(45) Papac, R., Jacobs, E., Foye, L., and Donohue, D. Systemic
      therapy with amethopterin in squamous carcinoma of the head
      and neck. Cancer Chemother Rep 32: 47, 1963.

(46) Hertz, R., Ross, G., and Lipsett, M. Primary chemotherapy
      of non-metastatic trophoblastic disease in women. Amer J
      Obstet Gyn 86: 808, 1963.

(47) Bellman, S., Hugosson, R., Johansson, B., and Sjogren, S.
      Chemotherapy of five supratentorial malignant gliomas with
      intra-arterial infusion of methotrexate. Acta Chir Scand
      127: 569, 1964.

(48)   Hreshchyshyn, M.   Experience with chemotherapy in gynecologic
       cancer.   New York State J Med 64: 2431, 1964.

(49)   Bagshawe, K., and Wilde, C.   Infusion therapy ·for pelvic
       trophoblastic tumors.   J Obstet Gynec Brit Comm 71: 565, 1964.

(50)   Acquarelli, M., Feder, R., and Gordon, H.   Continuous intra-
       arterial infusion of methotrexate for recurrent squamous
       cell carcinoma of the head and neck.   Amer Surg 30: 423, 1964.

(51)   Hayes, D., Wilkins, F., and Meredith, J.   Regional arterial
       infusion for localized malignancies.   Arch Surg 88: 1070, 1964.

(52)   Jesse, R., Villarreal, R., Letayf, V., et al.   Intra-arterial
       infusion for head and neck cancer.   Arch Surg 88: 618, 1964.

(53)   Hertz, R., Ross, G., and Lipsett, M.   Chemotherapy in women
       with trophoblastic disease: choriocarcinoma, chorioadenoma
       destruens, and complicated hydatidiform mole.   Ann N Y Acad
       Sci 114: 881, 1964.

(54)   Vogler, W.R., Huguley, C., Lea, J., et al.   Treatment of
       acute leukemia in adults with repeated 5-day courses of
       methotrexate in multiple small oral doses.   Proc Amer Assoc
       Cancer Res 5: 66, 1964.

(55)   Evans, A., D'Angio, G., and Mitus, A.   Central nervous system
       complications of children with acute leukemia.   J Pediat 64:
       94, 1964.

(56)   Brewer, J., Gerbie, A., Dolkart, R., et al.   Chemotherapy in
       trophoblastic diseases.   Amer J Obstet Gyn 90: 566, 1964.

(57)   Lamb, E., Morton, D., and Byron, R.   Methotrexate therapy of
       choriocarcinoma and allied tumors.   Amer J Obstet Gyn 90:
       317, 1964.

(58)   Condit, P., Ridings, G., Coin, J., et al.   Methotrexate and
       radiation in the treatment of patients with cancer.   Cancer
       Res 24: 1524, 1964.

(59)   Espiner, H., and Westbury, G.   Continuous chemotherapy by
       intra-arterial infusion.   Acta Un Int Cancr 20: 475, 1964.

(60)   Hellman, S., Ianotti, A., and Bertino, J.   Determinations
       of the levels of serum folate in patients with carcinoma of
       the head and neck treated with methotrexate.   Cancer Res 24:
       105, 1964.

(61) Watkins, E., and Sullivan, R. Cancer chemotherapy by
      prolonged arterial infusion. Surg Gyn and Obstet 118: 1,
      1964.

(62) Beahrs, O., Caldarola, V., and Harrison, E. Treatment of
      cancer of the head and neck by chemotherapy. JAMA 189:
      163, 1964.

(63) Frei, E., Speers, C., Brindley, C., et al. Clinical studies
      of dichloromethotrexate (NSC 29630). Clin Pharm Ther 6:
      160, 1965.

(64) Baker, R., and Gaertner, R. Regional arterial infusion of
      antimetabolites. J Surg Res 5: 132, 1965.

(65) Wilson, H., and Louis, J. The use of low dosage drug
      regimens in the treatments of neoplastic disease. Ann
      Intern Med 63: 918, 1965.

(66) Vogler, W., Huguley, C., and Kerr, W. Toxicity and anti-
      tumor effect of divided doses of methotrexate. Arch Intern
      Med 115: 285, 1965.

(67) Ross, G., Goldstein, D., Hertz, R., et al. Sequential use
      of methotrexate and actinomycin D in the treatment of
      metastatic choriocarcinoma and related trophoblastic
      diseases in women. Amer J Obstet Gyn 93: 223, 1965.

(68) Selawry, O. (Acute Leukemia Group B). New treatment
      schedule with improved survival in childhood leukemia.
      Intermittent parenteral vs daily oral administration of
      methotrexate for maintenance of induced remission. JAMA
      194: 75, 1965.

(69) Burkitt, D., Hutt, M., and Wright, D. The African lymphoma.
      Preliminary observations on response to therapy. Cancer 18:
      399, 1965.

(70) Hodgkinson, C., and Boyce, C. Prolonged intra-arterial
      therapy for advanced pelvic malignancy. Cancer 18: 1536,
      1965.

(71) Ross, C., and Selawry, O. Comparison of three dose schedules
      of methotrexate in lung cancer. Proc Amer Assoc Cancer Res
      6: 54 (#214), 1965.

(72) Burn, J., Johnston, I., Davies, A., and Sellwood, R. Cancer
      chemotherapy by continuous intra-arterial infusion of
      methotrexate. Brit J Surg 53: 329, 1966.

(73) Selawry, O., and James, D. Therapeutic index of methotrexate as related to dose schedule and route of administration in children with acute lymphocytic leukemia. Proc Amer Assoc Cancer Res 6: 56 (#224), 1965.

(74) Kligerman, M., Hellman, M., von Essen, C., and Bertino, J. Sequential chemotherapy and radiotherapy. Preliminary results of clinical trial with methotrexate in head and neck cancer. Radiology 86: 247, 1966.

(75) Rubin, R., Ommaya, A., Henderson, E., Bering, E., and Rall, D. Cerebrospinal fluid perfusion for central nervous system neoplasms. Neurology 16: 680, 1966.

(76) Luyendijk, W., and van Beusekom, G. Chemotherapy of cerebral gliomas with intra-carotid methotrexate-infusion. Acta Neurochir 15: 234, 1966.

(77) Gorgun, B., and Watne, A. Infusion chemotherapy in head and neck tumors. Arch Surg 92: 951, 1966.

(78) Dietzel, H., and Schwarz, R. Primary treatment of chorio-carcinoma with methotrexate. Arch Surg 92: 301, 1966.

(79) Krivit, W., Brubaker, C., Hartmann, J., et al. Induction of remission in acute leukemia of childhood by combination of prednisone and either 6-mercaptopurine or methotrexate. J Pediat 68: 965, 1966.

(80) Laufe, L., Blockstein, R., Parsi, F., and Lowy, A. Infusion through inferior gluteal artery for pelvic cancer. Obstet Gyn 28: 650, 1966.

(81) Bateman, J., Hazen, J., Stolinsky, D., and Steinfeld, J. Advanced carcinoma of the cervix treated by intra-arterial methotrexate. Amer J Obstet Gyn 96: 181, 1966.

(82) Roy, D. Treatment of advanced or recurrent carcinoma of the cervix by cytotoxic drugs. Indian J Cancer 4: 32, 1967.

(83) Hardisty, R., and Norman, P. Meningeal leukemia. Arch Dis Childh 42: 441, 1967.

(84) Eastern Cooperative Group in Solid Tumor Chemotherapy. Comparison of antimetabolites in the treatment of breast and colon cancer. JAMA 200: 770, 1967.

(85) Wei, P., and Ouyang, P. The use of methotrexate in the treatment of trophoblastic disease, especially chorio-

carcinoma. Amer J Obstet Gyn 98: 79, 1967.

(86) Hammond, C., Hertz, R., Ross, G., et al. Primary chemo-
      therapy for non-metastatic gestational trophoblastic
      neoplasms. Amer J Obstet Gyn 98: 71, 1967.

(87) Vogler, W., Huguley, C., and Rundles, R. Comparison of
      methotrexate with 6-mercaptopurine-prednisone in treatment
      of acute leukemia in adults. Cancer 20: 1221, 1967.

(88) Djerassi, I. Methotrexate infusions and intensive
      supportive care in the management of children with acute
      lymphocytic leukemia: follow-up report. Cancer Res 27:
      2561, 1967.

(89) Norrell, H., and Wilson, C. Brain tumor chemotherapy with
      methotrexate given intrathecally. JAMA 201: 15, 1967.

(90) Sullivan, R., Miller, E., Zurek, W., Oberfield, R., and
      Ojima, Y. Re-evaluation of methotrexate as an anticancer
      drug. Surg Gyn and Obstet 125: 819, 1967.

(91) Tindel, S. Intra-arterial chemotherapy for recurrent
      neoplasms. JAMA 200: 913, 1967.

(92) Lefkowitz, E., Papac, R., and Bertino, J. Head and neck
      cancer. III. Toxicity of 24-hour infusions of methotrexate
      (NSC 740) and protection by leucovorin (NSC 3590) in
      patients with epidermoid carcinomas. Cancer Chemother Rep
      51: 305, 1967.

(93) Wyatt, J., and McAninch, L. A chemotherapeutic approach to
      advanced testicular carcinoma. Canad J Surg 10: 421, 1967.

(94) Papac, R., Lefkowitz, E., and Bertino, J. Methotrexate
      (NSC 740) in squamous cell carcinoma of the head and neck.
      II. Intermittent intravenous therapy. Cancer Chemother Rep
      51: 69, 1967.

(95) Reed, L., Muggia, F., Klipstein, F., and Gellhorn, A.
      Intermittent parenteral methotrexate (NSC 740) therapy for
      carcinoma of the lung. Cancer Chemother Rep 51: 475, 1967.

(96) Andrews, N., and Wilson, W. Phase II study of methotrexate
      in solid tumors. Cancer Chemother Rep 51: 471, 1967.

(97) Johnson, F., Jacobs, E., and Silliphant, W. Trophoblastic
      tumors of the uterus. Problems of methotrexate therapy.
      Calif Med 108: 1, 1968.

(98) Newton, W., Sayers, M., and Samuels, L.   Intrathecal
      methotrexate (NSC 740) therapy for brain tumors in children.
      Cancer Chemother Rep 52: 257, 1968.

(99) Brubaker, C., Gilchrist, G., Hammond, D., et al.   Induction
      of remission in acute leukemia with prednisone and
      intravenous methotrexate.   J Pediat 73: 623, 1968.

(100) Couture, J.   Intra-arterial infusion therapy for oral cancer.
      Canad J Surg 11: 420, 1968.

(101) Lane, M., Moore, J., Levin, H., et al.   Methotrexate therapy
      for squamous cell carcinomas of the head and neck.   JAMA
      204: 561, 1968.

(102) Selawry, O., and Odom, S.   On eradication of leukemic
      meningiopathy.   Proc Amer Assoc Cancer Res 9: 62 (#246),
      1968.

(103) Nevinny, H., Hall, T., Haines, C., et al.   Comparison of
      methotrexate (NSC 740) and testosterone propionate (NSC
      9166) in the treatment of breast cancer.   J Clin Pharm 8:
      126, 1968.

(104) Vogler, W., Furtado, V., and Huguley, C.   Methotrexate for
      advanced cancer of the breast.   Cancer 21: 26, 1968.

(105) Leone, L., Albala, M., and Rege, V.   Treatment of carcinoma
      of the head and neck with intravenous methotrexate.   Cancer
      21: 828, 1968.

(106) Weiss, S., and Raskind, R.   Treatment of malignant brain
      tumors by local methotrexate.   A preliminary report.   Int
      Surg 51: 149, 1969.

(107) Hsu, C., and Cheng, Y.   Methotrexate therapy in trophoblastic
      disease at the Provincial Taipei Hospital (1955-1966).   A
      re-evaluation and proposals.   Amer J Obstet Gyn 103: 60,
      1969.

(108) Wilson, C., and Norrell, H.   Brain tumor chemotherapy with
      intrathecal methotrexate.   Cancer 23: 1038, 1969.

(109) Acute Leukemia Group B.   Acute lymphocytic leukemia in
      children.   Maintenance therapy with methotrexate administered
      intermittently.   JAMA 207: 923, 1969.

(110) Sullivan, M., Haggard, M., Donaldson, M., et al. Comparison
      of the prolongation of remission in meningeal leukemia with
      maintenance intrathecal methotrexate and intravenous bis-
      nitrosourea (BCNU). Proc Amer Assoc Cancer Res 11: 77
      (#306), 1970.

(111) VA Lung Group, unpublished data. (Personal communication,
      Dr. Julius Wolf).

(112) Goldin, A., Venditti, J., Kline, I., et al. Eradication of
      leukemic cells (L1210) by methotrexate and methotrexate plus
      citrovorum factor. Nature 212: 1548, 1966.

(113) Selawry, O. Tolerance to sequential use of methotrexate and
      leukovorin in cancer patients. Proc Amer Assoc Cancer Res
      11: 72 (#283), 1970.

(114) Moertel, C., Reitemeier, R., and Hahn, R. Oral methotrexate
      therapy of gastrointestinal carcinoma. Surg Gyn Obstet 130:
      292, 1970.

6-Mercaptopurine

Synonyms: Purinethol, 6 MP

Structure:

$\cdot\ H_2O$

Dosage: Usual dose for 6 MP (used alone) is 2.5–3.0 mg/kg/day,
               PO as a single daily dose, to response or limiting
               toxicity.

Toxicity: I.   Hematological – usually gradual in onset at
                    recommended schedule
                    A. Leukopenia
                    B. Thrombocytopenia
                    C. Anemia

               II. Gastrointestinal
                    A. Anorexia, nausea, or vomiting–seen in about
                        25% of adults, less commonly in children
                    B. Stomatitis – rare
                    C. Diarrhea – rare

               III. Hepatic
                    A. Clinical – jaundice occurs in about one-third
                        of adult patients, less commonly in children
                        1. Usually reversible with cessation of
                            therapy
                    B. Pathologic – bile stasis and hepatic necrosis
                        have been described

               IV. Dermatological – uncommon

Mechanism of Action:[1,2,3,4]   6 MP must be converted intracellularly
               to its corresponding ribonucleotide, the thio analog
               of inosinic acid, to exert its biological effects.
               Once this ribonucleotide (6-thioinosinic acid) is
               formed, it may have a number of actions of importance,
               including (1) suppression of de novo purine biosynthesis
               via "pseudofeedback inhibition" of the formation of
               ribosylamine 5-phosphate from glutamine and PRPP (5-
               phosphoribosyl-1-pyrophosphate); (2) inhibition of the
               formation of adenylic and guanylic acid from inosinic
               acid; and (3) inhibition of interconversion reactions
               among intermediate compounds in purine metabolism.

                          Role in Cancer Therapy

     6 MP has been in clinical use for 17 years. During that time
it has received a reasonably adequate trial in each of the common
tumors of man. It has demonstrated a response rate >20% in only
ALL–AUL, AML–AMoL, and lymphoma. The 37% response in lymphoma is
based on an evaluation of only 35 patients, and the scanty literature
suggests that 6 MP may be especially active in reticulum-cell
sarcoma. A definitive study of 6 MP remains to be done in this
disease.

In ALL-AUL, two-thirds of approximately 600 reported patients demonstrated an objective response to the administration of 6 MP alone, and the overall complete response rate appears to be about 35%. For previously untreated patients, the CR rate in 81 evaluated is 38%, about the same as the 40% obtained in a relatively small series by Holcomb with CTX (Cancer Chemother Rep 51: 389, 1967). The effectiveness of 6 MP as a remission maintenance drug after induction with prednisone or vincristine + prednisone has also been amply demonstrated in studies by both ALGB and the SWCCG, although that is beyond the scope of this review.

In AML-AMoL (including promyelocytic and erythroleukemias), the overall response rate is 28% of 521 cases, with 11.5% of 445 evaluated for CR obtaining this status. The results of different investigators and groups have varied markedly. In a study carried out for the Medical Research Council of the United Kingdom by a large working party[34,38], the median survival time for patients treated with 6 MP alone was only 61 days from the start of treatment, as compared to 71.5 days for patients who received only prednisone, 40 mg/day; 40 days for those who received 6 MP + this "low dose" of prednisone; and 21 days for those who received 6 MP + "high dose" prednisone. (In this series, 6/39 patients with AML remitted on low-dose steroid alone). These results are in marked contrast to the median survival of 6.5 months for 6 MP-treated patients obtained by Ellison et al[22] in this country, and imply (although these figures are not given for the British study) a very low response rate to 6 MP: Ellison and, more recently, Boggs et al, have shown that survival time is definitely and considerably prolonged for patients with AML who obtain a 6 MP remission, even a PR. The latter authors, in the largest single series reported for 6 MP alone against AML,[40] found that one-fourth of patients treated obtained CR or PR, and that median duration of CR was 8 months, and of PR, 4 months. Lifespan was not felt to be shortened in non-responders by the treatment. Considering only the 76 patients they had treated since 1961, Boggs et al found a 30% overall response rate for 6 MP, which is close to what can be obtained with ara-C or daunorubicin alone, if not actually as good.

It should be noted that, although slightly more than half of reported patients with CML in "blast crisis" have responded to 6 MP, most if not all of these were PR, and they were usually transient. The value of 6 MP in combination with other agents in the treatment of this condition remains to be explored. In the "chronic" form of CML, 6 MP has definite activity, but is probably inferior to busulfan as a first-line drug, as shown by Huguley et al[33]. Ellison et al found 6 MP, thioguanine, and 6-chloropurine (6-CP) to be essentially of equal activity in this disease, with 25/33 patients "improved"[24].

6 MP has given occasional responses in patients with multiple myeloma, hypernephroma, and head and neck cancer. In none of these does the response rate approach 20%.

It appears that the future role of 6 MP in cancer therapy probably lies in combination (concomitant or sequential) chemotherapy with other drugs, especially in the acute leukemias, and possibly also in the undifferentiated lymphomas.

Tumor Type or Site

Breast

Ref #	# Pts Evaluated	# Pts Responding	% Response	Dose Schedule and Remarks
11	1	0		2 mg/kg/day, PO as tolerated. Gradually increased in patients who failed to respond.
39	44	6		1 mg/kg/day x 60, PO (0.5 mg/kg bid). All PR. Eastern CDEP study
	45	6	13	Total.

Colorectal

Ref #	# Pts Evaluated	# Pts Responding	% Response	Dose Schedule and Remarks
11	1	0		2 mg/kg/day, PO as tolerated. Gradually increased in patients who failed to respond.
35	4	0		(1) Continuous daily infusion – 0.125–1 mg/kg/day x 6–10, IV (6 MP); 0.125–2 mg/kg/day x 5–14, IV (6 MP). (2) Single daily rapid injection – 2–6 mg/kg/day x 6–7, IV (6 MP); 1–8 mg/kg/day x 5–7, IV (6 MPR). (3) Single rapid weekly injection – 10 or 15 mg/kg/wk x 1–5, IV (6 MP); 8.5 or 10 mg/kg/wk x 1, IV (6 MPR).
39	45	2		1 mg/kg/day x 60, PO (0.5 mg/kg bid). Eastern CDEP study.

Colorectal (cont.)

Ref #	# Pts Evaluated	# Pts Responding	% Response	Dose Schedule and Remarks
41	25	2		6 mg/kg/day x 4, off drug 10 days, repeat as tolerated (PO). Pacific VACCG study. Transient PR's.
	$\overline{75}$	$\overline{4}$	5	Total.

Melanoma

Ref #	# Pts Evaluated	# Pts Responding	% Response	Dose Schedule and Remarks
11	1	0		2 mg/kg/day, PO as tolerated. Gradually increased in patients who failed to respond.
39	20	2	10	1 mg/kg/day x 60, PO (0.5 mg/kg bid). Both PR. Eastern CDEP study.
41	6	0		6 mg/kg/day x 4, off drug 10 days, repeat as tolerated (PO). Pacific VACCG study. 18 patients placed on study.
	$\overline{27}$	$\overline{2}$	7	Total.

Lung

Ref #	# Pts Evaluated	# Pts Responding	% Response	Dose Schedule and Remarks
6	3	0		1.5-6.7 mg/kg/day, PO as tolerated (often initial high-dose "loading" therapy, followed by low-dose daily maintenance).

Lung (cont.)

Ref #	# Pts Evaluated	# Pts Responding	% Response	Dose Schedule and Remarks
11	5	0		2 mg/kg/day, PO as tolerated. Gradually increased in patients who failed to respond.
35	2	1		(1) Continuous daily infusion − 0.125−1 mg/kg/day x 6-10, IV (6 MP); 0.125−2 mg/kg/day x 5-14, IV (6 MPR). (2) Single daily rapid injection − 2-6 mg/kg/day x 6-7, IV (6 MP); 1-8 mg/kg/day x 5-7, IV (6 MPR). (3) Single rapid weekly injection − 10 or 15 mg/kg/wk x 1-5, IV (6 MP); 8.5 or 10 mg/kg/wk x 1, IV (6 MPR).
39	25	1		1 mg/kg/day x 60, PO (0.5 mg/kg bid). Eastern CDEP study.
41	44	2		6 mg/kg/day x 4, off drug 10 days, repeat as tolerated (PO). Pacific VACCG study.
	79	4	5	Total.

Lymphoma

Ref #	# Pts Evaluated	# Pts Responding	% Response	Dose Schedule and Remarks
11	15	4		2 mg/kg/day, PO as tolerated. Gradually increased in patients who failed to respond. All reticulum−cell sarcoma; one of 14 mo duration.

Lymphoma (cont.)

Ref #	# Pts Evaluated	# Pts Responding	% Response	Dose Schedule and Remarks
11	5	0		2 mg/kg/day, PO as tolerated. Gradually increased in patients who failed to respond. All lymphosarcoma and Hodgkin's.
12	1	1		2-3 mg/kg/day, PO as tolerated. Reticulum-cell sarcoma; PR.
39	14	8		1 mg/kg/day x 60, PO (0.5 mg/kg bid). All PR; no breakdown as to tumor types. Eastern CDEP study.
	$\overline{35}$	$\overline{13}$	37	Total.

ALL-AUL

Ref #	# Pts Evaluated	# Pts Responding	% Response	Dose Schedule and Remarks
5	87	57		2.5 mg/kg/day, PO, as tolerated. 41 CR, 16 PR.
6	10	7		1.5-6.7 mg/kg/day, PO as tolerated (often initial high-dose "loading" therapy, followed by low-dose daily maintenance). Remission duration 2-7.5+ mo.
7	23	12		2.5 mg/kg/day, PO (usual) 8 CR, 4 PR - previously untreated.
7	11	4		2.5 mg/kg/day, PO (usual). 3 CR, 1 PR - previously treated.

ALL-AUL (cont.)

Ref #	# Pts Evaluated	# Pts Responding	% Response	Dose Schedule and Remarks
8	19	7		12.5-200 mg/day, PO as tolerated. 1 CR, 6 PR - previously treated.
9	18	9		2.5 mg/kg/day, PO as tolerated. 2 "good", 7 PR; 2/3 lymphosarcoma→ALL had PR.
10	8	5		2-4 mg/kg/day, PO as tolerated. 3 CR, 2 PR (in acute "childhood" leukemia).
11	22	13		2 mg/kg/day, PO as tolerated. Gradually increased in patients who failed to respond. 7 "good", 6 PR; (acute "childhood" leukemia).
12	7	7		2-3 mg/kg/day, PO as tolerated. 4 "good", 3 PR.
13	4	2		2.5 mg/kg/day, PO as tolerated. 1 CR, 1 PR.
14	4	2		2.5 mg/kg/day, PO as tolerated. Some patients also received steroids. 25-75 mg/day. 1 CR, 1 PR.
15	19	15		2 mg/kg/day, PO as tolerated. 10 "good", 5 PR; (acute "childhood" leukemia).
16	10	3		2.5 mg/kg/day, PO as tolerated. 3 "good" (previously treated patients).
17	4	2		2.5 mg/kg/day PO as tolerated. 1 CR, 1 PR - all adults. CR = 8+ mo.

ALL—AUL (cont.)

Ref #	# Pts Evaluated	# Pts Responding	% Response	Dose Schedule and Remarks
21	13	11		(1) 6.6 mg/kg/day, PO, to toxicity; repeated as tolerated. (2) 2.2 mg/kg/day, PO, as tolerated. "High"-dose interrupted. More rapid onset of remission.
21	22	20		(1) 6.6 mg/kg/day, PO, to toxicity; repeated as tolerated. (2) 2.2 mg/kg/day, PO, as tolerated. "Low"-dose continuous; longer remission duration.
23	67	46		2.5 mg/kg/day, PO as tolerated (6 MP) -- vs 2.5 mg/kg/day, PO as tolerated (6 MP) + 2.5 mg/kg/day, PO as tolerated (azaserine). All patients previously untreated. 30 CR, 16 PR. 6 MP+ azaserine→43/58 (28 CR, 15 PR). Median remission duration = 2.8 mo for 6 MP alone, 4.1 mo for 6 MP+ azaserine induction.
26	54	22	44	(1) MTX, 1.25 mg/day for patients <1 year; 2.5 mg/day for patients 2-10 years old; 5 mg/day for patients >10 (PhaseI) - PO as tolerated; followed by (Phase II) - 6 MP, 3 mg/kg/day, PO as tolerated. (2) (Phase I) 6 MP, followed by (Phase II) MTX (same doses). (3) 6 MP + MTX (same doses). [Prednisone used for "serious clinical situations" but not electively]. ALGB study. 12 CR, 12 PR. Some patients previously treated with steroids. MTX→15/55 (27%), with 12 CR, 3 PR. MTX + 6 MP →23/40 (58%), with 17 CR, 6 PR.

ALL-AUL (cont.)

Ref #	# Pts Evaluated	# Pts Responding	% Response	Dose Schedule and Remarks
27	59	50		(1) 2.5 mg/kg/day, PO as tolerated (standard 6 MP). (2) 2.5 mg/kg/day, PO - 6 MP + 0.25 mg/kg/day, PO - DON, as tolerated. (3) 6.6 mg/kg/day, PO - 6 MP, for 14-21 days, followed by standard dose therapy. 21 CR, 29 PR. 31/59→M_1 marrow. All patients previously untreated. "Standard" regimen.
27	64	57		(1) 2.5 mg/kg/day, PO as tolerated (standard 6 MP). (2) 2.5 mg/kg/day, PO - 6 MP + 0.25 mg/kg/day, PO - DON, as tolerated. (3) 6.6 mg/kg/day, PO - 6 MP, for 14-21 days, followed by standard dose therapy. 22 CR, 35 PR. 37/64→M_1 marrow. "High dose" regimen. 6 MP (standard) + DON→65/71, with 30 CR, 50/71 →M_1 marrow (significantly better).
31	2	1		2.5 mg/kg/day to total dose 6-8 gm in 4-6 wks (6 MP) -- vs same dose of 6 MP + 60-100 mg/day x 14-28 (prednisone). 6 MP + prednisone →6/8, with 5 CR, 1 PR.
32	64	37		2.5 mg/kg/day, PO as tolerated. All patients refractory to steroids. 19 CR, 18 PR. SWCCG study.
	591	391	66	Total. CR+ "good" = 189/544 = 35%.

ALL-AUL (cont.)

Ref #	# Pts Evaluated	# Pts Responding	% Response	Dose Schedule and Remarks
	213	165	77	Total, previously untreated patients. 81 CR = 38%.
	104	51	49	Total, previously treated patients. 26 CR = 25%. 25%.
AML-AMoL				
5	50	17		2.5 mg/kg/day, PO, as tolerated. 7 CR, 10 PR ("adult" acute leukemia).
6	15	7		1.5-6.7 mg/kg/day, PO as tolerated (often initial high-dose "loading" therapy, followed by low-dose daily maintenance). 1 CR; duration remissions, 0.5-6+ mo.
7	8	1		2.5 mg/kg/day, PO (usual). PR; ("adult" acute leukemia).
9	4	4		2.5 mg/kg/day, PO as tolerated. All 4 "good", all in AMoL.
10	10	8		2-4 mg/kg/day, PO as tolerated. 2 CR, 6 PR ("adult" acute leukemia).
11	12	4		2 mg/kg/day, PO as tolerated. Gradually increased in patients who failed to respond. 2 "good", 2 PR ("adult" acute leukemia).

AML-AMoL (cont.)

Ref #	# Pts Evaluated	# Pts Responding	% Response	Dose Schedule and Remarks
12	20	12		2-3 mg/kg/day, PO as tolerated. 2 "good", 10 PR.
13	5	3		2.5 mg/kg/day, PO as tolerated. 2 CR, 1 PR ("adult" acute leukemia).
14	43	16		2.5 mg/kg/day, PO as tolerated. Some patients also received steroids, 25-75 mg/day. 5 CR, 11 PR.
15	13	2		2 mg/kg/day, PO as tolerated. 2 PR ("adult" acute leukemia).
16	5	2		2.5 mg/kg/day, PO as tolerated. 2 PR - all patients previously treated.
17	12	5		2.5 mg/kg/day, PO x 3-21 days. 1 CR, 4 PR. CR = 3 mo duration.
19	21	4		150 mg/day, PO, adjusted as tolerated. 6 MP + steroids →3/8 CR. 4 CR ("adult" acute leukemia).
22	18	5		2.5 mg/kg/day, PO as tolerated (6 MP); 15-20 mg/kg/day, PO as tolerated (6 CP). MST = 5 mo for 6 CP, 6.5 mo for 6 MP. 1 CR, 4 PR. 6 CP →3/16, with 1 CR, 2 PR. MST = 12 mo for patients who obtained CR or PR, 7.5 mo for non-responders who had 3 wks treatment.

AML-AMoL (cont.)

Ref #	# Pts Evaluated	# Pts Responding	% Response	Dose Schedule and Remarks
26	42	8		(1) MTX, 1.25 mg/day for patients <1 year; 2.5 mg/day for patients 2-10 years old; 5 mg/day for patients >10 (Phase I) - PO as tolerated; followed by (Phase II) - 6 MP, 3 mg/kg/day; PO as tolerated. (2) (Phase I) - 6 MP followed by (Phase II) - MTX (same doses). (3) 6 MP + MTX (same doses). [Prednisone used for "serious clinical situations" but not electively]. ALGB study. 4 CR, 4 PR. MTX →4/43, with 2 CR, 2 PR. 6 MP + MTX →6/46, with 5 CR, 1 PR.
30	47	7		2.5 mg/kg/day, PO as tolerated - (6 MP) -- vs 11-20 mg/kg/day, PO as tolerated - (6 CP). 1 CR, 6 PR. 6 CP →2 CR, 7 PR of 50. VACCG study.
31	10	3		2.5 mg/kg/day to total dose 6-8 gm in 4-6 wks (6 MP) -- vs same dose of 6 MP + 60-100 mg/day x 14-28 (prednisone). 2 CR, 1 PR. 6 MP + steroid →11/21, with 4 CR.
34,38	-	-		2.5 mg/kg/day, PO x 8 wks or to remission (6 MP) -- vs same dose regimen 6 MP + prednisone 40 mg/day, PO x 3 wks -- vs same dose regimen 6 MP + prednisone 250 mg/day, PO x 2 wks. (1) 6 MP, 2.5 mg/kg/day, PO -- vs (2) 6 MP, 2.5 mg/kg/day, PO + prednisone, 40 mg/day, PO -- vs (3) prednisone, 40 mg/day, PO. See discussion.

AML–AMoL (cont.)

Ref #	# Pts Evaluated	# Pt's Responding	% Response	Dose Schedule and Remarks
37	18	3		400 mg/m^2 x 2/wk or 800 mg/m^2/wk (6 MP) — vs 30 mg/m^2 x 2/wk or 80 mg/m^2/wk (MTX). ALGB study. Twice weekly schedule. MTX →2/19.
37	22	0		400 mg/m^2 x 2/wk or 800 mg/m^2/wk (6 MP) — vs 30 mg/m^2 x 2/wk or 80 mg/m^2/wk (MTX). ALGB study. Once weekly schedule. MTX →1/19.
40	146	33	23	2.5 mg/kg/day, PO to $\stackrel{>}{-}$ 6 wks or remission if possible, as tolerated. 21 CR, 12 PR. CR = 15% of total treated. See discussion.
	$\overline{521}$	$\overline{144}$	28	Total. 51/445 CR = 11.5%.

CML, Blast Crisis

5	6	2		2.5 mg/kg/day, PO, as tolerated. Both PR.
7	8	4		2.5 mg/kg/day, PO (usual). 3 CR, 1 PR.
10	2	2		2-4 mg/kg/day, PO as tolerated. Both PR.
12	6	6		2-3 mg/kg/day, PO as tolerated. All PR.
15	2	0		2 mg/kg/day, PO as tolerated.
25	5	2		150-200 mg/day, PO as tolerated. PR "up to 6 mo".
	$\overline{29}$	$\overline{16}$	55	Total. 3/29 = 10% CR.

CML

Ref #	# Pts Evaluated	# Pts Responding	% Response	Dose Schedule and Remarks
5	12	11		2.5 mg/kg/day, PO, as tolerated. All PR.
6	5	4		1.5-6.7 mg/kg/day, PO as tolerated (often initial high-dose "loading" therapy, followed by low-dose daily maintenance).
7	3	2		2.5 mg/kg/day, PO (usual). Both CR.
11	1	0		2 mg/kg/day, PO as tolerated. Gradually increased in patients who failed to respond.
14	10	6		2.5 mg/kg/day, PO as tolerated. Some patients also received steroids, 25-75 mg/day.
15	4	2		2 mg/kg/day, PO as tolerated. Both PR.
16	5	5		2.5 mg/kg/day, PO as tolerated.
18	17	11		2.5 mg/kg/day, PO as tolerated. All "CR", varied from 6-30 mo duration.
24	–	–		2.5 mg/kg/day, PO (6 MP) -- vs 2 mg/kg/day, PO (TG) -- vs 15-20 mg/kg/day, PO (6 CP). See discussion.
25	25	18		150-200 mg/day, PO as tolerated. All "good" responses. 1/3 "radioresistant".

CML (cont.)

Ref #	# Pts Evaluated	# Pts Responding	% Response	Dose Schedule and Remarks
33	15	5	33	3 mg/kg/day, PO as tolerated (6 MP) -- vs 6 mg/day, PO as tolerated (busulfan). 5/15 "good" response to 6 MP. 30/47 "good" response to busulfan, with 12/47 "excellent".
	100	64	64	Total.

CLL

Ref #	# Pts Evaluated	# Pts Responding	% Response	Dose Schedule and Remarks
6	1	0		1.5-6.7 mg/kg/day, PO as tolerated (often initial high-dose "loading" therapy, followed by low-dose daily maintenance).
13	2	0		2.5 mg/kg/day, PO as tolerated.
15	1	0		2 mg/kg/day, PO as tolerated.
	4	0		Total.

Multiple Myeloma

Ref #	# Pts Evaluated	# Pts Responding	% Response	Dose Schedule and Remarks
10	2	0		2-4 mg/kg/day, PO as tolerated.
11	15	2		2 mg/kg/day, PO as tolerated. Gradually increased in patients who failed to respond.
13	2	0		2.5 mg/kg/day, PO as tolerated.
	19	2	10	Total.

Kidney

Ref #	# Pts Evaluated	# Pts Responding	% Response	Dose Schedule and Remarks
11	2	0		2 mg/kg/day, PO as tolerated. Gradually increased in patients who failed to respond.
36	1	1		150 mg/day as tolerated; total dose 2100 mg. Good PR x 5 mo.
39	3	0		1 mg/kg/day x 60, PO (0.5 mg/kg bid).
41	6	0		6 mg/kg/day x 4, off drug 10 days, repeat as tolerated (PO).
	$\overline{12}$	$\overline{1}$	8.5	Total.

Head and Neck

Ref #	# Pts Evaluated	# Pts Responding	% Response	Dose Schedule and Remarks
35	3	0		(1) Continuous daily infusion - 0.125-1 mg/kg/day x 6-10, IV (6 MP); 0.125-2 mg/kg/day x 5-14, IV (6 MPR). (2) Single daily rapid injection - 2-6 mg/kg/day x 6-7, IV (6 MP); 1-8 mg/kg/day x 5-7, IV (6 MPR). (3) Single rapid weekly injection - 10 or 15 mg/kg/wk x 1-5, IV (6 MP); 8.5 or 10 mg/kg/wk x 1, IV (6 MPR).
39	32	5		1 mg/kg/day x 60, PO (0.5 mg/kg bid). Eastern CDEP study.
41	10	1		6 mg/kg/day x 4, off drug 10 days, repeat as tolerated (PO). Pacific VACCG study. 21 patients entered.
	$\overline{45}$	$\overline{6}$	12	Total.

References

(1)   Burchenal, J., and Ellison, R. The pyrimidine and purine
        antagonists. Clin Pharmacol Ther 2: 523, 1961.

(2)   Calabresi, P., and Welch, A. Chemotherapy of neoplastic
        diseases. Ann Rev Med 13: 147, 1962.

(3)   Elion, G., Callahan, S., Rundles, R., et al. Relationship
        between metabolic fates and antitumor activities of thiopurines.
        Cancer Res 23: 1207, 1963.

(4)   Brockman, R. Biochemical aspects of mercaptopurine inhibition
        and resistance. Cancer Res 23: 1191, 1963.

(5)   Burchenal, J., Ellison, R., Murphy, M., et al. Clinical
        studies on 6-mercaptopurine. Ann N Y Acad Sci 60: 359, 1954.

(6)   Hall, B., Richards, M., Willett, F., et al. Clinical
        experience with 6-mercaptopurine in human neoplasia. Ann N Y
        Acad Sci 60: 374, 1954.

(7)   Bernard, J., and Seligmann, M. A study of 61 leukemias
        treated with 6-mercaptopurine. Ann N Y Acad Sci 60: 385, 1954.

(8)   Farber, S. Summary of experience with 6-mercaptopurine. Ann
        N Y Acad Sci 60: 412, 1954.

(9)   Pierce, M. Leukemia in children: treatment of 22 cases with
        6-mercaptopurine. Ann N Y Acad Sci 60: 415, 1954.

(10)   Rundles, R., and Crago, J. 6-mercaptopurine therapy in
        neoplastic disease. Ann N Y Acad Sci 60: 425, 1954.

(11)   Hyman, G., Gellhorn, A., and Wolff, J. The therapeutic
        effect of mercaptopurine in a variety of human neoplastic
        diseases. Ann N Y Acad Sci 60: 430, 1954.

(12)   Bethell, F., and Thompson, D. Treatment of leukemia and
        related disorders with 6-mercaptopurine. Ann N Y Acad Sci
        60: 436, 1954.

(13)   Fountain, J. Clinical observations of the treatment of
        leukemia and allied disorders with 6-mercaptopurine. Ann N Y
        Acad Sci 60: 439, 1954.

(14)   Rosenthal, N., Rosenthal, R., and Lee, S. Role of
        mercaptopurine in the treatment of leukemia and related
        diseases. Ann N Y Acad Sci 60: 448, 1954.

(15)   Gaffney, P., and Cooper, W. A clinical study of 6-
       mercaptopurine. Ann N Y Acad Sci 60: 478, 1954.

(16)   Wilson, S. The clinical and hematologic response of
       previously treated leukemic subjects to the antimetabolite
       6-mercaptopurine. Ann N Y Acad Sci 60: 499, 1954.

(17)   Hayhoe, F. 6-mercaptopurine in acute leukemia. Lancet 3:
       903, 1955.

(18)   Fountain, J. Treatment of chronic myeloid leukemia with
       mercaptopurine. Brit Med J 2: 1345, 1956.

(19)   Whitelaw, D., Moffat, R., Perry, W., et al. Acute leukemia
       in adults treated with 6-mercaptopurine. Canad Med Assoc
       74: 423, 1956.

(20)   Greig, H., Metz, J., Laird, M., et al. Chemotherapy of
       leukemia. II. 6-mercaptopurine ("Purinethol") in the
       treatment of acute leukemia and some other neoplastic
       diseases of the reticuloendothelial system. South
       African Med J 30: 360, 1956.

(21)   Hyman, C., Brubaker, C., and Sturgeon, P. 6-mercaptopurine
       in childhood leukemia: comparison of large dose interrupted
       with small dose continuous therapy. Cancer Res 17: 851,
       1957.

(22)   Ellison, R., Silver, R., and Engle, R. Comparative study of
       6-chloropurine and 6-mercaptopurine in acute leukemia in
       adults. Ann Intern Med 51: 322, 1959.

(23)   Heyn, R., Brubaker, C., Burchenal, J., et al. The comparison
       of 6-mercaptopurine with the combination of 6-mercaptopurine
       and azaserine in the treatment of acute leukemia in children:
       Results of a cooperative study. Blood 15: 350, 1960.

(24)   Ellison, R., and Burchenal, J. Treatment of chronic
       granulocytic leukemia with the 6-substituted purines 6-
       mercaptopurine, thioguanine, and 6-chloropurine. Clin Pharm
       Ther 1: 631, 1960.

(25)   Fountain, J. Treatment of chronic myeloid leukemia with
       mercaptopurine. Acta Unio Int Cancer 16: 846, 1960.

(26)   Frei, E., Freireich, E., Gehan, E., et al. Studies of
       sequential and combination antimetabolite therapy in acute
       leukemia: 6-mercaptopurine and methotrexate. Blood 18:
       431, 1961.

(27) Sullivan, M., Beatty, E., Hyman, C., et al. A comparison
      of the effectiveness of standard dose 6-mercaptopurine,
      combination 6-mercaptopurine and DON, and high-loading
      6-mercaptopurine therapies in the treatment of acute leukemia
      in children: results of a cooperative study. Cancer Chemother
      Rep 16: 161, 1962, and Cancer Chemother Rep 18: 83, 1962.

(28) Shullenberger, C. Evaluation of the comparative effectiveness
      of Myleran and 6 MP in the management of patients with chronic
      myelocytic leukemia. Cancer Chemother Rep 16: 203, 1962.

(29) Shullenberger, C. Long-range treatment of polycythemia vera
      with 6-mercaptopurine. Cancer Chemother Rep 16: 251, 1962.

(30) Whittington, R., Rivers, S., Doyle, R., et al. Acute
      leukemia in the adult male. I. Comparative effect of 6-
      mercaptopurine and 6-chloropurine. Cancer Chemother Rep
      18: 73, 1962.

(31) Bridges, J., Hayes, D., and Nelson, M. Therapy of acute
      leukemia: comparison of initial treatment with 6-mercaptopurine
      alone and of combination with steroids. Brit J Cancer 16:
      46, 1962.

(32) Sutow, W., Haggard, M., Blattner, R., et al. Studies of ACTH,
      hydrocortisone, and 6-mercaptopurine in the treatment of
      children with acute leukemia. J Pediat 61: 693, 1962.

(33) Huguley, C., Grizzle, J., Rundles, R., et al. Comparison of
      6-mercaptopurine and busulfan in chronic granulocytic leukemia.
      Blood 21: 89, 1963.

(34) Working party on the evaluation of different methods of
      therapy in leukemia. Brit Med J 1: 7, 1963.

(35) Regelson, W., Holland, J., Frei, E., et al. Comparative
      clinical toxicity of 6-mercaptopurine and 6-mercaptopurine
      ribonucleoside administered intravenously to patients with
      advanced cancer. Cancer Chemother Rep 36: 41, 1964.

(36) Lemon, H., Miller, D., Smith, J., et al. Remission of
      metastases of erythropoietin - secreting renal cell
      adenocarcinoma after 6-mercaptopurine therapy. Cancer
      Chemother Rep 36: 49, 1964.

(37) Ellison, R., and Hoogstraten, B. Intravenous 6-mercaptopurine
      and methotrexate in adults with acute leukemia. Proc Amer
      Assoc Cancer Res 6: 17, 1965.

(38)   Working party on the evaluation of different methods of
       therapy in leukemia. Brit Med J 1: 1383, 1966.

(39)   Moore, G., Bross, I., Ausman, R. Effects of 6-mercaptopurine
       in 290 patients with advanced cancer. Cancer Chemother Rep
       52: 655, 1968.

(40)   Boggs, D., Wintrobe, M., and Cartwright, G. To treat or not
       to treat acute granulocytic leukemia. II. Arch Intern Med
       123: 568, 1969.

(41)   Fink, D., and Foye, L., Jr. 6-mercaptopurine (NSC 755)
       given intermittently in high doses: Phase II study.
       Cancer Chemother Rep 54: 31, 1970.

5-Fluorouracil

Synonyms: 5-FU, FU

Structure:

Dosage: 1.   15 mg/kg/wk x 4, IV; then (if neither mild toxicity
                    nor antitumor effect seen) increased to 20
                    mg/kg/wk, as tolerated. Minimum course of
                    treatment = 6 wks, or
               2.   15 mg/kg/day x 3-5, IV, followed by 7.5 mg/kg
                    every other day to mild toxicity. Subsequent
                    courses ordinarily given at monthly intervals, or
               3.   12 mg/kg/day x 4-5, then 6 mg/kg every other day
                    to mild toxicity. Subsequent courses ordinarily
                    given at monthly intervals.

Toxicity: I.   Gastrointestinal
                    A.   Anorexia, nausea and vomiting
                    B.   Diarrhea, stomatitis - the appearance of
                         either of these is an indication to stop
                         drug until the toxic manifestation subsides
                         completely.

              II.   Hematological
                    A.   Leukopenia
                    B.   Thrombocytopenia

             III.   Alopecia - uncommon

              IV.   Neurological
                    A.   Cerebellar signs - uncommon

               V.   Dermatological - skin eruptions occur uncommonly

Mechanism of Action: Thymidylic acid is the deoxyribonucleotide of
               thymine (5-methyluracil), the pyrimidine base unique to
               DNA. The methylation of 2-deoxyuridine-5'-phosphate to
               yield this nucleic acid is ultimately catalyzed by the
               enzyme thymidylate synthetase. 5-FU, when converted
               in vivo to the deoxynucleotide, has an affinity for the
               thymidylate synthetase system, and is not itself
               incorporated into DNA. It thus blocks thymidylate
               (and thereby DNA) synthesis.[1,2] This effect is thought
               to be primiiily responsible for the cytotoxic action of
               the drug. In addition, 5-FU is incorporated as the
               nucleotide into RNA, probably thereby depressing RNA
               synthesis directly by blocking incorporation of uracil
               and orotic acid into RNA.[3]

Role in Cancer Therapy

5-FU has been used against human malignancy since 1957. The
vast majority of patients treated with this agent have received it
according to the "loading-dose" schedule advocated initially by

Curreri and Ansfield.[5] A standard course, according to this
schedule, consists of rapid injection of 15 mg/kg/day for 4 to 5
days, followed by 7.5 mg/kg every 2 or 3 days until mild toxicity
(usually gastrointestinal) is evident. Subsequent courses are
ordinarily given at monthly intervals. More recently, Ansfield
recommended a lowered-dose loading schedule as less toxic:[35] 12
mg/kg/day x 4-5, then 6 mg/kg every other day to slight toxicity.
With this modified dose schedule, among 206 patients evaluated for
toxicity, 61% had diarrhea, 30% had stomatitis, and 39% had a WBC
count <2000/mm^3 as a result of therapy. The mortality rate was
0.5%. This did represent a considerable improvement over the
toxicity encountered with the "standard" regimen, in which 32% of
1091 evaluable patients developed a WBC <2000 and there was a 2.9%
overall mortality.[5,35]

In 1968, Jacobs et al[45] reported results of treatment of
patients with 5-FU, without a loading dose, on a weekly basis:
129 patients with disseminated cancer were treated on a dose
schedule of 15 mg/kg/wk x 4, then increased to 20 mg/kg/wk (if
necessary) to levels producing mild toxicity or an antitumor effect.
Only 11 of the 129 (8.5%) developed a WBC count <3000 while on
5-FU therapy, and none had a WBC of <2000/mm^3. There were no drug
deaths. At the same time, the proportion of patients achieving a
tumor response was at least as great as that obtained using a
loading-dose regimen. It would seem that Jacobs' regimen therefore
has a great deal to recommend it, particularly with regard to the
possible future use of 5-FU in combination with other myelosuppressive
or enterotoxic agents. It should be noted that a weekly dose of
5-FU less than 15 mg/kg is probably too low: Horton et al saw no
responses in 44 patients who received the drug alone at a dose of
10 mg/kg/wk, including 16 with colon and 5 with breast cancer.[41]

A vast accumulated experience with 5-FU in carcinoma of the
breast indicates that 28% of patients treated with this agent may
be expected to respond. 5-FU has been the single most commonly
used cytotoxic agent in this tumor type, although MTX and
cyclophosphamide appear to be agents of at least equivalent
activity. Those who responded to 5-FU therapy, in a large series
reported by Ansfield et al, had a median survival time of 29 months
after treatment was initiated, as opposed to only 9 months for
patients whose disease progressed on therapy.[46] Interestingly,
in the same series, a group of patients whose disease was "unchanged"
while on therapy with 5-FU had a median survival almost as good as
that of the "responders": 26 months. The implication of these
data seems to be that a patient is best kept on therapy with 5-FU,
and may actually be deriving significant benefit from it, even if
there is no measurable regression of tumor, so long as there is not
actual progression.

5-FU is at present clearly the most effective single chemotherapeutic agent in the treatment of carcinoma of the colon and rectum. About 1 in 4 patients will have an objective tumor response, lasting in most cases for a period of a few months, although some responses in excess of a year's duration have been seen.[49]

Against lung cancer the overall reported response rate with 5-FU is only 6% of 143 patients. It thus appears to be less active than cyclophosphamide, HN_2, or procarbazine. In a relatively small number of patients treated with malignant melanoma, the response rate to 5-FU was negligible.

Treatment with 5-FU, on the basis of the reported data, may be expected to result in an objective response in 25-30% of patients with carcinoma of the pancreas, cervical and uterine cancer, gastric carcinoma, and ovarian tumors. It is probably inferior to alkylating agents for initial chemotherapy in ovarian cancer; in the other categories, 5-FU appears to be the most effective available drug. It may also be the most useful single cytotoxic agent in patients with carcinoma of the prostate (9/24 responses reported), carcinoma of the bladder (27/78 responses reported), and hepatoma (11/28 responses reported). Responses have been reported to 5-FU in patients with metastatic neuroblastoma and Ewing's sarcoma. Definite conclusions as to its value in these tumor types cannot be drawn, due to the small number of cases reported and the known activity of other drugs (e.g., CTX and vincristine) against them.

There are two major tumor categories in which 5-FU has received an inadequate trial, based on published reports: lymphoma and acute leukemia. In lymphomas, the overall response rate of 26% (6/23) for 5-FU becomes more respectable if one notes that almost all patients treated had the relatively drug-resistant reticulum-cell sarcoma or lymphosarcoma, rather than Hodgkin's disease. Further efforts to explore the value of this agent in lymphomas may be indicated. In acute leukemia, 5-FU might be expected to have some effect on the basis of its activity in animal leukemia systems.[4] The only group effort to study 5-FU in acute leukemia[33] foundered on the occurrence of early, very severe gastrointestinal toxicity. Both this side effect and that of severe bone-marrow toxicity might be at least partially circumvented by use of the weekly dose schedule. Certainly, 5-FU remains an agent of undetermined potential in this tumor type.

Tumor Type or Site

Breast

Ref #	# Pts Evaluated	# Pts Responding	% Response	Dose Schedule and Remarks ("Standard" = 15 mg/kg daily by IV push x 4-5, then 7.5 mg/kg q 2-3 days to toxicity, repeated monthly).
6	9	1		(1) 4-8 mg/kg/day x 14-42 (IV or PO). (2) 10-15 mg/kg/wk. (3) 16-34 mg/kg x 1 (single-dose). (4) 15 mg/kg/day x 5, repeat every 28 days. ECOG study. Response seen at 15 mg/kg/wk schedule.
7	9	2		"Standard". PR, durations 4 and 12 mo. Two of 9 had drug-related deaths.
8	2	1		1 gm/day x 5 by daily 8 hr IV infusion.
9	6	1		"Standard". Only "marked" objective response included.
10	8	1		"Standard". One of 8 had life-threatening toxicity.
11	10	7		"Standard".
12	5	2		15 mg/kg/day x 5, monthly. Response durations 2 and 3 mo.
14	43	18		"Standard". Median response duration = 6 mo. 4 remissions >1 year.
15	38	15		"Standard". In this series, 7/144 deaths were drug-related.

Breast (cont.)

Ref #	# Pts Evaluated	# Pts Responding	% Response	Dose Schedule and Remarks ("Standard" = 15 mg/kg daily by IV push x 4–5, then 7.5 mg/kg q 2–3 days to toxicity, repeated monthly).
17	3	3		"Standard". In this series, 2/50 deaths were drug-related.
18	28	7		"Standard". 4 "good" responses. In this series, 15/170 patients had drug-related deaths.
24	–	–		"Standard". 5-FU→52/158 responses (included in reference 46); FUDR→18/39.
25	22	15		"Standard" or 15 mg/kg/day x 3, then 7.5 mg/kg on days 4 and 5, followed by 7.5 mg/kg x 2/wk for 4–6 wks.
26	10	2		15 mg/kg/day x 3; 7.5 mg/kg on day 5.
27	2	0		"Standard".
28	3	1		1 gm/day x 5, then 0.5 gm q 2 days to toxicity.
30	25	14		"Standard", except 7.5–10 mg/kg/wk given as maintenance. Ambulatory patients only. Includes 13 patients who received 5-FU + steroids. (7/12 responded to 5-FU alone).
31	10	0		"Standard".
31	13	6		7.5 mg/kg/day to toxicity.
36	30	11		"Standard". Comparison study with CTX, which gave 7/32 responses.

Breast (cont.)

Ref #	# Pts Evaluated	# Pts Responding	% Response	Dose Schedule and Remarks ("Standard" = 15 mg/kg daily by IV push x 4-5, then 7.5 mg/kg q 2-3 days to toxicity, repeated monthly).
38	8	1		15 mg/kg/day x 3; off 4 days, then 7.5 mg/kg/wk x 2, to toxicity.
40	30	8		5-FU, "Standard". FUDR, 30 mg/kg/day x 4, then 15 mg/kg q 2 days x 4. MTX, 0.4 mg/kg/day x 4, then 0.2 mg/kg q 2 days x 4. Repeated after 4 wks. Median response = 8 wks. FUDR →9/31, MTX →5/35 responses. Frequency of WBC <3000 was twice as great with 5-FU and FUDR as with MTX. Difference in response rates not statistically significant among the 3 drugs. ECOG study.
41	5	0		10 mg/kg/wk. Combination of 5-FU, Mitomycin C, Thio-TEPA and fluoxymesterone →3/12 responses.
42	44	13	30	2.5 mg/kg q 6 hrs →15 mg/kg/day x 5, then 1.25 mg/kg q 6 hrs →7.5 mg/kg q 2 days to toxicity. No deaths or serious toxic reactions reported with this modified dose schedule.
43	56	18		"Standard". Eastern CDEP study.
45	20	9	45	15 mg/kg/wk x 4; then, if tolerated, 20 mg/kg/wk x 4. Only >50% regressions included as responses.

Breast (cont.)

Ref #	# Pts Evaluated	# Pts Responding	% Response	Dose Schedule and Remarks ("Standard" = 15 mg/kg daily by IV push x 4–5, then 7.5 mg/kg q 2–3 days to toxicity, repeated monthly).
46	676	156	23	"Standard" or 12 mg/kg/day x 5, then 6 mg/kg q 2 days to toxicity. Median survival of responders = 29 mo. Median survival of 156 patients who were "unchanged" objectively = 26 mo. Median survival of 364 patients whose disease progressed on therapy = 9 mo.
48	27	8	30	15 mg/kg/day to mild toxicity by IV infusion of 1, 2, 4, or 8 hrs/day. Two of 86 patients = 3% had drug-related deaths in this overall series.
	1142	320	28	Total.

Colorectal

Ref #	# Pts Evaluated	# Pts Responding	% Response	Dose Schedule and Remarks
6	8	1		(1) 4–8 mg/kg/day x 14–42 (IV or PO). (2) 10–15 mg/kg/wk, IV. (3) 16–34 mg/kg, single dose. (4) 15 mg/kg/day x 5, repeat every 28 days. ECOG study.
7	12	1		"Standard". 2 mo remission duration.
8	6	1		12–15 mg/kg/day x 3–6, IV push.
8	6	2		1 gm/day x 5 by daily 9 hr IV infusion.

Colorectal (cont.)

Ref #	# Pts Evaluated	# Pts Responding	% Response	Dose Schedule and Remarks ("Standard" = 15 mg/kg daily by IV push x 4-5, then 7.5 mg/kg q 2-3 days to toxicity, repeated monthly).
9	9	3		"Standard". Only "marked" objective responses included.
10	36	5	14	"Standard". 3 deaths in 36 patients related to drug toxicity.
11	17	8		"Standard".
12	12	5		15 mg/kg/day x 5, monthly. 2/12 drug-related deaths. Response duration range, 1.5-5 mo.
14	12	1		"Standard". Response duration >6 mo.
15	37	10	27	"Standard". In this series, 7/144 deaths were drug-related.
16	11	1		"Standard". In this series, 4/40 drug-related deaths occurred.
17	9	2		"Standard". In this series, 2/50 drug-related deaths occurred.
18	45	9	20	"Standard". In this series, 15/170 drug-related deaths occurred. 3 "good" and 6 "moderate" objective responses.
19,20	130	40	31	"Standard". 6/104 drug-related deaths.[19] HN_2 →3/26, CTX →4/16 responses in same series. Mean response duration with 5-FU = 5.8 mo.

Colorectal (cont.)

Ref #	# Pts Evaluated	# Pts Responding	% Response	Dose Schedule and Remarks ("Standard" = 15 mg/kg daily by IV push x 4–5, then 7.5 mg/kg q 2–3 days to toxicity, repeated monthly).
21	115	18	16	"Standard". In this series, 23/1091 = 2.9% of patients had definitely drug-related deaths.
22	87	10	11	"Standard". In this series, about 5% of patients had drug-related deaths. Data may include those in Reference #10.
23	30	6		"Standard".
24	-	-		"Standard". FUDR →20/44 responses in this comparative study, -- vs 18/115 for 5-FU.
25	19	12		"Standard" or 15 mg/kg/day x 3, then 7.5 mg/kg on days 4 and 5, followed by 7.5 mg/kg x 2/wk for 4–6 wks.
26	12	5		15 mg/kg/day x 3, then 7.5 mg/kg on day 5.
27	8	1		"Standard".
28	9	2		1 gm/day x 5, then 0.5 gm q 2 days to toxicity.
29	10	1		"Standard".
30	37	14	38	"Standard", except 7.5-10 mg/kg/wk given as maintenance. Ambulatory patients only. 5 patients had response >6 mo in duration. Some patients classed as response who had stable disease without progression.

Colorectal (cont.)

Ref #	# Pts Evaluated	# Pts Responding	% Response	Dose Schedule and Remarks ("Standard" = 15 mg/kg daily by IV push x 4-5, then 7.5 mg/kg q 2-3 days to toxicity, repeated monthly).
35	41	7	17	12 mg/kg/day x 4-5, then 6 mg/kg/day to slight toxicity. FUDR →25/57 in this series. 1/206 = 0.5% of patients had drug-related deaths.
37	144	56	39	"Standard". 16 complete and 40 partial responses reported.
38	12	4	15	15 mg/kg/day x 3; off 4 days, then 7.5 mg/kg/wk x 2, to toxicity.
40	48	13	27	5-FU, "Standard". FUDR, 30 mg/kg/day x 4, then 15 mg/kg q 2 days x 4. MTX, 0.4 mg/kg/day x 4, then 0.2 mg/kg q 2 days x 4. Repeated after 4 wks. ECOG study. Median duration response = 11 wks. Comparison study with MTX →4/40 responses, and FUDR →2/46 responses. Median duration MTX response = 22 wks. Difference in response rates not statistically significant among the three drugs.
41	16	0		10 mg/kg/wk. Comparison with combination of 5-FU, Mitomycin C, Thio-TEPA and fluoxymesterone →4/22 responses.
43	80	15	18.5	"Standard". 2 CR, 13 PR. 13/54 colon, 2/26 rectum responses.
45	33	9	27	15 mg/kg/wk x 4; then, if tolerated, 20 mg/kg/wk x 4. Only >50% regressons included as responses.

Colorectal (cont.)

Ref #	# Pts Evaluated	# Pts Responding	% Response	Dose Schedule and Remarks ("Standard" = 15 mg/kg daily by IV push x 4–5, then 7.5 mg/kg q 2–3 days to toxicity, repeated monthly).
47	132	22	17	"Standard". FUDR →32/145 = 22% responses. No difference seen in response rates of patients with colon -- vs rectal primary to either 5-FU or FUDR.
50	37	9	24	15 mg/kg/day to mild toxicity by IV infusion of 1, 2, 4, or 8 hrs/day. 2/87 patients in this series had drug-related deaths (3%).
51	35	7	20	Loading course (all patients) = 12 mg/kg/day x 4–5, then 6 mg/kg q 2 days to toxicity. Maintenance = monthly "loading course" -- vs 1 gm/wk. Responses in group on weekly maintenance (4/20): 7, 8, 14, and 17 mo duration. Responses in group on monthly maintenance (3/15): 3, 6, and 10 mo duration.
	1255	300	24	Total.

Melanoma

Ref #	# Pts Evaluated	# Pts Responding	% Response	
8	2	0		(1) 12–15 mg/kg/day x 3–6. (2) 1 gm/day x 5 by daily 8 hr IV infusion.
10	4	0		"Standard".
13	1	0		15 mg/kg/day x 5, repeated as tolerated.

Melanoma (cont.)

Ref #	# Pts Evaluated	# Pts Responding	% Response	Dose Schedule and Remarks ("Standard" = 15 mg/kg daily by IV push x 4-5, then 7.5 mg/kg q 2-3 days to toxicity, repeated monthly).
14	4	0		"Standard".
15	1	0		"Standard".
17	3	0		"Standard".
18	1	0		"Standard".
21	8	0		"Standard".
43	13	1		"Standard".
	37	1	2.5	Total.

Lung

Ref #	# Pts Evaluated	# Pts Responding	% Response	Dose Schedule and Remarks
6	28	2		(1) 4-8 mg/kg/day x 14-42 (IV or PO). (2) 10-15 mg/kg/wk, IV. (3) 16-34 mg/kg, single dose. (4) 15 mg/kg/day x 5, repeat every 28 days.
7	4	0		"Standard".
8	2	0		12-15 mg/kg/day x 3-6.
9	9	1		"Standard".
10	14	1		"Standard".
11	2	0		"Standard".

Lung (cont.)

Ref #	# Pts Evaluated	# Pts Responding	% Response	Dose Schedule and Remarks ("Standard" = 15 mg/kg daily by IV push x 4-5, then 7.5 mg/kg q 2-3 days to toxicity, repeated monthly).
14	2	0		"Standard".
15	10	0		"Standard".
16	6	0		"Standard". Adenocarcinoma.
17	5	0		"Standard".
18	7	0		"Standard".
21	16	0		"Standard".
25	3	0		"Standard" or 15 mg/kg/day x 3, then 7.5 mg/kg on days 4 and 5, followed by 7.5 mg/kg x 2/wk for 4-6 wks.
27	2	0		"Standard".
38	3	0		15 mg/kg/day x 3; off 4 days, then 7.5 mg/kg x 2/wk for 2 wks or to toxicity.
43	26	4		"Standard".
45	4	1		15 mg/kg/wk x 4; then, if tolerated, 20 mg/kg/wk x 4. Only >50% regressions included as response.
	143	9	6	Total.

Lymphoma

Ref #	# Pts Evaluated	# Pts Responding	% Response	Dose Schedule and Remarks ("Standard" = 15 mg/kg daily by IV push x 4-5, then 7.5 mg/kg q 2-3 days to toxicity, repeated monthly).
7	1	0		"Standard". Reticulum-cell sarcoma.
9	2	1		"Standard". Hodgkin's disease.
13	2	2		15 mg/kg/day x 5, repeated as tolerated. Both PR; both patients had lymphosarcoma in childhood.
14	7	1		"Standard". PR, >2 mo and <6 mo duration.
15	2	0		"Standard".
21	7	1		"Standard". All patients had reticulum-cell sarcoma. Response was a complete regression of >5 years' duration.
43	2	1		"Standard".
	23	6	26	Total. Probably includes only 2 cases of Hodgkin's disease.

"Acute Leukemia"

5	7	0		"Standard". No details on morphologic type.
15	1	0		"Standard". Patient with ALL.

"Acute Leukemia" (cont.)

Ref #	# Pts Evaluated	# Pts Responding	% Response	Dose Schedule and Remarks ("Standard" = 15 mg/kg daily by IV push x 4–5, then 7.5 mg/kg q 2–3 days to toxicity, repeated monthly).
33	13	1		10 mg/kg/day x 5, off 5 days, then 10 mg/kg/day x 5, etc., (10 patients). 3 patients received 15 mg/kg x 1, then 7.5 mg/kg/day x 3, off 3 days, and repeated cycle. Minimum of 2 courses in 21 days considered adequate trial. 4 of 13 received an "adequate trial". Remission classed as CR, but only 2 wks in duration. All patients had ALL, advanced and refractory. Severe GI toxicity limited study. Note dose schedule used.
	21	1		Total. See discussion.

Stomach

Ref #	# Pts Evaluated	# Pts Responding	% Response	Dose Schedule and Remarks
7	4	1		"Standard".
9	3	1		"Standard". Only "marked" objective responses included.
10	12	3		"Standard". 1/12 had drug-related death.
11	4	1		"Standard".
12	3	3		15 mg/kg/day x 5, monthly. Durations 3, 3, and 1+ mo.
14	7	3		"Standard". All responses <2 mo duration.

Stomach (cont.)

Ref #	# Pts Evaluated	# Pts Responding	% Response	Dose Schedule and Remarks ("Standard" = 15 mg/kg daily by IV push x 4-5, then 7.5 mg/kg q 2-3 days to toxicity, repeated monthly).
15	9	3		"Standard". Most responses of short duration.
16	9	2		"Standard".
17	6	0		"Standard".
18	19	2		"Standard". 4 other patients had ↓ in tumor size, but without clinical benefit.
19	30	10	33	"Standard". Mean duration response = 4.7 mo. 3 drug deaths of 30.
21	8	2		"Standard".
25	2	1		"Standard" or 15 mg/kg/day x 3, then 7.5 mg/kg on days 4 and 5, followed by 7.5 mg/kg x 2/wk for 4-6 wks.
26	14	4		15 mg/kg/day x 3, then 7.5 mg/kg on day 5.
27	2	0		"Standard".
28	1	0		1 gm/day x 5, then 0.5 gm q 2 days to toxicity.
29	3	2		"Standard".
30	10	2		"Standard", except 7.5-10 mg/kg/wk given as maintenance. One remission >6 mo duration. Ambulatory patients only.
34	27	5	19	"Standard".

Stomach (cont.)

Ref #	# Pts Evaluated	# Pts Responding	% Response	Dose Schedule and Remarks ("Standard" = 15 mg/kg daily by IV push x 4-5, then 7.5 mg/kg q 2-3 days to toxicity, repeated monthly).
37	49	15	31	"Standard". 8 complete and 7 partial regressions reported.
38	5	0		15 mg/kg/day x 3; off 4 days, then 7.5 mg/kg x 2/wk for 2 wks or to toxicity.
39	250	>125	>50	15 mg/kg q 2 days to toxicity (total dose, 3-7 gm/course). Russian study.
43	25	6		"Standard". Eastern CDEP study.
45	9	4		15 mg/kg/wk x 4; then 20 mg/kg/wk x 4, if tolerated. Only regressions >50% included as responses.
	$\overline{511}$	$\overline{>195}$	~40	Total.
	261	70	27	Total, minus Russian data.
Pancreas				
7	1	0		"Standard".
8	3	1		12-15 mg/kg/day x 3-6.
9	1	0		"Standard".
12	6	3		15 mg/kg/day x 5, monthly. Remission durations: 1, 2, and 8+ mo.

Pancreas (cont.)

Ref #	# Pts Evaluated	# Pts Responding	% Response	Dose Schedule and Remarks ("Standard" = 15 mg/kg daily by IV push x 4-5, then 7.5 mg/kg q 2-3 days to toxicity, repeated monthly).
14	1	1		"Standard". Remission duration <2 mo.
15	5	1		"Standard". Remission duration <13 wks.
16	6	0		"Standard".
17	3	0		"Standard".
18	3	0		"Standard".
19	26	11	42	"Standard". Mean response duration = 6.8 mo.
21	6	0		"Standard".
25	2	1		"Standard" or 15 mg/kg/day x 3, then 7.5 mg/kg on days 4 and 5, followed by 7.5 mg/kg x 2/wk for 4-6 wks.
27	1	0		"Standard".
30	5	0		"Standard", except 7.5-10 mg/kg/wk given as maintenance.
34	20	3	16	"Standard".
37	17	5		"Standard". 3 complete and 2 partial regressions reported.
38	4	1		15 mg/kg/day x 3, off 4 days, then 7.5 mg/kg x 2/wk for two wks or to toxicity.

Pancreas (cont.)

Ref #	# Pts Evaluated	# Pts Responding	% Response	Dose Schedule and Remarks ("Standard" = 15 mg/kg daily by IV push x 4–5, then 7.5 mg/kg q 2–3 days to toxicity, repeated monthly).
43	11	2		"Standard". Eastern CDEP study.
45	4	0		15 mg/kg/wk x 4; then 20 mg/kg/wk x 4, if tolerated.
	125	29	23	Total.
				Ovary
9	4	2		"Standard". Only "marked" objective regressions included.
10	7	2		"Standard".
11	4	2		"Standard".
14	8	2		"Standard". One response >6 mo duration.
15	4	2		"Standard". One response >13 wks duration.
18	12	4		"Standard".
21	21	4		"Standard".
25	5	4		"Standard" or 15 mg/kg/day x 3, then 7.5 mg/kg on days 4 and 5 followed by 7.5 mg/kg x 2/wk for 4–6 wks.
30	7	4		"Standard", except 7.5–10 mg/kg/wk given as maintenance. Two responses >1 year duration. Ambulatory patients only.

Ovary (cont.)

Ref #	# Pts Evaluated	Responding	Response	Dose Schedule and Remarks ("Standard" = 15 mg/kg daily by IV push x 4–5, then 7.5 mg/kg q 2–3 days to toxicity, repeated monthly).
44	21	6		"Standard". All responses >3 mo; one response >40 mo.
45	8	0		15 mg/kg/wk x 4; then 20 mg/kg/wk x 4, if tolerated.
	101	32	32	Total.
Prostate				
9	1	0		"Standard".
15	4	1		"Standard". Response <13 wks duration.
18	1	0		"Standard".
21	7	1		"Standard".
25	3	2		"Standard" or 15 mg/kg/day x 3, then 7.5 mg/kg on days 4 and 5, followed by 7.5 mg/kg x 2/wk for 4–6 wks.
38	1	1		15 mg/kg/day x 3, off 4 days, then 7.5 mg/kg x 2/wk for 2 wks or to toxicity.
43	7	4		"Standard".
	24	9	37.5	Total.

Bladder

Ref #	# Pts Evaluated	# Pts Responding	% Response	Dose Schedule and Remarks ("Standard" = 15 mg/kg daily by IV push x 4-5, then 7.5 mg/kg q 2-3 days to toxicity, repeated monthly).
7	3	1		"Standard".
8	3	1		12-15 mg/kg/day x 3-6.
8	2	0		1 gm/day x 5 by daily 8 hr IV infusion.
9	12	9		"Standard". Only "marked" objective regressions included.
10	4	1		"Standard".
14	2	0		"Standard".
15	6	0		"Standard".
17	3	1		"Standard".
18	3	0		"Standard".
21	7	1		"Standard".
25	2	0		"Standard" or 15 mg/kg/day x 3, then 7.5 mg/kg on days 4 and 5, followed by 7.5 mg/kg x 2/wk for 4-6 wks.
27	1	0		"Standard".
30	9	1		"Standard", except 7.5-10 mg/kg/wk given as maintenance. Response >1 year in duration.
32	7	4		"Standard". "Patients with superficial lesions showed significant improvement, while those with invasive tumors did not respond."

Bladder (cont.)

Ref #	# Pts Evaluated	# Pts Responding	% Response	Dose Schedule and Remarks ("Standard" = 15 mg/kg daily by IV push x 4-5, then 7.5 mg/kg q 2-3 days to toxicity, repeated monthly).
38	1	1		"Standard".
43	9	6		"Standard". 1 complete and 5 partial responses reported.
	$\overline{74}$	$\overline{26}$	35	Total.

Testicular Tumors

7	1	0		"Standard". Embryonal carcinoma.
9	3	1		"Standard". All seminomas.
11	3	1		"Standard". 1/2 embryonal cell, 0/1 seminoma.
14	1	1		"Standard". Response <2 mo duration.
15	2	0		"Standard".
17	1	0		"Standard". Seminoma.
	$\overline{11}$	$\overline{3}$	28	Total.

Hepatoma

15	4	1		"Standard". Includes "tumors of liver and biliary tract".

Hepatoma (cont.)

Ref #	# Pts Evaluated	# Pts Responding	% Response	Dose Schedule and Remarks ("Standard" = 15 mg/kg daily by IV push x 4-5, then 7.5 mg/kg q 2-3 days to toxicity, repeated monthly).
18	5	1		"Standard".
21	4	2		"Standard".
25	4	2		"Standard" or 15 mg/kg/day x 3, then 7.5 mg/kg on days 4 and 5, followed by 7.5 mg/kg x 2/wk for 4-6 wks.
28	1	1		1 gm/day x 5, then 0.5 gm q 2 days to toxicity.
34	2	0		"Standard".
43	4	1		"Standard". Includes tumors of "liver and bile passage".
45	4	3		15 mg/kg/wk x 4; then 20 mg/kg/wk x 4, if tolerated. Only regressions >50% included as response.
	28	11	40	Total.

Head and Neck

6	12	1		(1) 4-8 mg/kg/day x 14-42 days, IV or PO. (2) 10-15 mg/kg/wk, IV. (3) 16-34 mg/kg, single dose. (4) 15 mg/kg/day x 5, repeated every 29 days. ECOG study.

Head and Neck (cont.)

Ref #	# Pts Evaluated	# Pts Responding	% Response	Dose Schedule and Remarks ("Standard" = 15 mg/kg daily by IV push x 4-5, then 7.5 mg/kg q 2-3 days to toxicity, repeated monthly).
7	8	1		"Standard". Response in laryngeal carcinoma.
10	5	1		"Standard".
14	1	0		"Standard".
15	3	1		"Standard". Laryngeal carcinoma.
17	12	5		"Standard".
21	23	1		"Standard". 1/6 responses in transitional cell carcinoma of nasopharynx.
25	3	1		"Standard" or 15 mg/kg/day x 3, then 7.5 mg/kg on days 4 and 5, followed by 7.5 mg/kg x 2/wk for 4-6 wks.
28	33	1		1 gm/day x 5, then 0.5 gm q 2 days to toxicity.
43	36	5		"Standard". 1/7 tongue, 4/29 in mouth, pharynx and larynx group.
45	12	1		"Standard". Only regressions >50% included as response.
	118	18	15	Total.

Esophagus

9	1	0		"Standard".

Esophagus (cont.)

Ref #	# Pts Evaluated	# Pts Responding	% Response	Dose Schedule and Remarks ("Standard" = 15 mg/kg daily by IV push x 4-5, then 7.5 mg/kg q 2-3 days to toxicity, repeated monthly).
17	1	0		"Standard".
18	2	0		"Standard".
28	1	1		1 gm/day x 5, then 0.5 gm q 2 days to toxicity.
29	1	0		"Standard".
43	9	2		"Standard".
45	3	0		15 mg/kg/wk x 4; then 20 mg/kg/wk x 4, if tolerated.
	18	3	11	Total.

Cervix and Uterus

Ref #	# Pts Evaluated	# Pts Responding	% Response	Dose Schedule and Remarks
7	5	2		"Standard". 2/3 uterus, 0/2 cervix responses.
9	4	0		"Standard". 0/2 uterus, 0/2 cervix responses.
11	2	0		"Standard". Cervix.
14	2	0		"Standard". 0/1 uterus, 0/1 cervix responses.
15	5	1		"Standard". 1/3 uterus, 0/2 cervix responses.
18	5	1		"Standard".
21	25	6		"Standard". 1/8 uterus, 5/17 cervix responses.

Cervix and Uterus (cont.)

Ref #	# Pts Evaluated	# Pts Responding	% Response	Dose Schedule and Remarks ("Standard" = 15 mg/kg daily by IV push x 4-5, then 7.5 mg/kg q 2-3 days to toxicity, repeated monthly).
25	2	0		"Standard" or 15 mg/kg/day x 3, then 7.5 mg/kg on days 4 and 5, followed by 7.5 mg/kg x 2/wk for 4-6 wks.
27	6	3		"Standard".
30	6	4		"Standard", except 7.5-10 mg/kg/wk given as maintenance. All cervix; 3 responses <6 mo, 1 response >1 year.
38	1	1		15 mg/kg/day x 3, off 4 days, then 7.5 mg/kg x 2/wk for 2 wks or to toxicity.
43	22	7		"Standard". 2/8 uterus, 5/15 cervix responses.
44	110	23	21	"Standard". 8/21 uterus, 15/89 cervix responders. Mean remission duration 5 mo.
	$\overline{195}$	$\overline{48}$	25	Total. 14/46 uterus = 30% response; 29/136 cervix = 21% response.

Kidney

Ref #	# Pts Evaluated	# Pts Responding	% Response	Dose Schedule and Remarks
9	2	0		"Standard".
11	1	0		"Standard".
14	7	0		"Standard".

Kidney (cont.)

Ref #	# Pts Evaluated	# Pts Responding	% Response	Dose Schedule and Remarks ("Standard" = 15 mg/kg daily by IV push x 4-5, then 7.5 mg/kg q 2-3 days to toxicity, repeated monthly).
15	2	0		"Standard".
18	3	0		"Standard".
21	10	0		"Standard".
28	2	0		1 gm/day x 5, then 0.5 gm q 2 days to toxicity.
43	15	0		"Standard".
	42	0		Total.
			Ewing's Sarcoma	
7	1	0		"Standard".
13	4	3		15 mg/kg/day x 5, repeated as tolerated.
	5	3	60	Total.

References

(1)   Heidelberger, C., Chaudhuri, N., Danneburg, P., et al.
      Fluorinated pyrimidines, a new class of tumor-inhibitory
      compounds. Nature 179: 663, 1957.

(2)   Bosch, L., Harbers, E., and Heidelberger, C. Studies on
      fluorinated pyrimidines. V. Effects on nucleic acid
      metabolism in vitro. Cancer Res 18: 335, 1958.

(3)   Harbers, E., Chaudhuri, N., and Heidelberger, C. Studies on
      fluorinated pyrimidines. VIII. Further biochemical and
      metabolic investigations. J Biol Chem 234: 1255, 1959.

(4)   Burchenal, J. The effects of halogenated pyrimidine
      derivatives on a spectrum of transplanted mouse leukemias.
      Proc Amer Assoc Cancer Res 2: 285, 1958.

(5)   Curreri, A., Ansfield, F., McIver, F., et al. Clinical studies
      with 5-fluorouracil. Cancer Res 18: 478, 1958.

(6)   Gold, G., Hall, T., Shnider, B., et al. A clinical study of
      5-fluorouracil. Cancer Res 19: 935, 1959.

(7)   Olson, K., and Greene, J. Evaluation of 5-fluorouracil in
      treatment of cancer. J Nat Cancer Instit 25: 133, 1960.

(8)   Lemon, H. Reduction of 5-fluorouracil toxicity in man with
      retention of anticancer effect by prolonged intravenous
      administration in 5% dextrose. Cancer Chemother Rep 8: 97,
      1960.

(9)   Wilson, W. Chemotherapy of human solid tumors with 5-
      fluorouracil. Cancer 13: 1230, 1960.

(10) Young, C., Ellison, R., Sullivan, R., et al. The clinical
      evaluation of 5-fluorouracil and 5-fluoro-2'-deoxyuridine in
      solid tumors in adults. A progress report. Cancer Chemother
      Rep 6: 17, 1960.

(11) Allaire, F., Thieme, E., and Korst, D. Cancer chemotherapy
      with 5-fluorouracil alone and in combination with x-ray therapy.
      Cancer Chemother Rep 14: 59, 1960.

(12) Cornell, G., Cahow, C., Frey, C., et al. Clinical experience
      with 5-fluorouracil in the treatment of malignant disease.
      Cancer Chemother Rep 9: 23, 1960.

(13) Krivit, W., and Bentley, H. Use of 5-fluorouracil in the management of advanced malignancies in childhood. Am J Dis Childh 100: 217, 1960.

(14) Kennedy, B., and Theologides, A. The role of 5-fluorouracil in malignant disease. Ann Intern Med 55: 719, 1961.

(15) Weiss, A., Jackson, L., and Carabasi, R. An evaluation of 5-fluorouracil in malignant disease. Ann Intern Med 55: 731, 1961.

(16) Knoepp, L., Kastl, W., Rayburn, A., et al. Clinical experience with 5-fluorouracil. Cancer Chemother Rep 12: 89, 1961.

(17) Staley, C., Keith, J., Cortes, N., et al. Treatment of advanced cancer with 5-fluorouracil. Surg Gyn and Obstet 112: 185, 1961.

(18) Vaitkevicius, V., Brennan, M., Beckett, V., et al. Clinical evaluation of cancer chemotherapy with 5-fluorouracil. Cancer 41: 131, 1961.

(19) Hurley, J., Ellison, E., and Carey, L. Treatment of advanced cancer of the gastrointestinal tract with antitumor agents. Gastroenterology 41: 557, 1961.

(20) Hurley, J. Chemotherapy of colon tumors: panel discussion. (Cole, W.H., moderator). Am J Surg 103: 94, 1962.

(21) Ansfield, F., Schroeder, J., and Curreri, A. Five years' clinical experience with 5-fluorouracil. JAMA 181: 295, 1962.

(22) Ellison, R. Experience with fluorinated pyrimidines in adenocarcinoma of the lower intestinal tract. N Y J Med 14: 2364, 1962.

(23) Hyman, G., Ultmann, J., and Habif, D. Factors to be considered in the clinical evaluation of a new chemotherapeutic agent (5-fluorouracil). Cancer Chemother Rep 16: 397, 1962.

(24) Curreri, A., and Ansfield, F. Comparison of 5-fluorouracil and 5-fluoro-2'-deoxyuridine in the treatment of far-advanced breast and colon lesions. Cancer Chemother Rep 16: 387, 1962.

(25) Hall, B., and Good, J. Treatment of far-advanced cancer with 5-fluorouracil, used alone and in combination with irradiation. Incidence and duration of remission and survival-time data in 223 patients. Cancer Chemother Rep 16: 369, 1962.

(26) Eyerly, R. The effects of 5-fluorouracil in patients with incurable cancer. Cancer Chemother Rep 20: 89, 1962.

(27) Choy, D., Stylianou, S., and Hangul, A. Experience with 5-fluorouracil in a variety of solid tumors. Cancer Chemother Rep 24: 99, 1962.

(28) White, J., Ricketts, W., and Strudwick, W. A clinical study of 5-fluorouracil in a variety of far-advanced human malignancies. J Nat Med Assoc 54: 315, 1962.

(29) Baines, C., and Ley, D. A preliminary report on the use of 5-fluorouracil in malignant disease. Canad Med Assoc J 86: 207, 1962.

(30) Field, J. 5-fluorouracil treatment of advanced cancer in ambulatory patients. Cancer Chemother Rep 33: 45, 1963.

(31) Dao, T., and Grinberg, R. Fluorinated pyrimidines in treatment of breast cancer patients with liver metastases. Cancer Chemother Rep 27: 71, 1963.

(32) Glenn, J., Hunt, L., and Lathem, J. Chemotherapy of bladder carcinoma with 5-fluorouracil. Cancer Chemother Rep 27: 67, 1963.

(33) Hartmann, J., Origenes, M., Murphy, M., et al. Effects of 2'-deoxy-5-fluorouridine and 5-fluorouracil on childhood leukemia. Cancer Chemother Rep 34: 51, 1964.

(34) Moertel, C., Reitemeier, R., and Hahn, R. Fluorinated pyrimidine therapy of advanced gastrointestinal cancer. Gastroenterology 46: 371, 1964.

(35) Ansfield, F. A less toxic fluorouracil dosage schedule. JAMA 190: 234, 1964.

(36) Talley, R., Vaitkevicius, V., and Leighton, G. Comparison of cyclophosphamide and 5-fluorouracil in the treatment of patients with metastatic breast cancer. Clin Pharm Ther 6: 740, 1965.

(37) Rochlin, D., Smart, C., and Silva, A. Chemotherapy of malignancies of the gastrointestinal tract. Am J Surg 109: 43, 1965.

(38) Cressy, N., and Schell, H. 5-fluorouracil in glucose and saline: therapeutic effect and toxicity. Cancer Chemother Rep 9: 683, 1966.

(39)   Blokhina, N., and Blokhin, N.   5-fluorouracil therapy for
       cancer of the stomach.   Cancer 20: 668, 1967.

(40)   Eastern Cooperative Group in Solid Tumor Chemotherapy.
       Comparison of antimetabolites in the treatment of breast
       and colon cancer.   JAMA 200: 770, 1967.

(41)   Horton, J., Gehrt, P., Cunningham, T., et al.   A comparison
       of combination and single drug chemotherapy in cancer of the
       colon, breast, and other organs.   Proc Amer Assoc Cancer Res
       8: 120, 1967.

(42)   Mackman, S., Ramirez, G., and Ansfield, F.   Results of 5-
       fluorouracil given by the multiple daily dose method in
       disseminated breast cancer.   Cancer Chemother Rep 51: 483,
       1967.

(43)   Moore, G., Bross, I., Ausman, R., et al.   Effects of 5-
       fluorouracil (NSC 19893) in 389 patients with cancer.   Cancer
       Chemother Rep 52: 641, 1968.

(44)   Malkasian, G., Decker, D., Mussey, E., et al.   Observations
       on gynecologic malignancy treated with 5-fluorouracil.   Am J
       Ob Gyn 100: 1012, 1968.

(45)   Jacobs, E., Luce, J., and Wood, D.   Treatment of cancer
       with weekly intravenous 5-fluorouracil.   Cancer 22: 1233, 1968.

(46)   Ansfield, F., Ramirez, G., Mackman, S., et al.   A ten-year
       study of 5-fluorouracil in disseminated breast cancer with
       clinical results and survival times.   Cancer Res 29: 1062,
       1969.

(47)   Moertel, C., Reitemeier, R., and Hahn, R.   Comparative
       response of carcinoma of the rectum and carcinoma of the
       colon to fluorinated pyrimidine therapy.   Cancer Chemother
       Rep 53: 283, 1969.

(48)   Hall, T., Cavins, J., Khung, C., et al.   Time and vehicle
       studies of a safe and effective method for administration of
       5-fluorouracil.   Cancer 19: 1008, 1966.

Cytosine Arabinoside

Synonyms: ara-C, CA, cytarabine, 1-β-D-arabinofuranosyl-cytosine, Cytosar.

Structure:

227

Dosage: There is no established optimal dose schedule. See
                 discussion and tables.

Toxicity: I.   Hematological - usual dose-limiting toxicity
                      A.   Leukopenia
                      B.   Thrombocytopenia
                      C.   Anemia

                 II. Gastrointestinal - common
                      A.   Anorexia, nausea and vomiting - usually mild
                           and transient

                 III. Hepatic - uncommon
                      A.   Usually reversible, often subclinical

Mechanism of Action: Ara-C, when converted to its
        phosphorylated derivatives, is a direct and specific
        inhibitor of DNA synthesis. It was originally
        proposed that this inhibition occurred through
        blockade of the conversion of cytidine diphosphate to
        deoxycytidine diphosphate (ribonucleotide reductase
        inhibition).[1] Such a mechanism of action is known
        to exist for hydroxyurea. However, Moore and Cohen[2]
        demonstrated that a tumor cell reductase was very
        poorly inhibited by the diphosphate or triphosphate
        (ara-CTP) of ara-C. Subsequently, Furth and Cohen[3]
        demonstrated that ara-CTP was an effective inhibitor of
        mammalian DNA polymerase, probably acting as a
        competitive inhibitor of deoxycytidine triphosphate,
        rather than inhibiting its synthesis. Inhibition of
        DNA polymerase is now most generally accepted as
        representing the mechanism of action of ara-C.

                         Role in Cancer Therapy

     Ara-C is a relatively new agent in cancer chemotherapy,
recently made commercially available under the name "Cytosar".
Its chief effectiveness appears to be in the treatment of AML-AMoL.
Of 299 reported cases, 21% obtained CR when treated with ara-C
alone. This response rate compares favorably with the overall CR
rate for 6 MP, MTX, or high-dose prednisone used alone, and is
only slightly less than that reported for daunorubicin, an
investigational drug with a poorer therapeutic index. Ara-C
thus probably represents the most useful single drug available
today for the treatment of this form of acute leukemia.

     In the L1210 mouse leukemia, ara-C appears to be much more
effective on an intermittent schedule in which the doses are
given spaced closely together (every 3 hours x 8, every 4 days).[4]

Attempts have been made to exploit this apparent schedule dependency by giving ara-C on an intermittent infusion basis in man. It is not yet clear what clinical schedule is optimal, but the results of daily infusions of 50 or 100 mg/m^2 over one hour,[13] continuous infusions of 1000 mg/m^2 over 5 days, repeated at 9-day intervals,[15] or infusions of 75 mg/m^2 over 4 hours, daily x 4, with repeat courses after a 3-day rest period,[21] do not appear significantly different, in terms of response rate for adults. No comparative, controlled study has yet been done of the various schedules, nor have a large number of patients with AML-AMoL, treated according to a daily "push" schedule, been reported. It is of interest that the CR rate of 27% observed in earlier studies by Acute Leukemia Group B,[13] using daily one-hour infusions of 50 or 100 mg/m^2, had dropped to 17% for a larger, later series treated according to the same schedule.[17]

Ara-C is perhaps unique among antileukemic drugs, in that it appears more effective against AML-AMoL than against ALL-AUL. The overall reported CR rate in this disease with ara-C alone is only 7% (of 122 patients). Moreover, a study of high-dose, intermittent infusion by Wang et al[20] demonstrated CR in only 3 of 34 patients treated, so that the poor results obtained in this form of acute leukemia probably can not be attributed to the employment of daily "push" schedules. There is some evidence[18] that ara-C may be of use in patients with advanced disease when administered in combination with prednisone. In addition, it has been shown to have an effect on meningeal leukemia,[20] when administered intrathecally.

Ara-C, at least when used alone, does not appear to have major activity in other types of human cancer, although the evaluation of this agent in lymphomas has been inadequate.

Current investigations with ara-C focus largely on its use in combination with other drugs, either concomitantly or sequentially. It may find its greatest application in the future in such a role.

Tumor Type or Site

Breast

Ref #	# Pts Evaluated	# Pts Responding	% Response	Dose Schedule (IV) and Remarks
16	1	0		Varied – most therapy by 24–96 hr infusion q 2 wks.
22	20	3		3.5 mg/kg/day x 10, "push". All PR.
23	28	3		1–4 mg/kg/day x 10, "push"; maintenance = 5 mg/kg/day x 3, off 4 and repeat, or 3 mg/kg/day x 6, off 8 and repeat. (A few patients received 24-hr infusion).
	$\overline{49}$	$\overline{6}$	11	Total.

Colorectal

Ref #	# Pts Evaluated	# Pts Responding	% Response	Dose Schedule (IV) and Remarks
16	5	1		Varied – most therapy by 24–96 hr infusion q 2 wks. PR of 4 mo duration at 400–600 mg/m^2 by 96 hr infusion q 2 wks.
22	28	0		3.5 mg/kg/day x 10, "push". COG study.
23	49	9	18	1–4 mg/kg/day x 10, "push"; maintenance = 5 mg/kg/day x 3, off 4 and repeat, or 3 mg/kg/day x 6, off 8 and repeat. (A few patients received 24-hr infusion). 2 CR, 7 PR. 1 of 5 treated by 24 hr infusion had PR. COG—Phase I study.
	$\overline{77}$	$\overline{10}$	13	Total.

Melanoma

Ref #	# Pts Evaluated	# Pts Responding	% Response	Dose Schedule (IV) and Remarks
16	3	0		Varied — most therapy by 24–96 hr infusion q 2 wks.
22	15	0		3.5 mg/kg/day x 10, "push".
23	21	1		1–4 mg/kg/day x 10, "push"; maintenance = 5 mg/kg/day x 3, off 4 and repeat, or 3 mg/kg/day x 6, off 8 and repeat.
	39	1	2.5	Total.

Lung

Ref #	# Pts Evaluated	# Pts Responding	% Response	Dose Schedule (IV) and Remarks
16	13	0		Varied — most therapy by 24–96 hr infusion q 2 wks.
22	10	0		3.5 mg/kg/day x 10, "push".
23	20	0		1–4 mg/kg/day x 10, "push"; maintenance = 5 mg/kg/day x 3, off 4 and repeat, or 3 mg/kg/day x 6, off 8 and repeat. (A few patients received infusion).
	43	0	0	Total.

AML-AMoL

Ref #	# Pts Evaluated	# Pts Responding	% Response	Dose Schedule (IV) and Remarks
12	8	0	0	20-35 mg/m^2 q 3 hr, IV push x 8; rest 3 days and repeat as tolerated, cyclically. See discussion.
13	77	19 (12 CR)	25 (16% CR)	30 mg/m^2/day by 12 hr infusion or 30 mg/m^2/day by 24 hr infusion to response or prohibitive toxicity. Includes both 12 and 24 hr infusions at 30 mg/m^2/day. ALGB.
13	21	4 (4 CR)	19 (19% CR)	10 mg/m^2/day by 12 hr infusion or 10 mg/m^2/day by 24 hr infusion to response or prohibitive toxicity. Includes both 12 and 24 hr infusions at 10 mg/m^2/day. ALGB.
13	16	4 (3 CR)	25 (19% CR)	30 mg/m^2/day by 1 hr infusion to response or prohibitive toxicity (3 to 6 wks). ALGB.
13	20	6 (6 CR)	30 (30% CR)	50 mg/m^2/day by 1 hr infusion to response or prohibitive toxicity (3 to 6 wks). ALGB.
13	20	6 (5 CR)	30 (25% CR)	100 mg/m^2/day by 1 hr infusion to response or prohibitive toxicity (3 to 6 wks). ALGB.
13	26	4 (3 CR)	15 (12% CR)	30 mg/m^2/day by 4 hr infusion to response or prohibitive toxicity. ALGB.
14	6	2 (0 CR)	33	3 to 5 mg/kg/day, "push" x $\geq$ 10 days. Both PR in erythroleukemia.

AML–AMoL (cont.)

Ref #	# Pts Evaluated	# Pts Responding	% Response	Dose Schedule (IV) and Remarks
15	8	1 (1 CR)	12.5 (12.5% CR)	100–450 mg/m^2/day x 5, "push". Courses repeated after at least 9 day rest intervals. CR 8 months' duration.
15	36	14 (9 CR)	39 (25% CR)	200 mg/m^2/day x 5, continuous infusion. Repeat courses after at least 9 day intervals. Median duration CR = 9 and 3/4 mo. Range CR = 1 and 3/4 to 15+ mo.
17	–	–		100 mg/m^2/day by 1 hr infusion to M_1 marrow, or to $\geq$ 3 periods of hypoplasia without M_1, or to 8 wks. ALGB. See discussion.
19	12	3 (2 CR)		150–200 mg/m^2/day as 24 hr continuous infusion x 5 days q 2 wks. 5 patients had inadequate trials. All children.
21	49	21 (CR)	43+ (43% CR)	10–15 mg/m^2 "push", followed by 60 mg/m^2 immediately as a 4 hr infusion, daily x 4. Courses repeated, after at least 3 day rest intervals, to remission or limiting toxicity. CR in 14/37 adults = 38%, median duration 5 mo. CR in 7/12 children, median duration 4 mo.
	299	81+ (63 CR)	27 (21% CR)	Total.

Lymphoma (cont.)

Ref #	# Pts Evaluated	# Pts Responding	% Response	Dose Schedule (IV) and Remarks
22	4	1 (0 CR)	25	3.5 mg/kg/day x 10, "push".
23	1	0 (0 CR)		1-4 mg/kg/day x 10, "push", maintenance = 5 mg/kg/day x 3, off 4 and repeat, or 3 mg/kg/day, off 8 and repeat. (A few patients received 24-hr infusion).
	$\overline{5}$	$\overline{1}$	20	Total.
ALL-AUL				
10	10	5 (0 CR)		3 mg/kg/day x 10, "push". 4 patients had M_1 marrow.
12	2	0		20-30 mg/m^2 q 3 hr IV "push" x 8; rest 3 days and repeat as tolerated, cyclically.
13	15	3 (2 CR)		30 mg/m^2/day by 12 hr infusion; 30 mg/m^2/day by 24 hr infusion to response or prohibitive toxicity. Includes both 12 and 24 hr infusions at 30 mg/m^2/day. ALGB study.

ALL–AUL (cont.)

Ref #	# Pts Evaluated	# Pts Responding	% Response	Dose Schedule (IV) and Remarks
13	3	3 (2 CR)		10 mg/m^2/day by 12 hr infusion; 30 mg/m^2/day by 24 hr infusion to response or prohibitive toxicity. Includes both 12 and 24 hr infusions at 10 mg/m^2/day. ALGB study.
13	19	3 (2 CR)		30 mg/m^2/day by 4 hr infusion; 30, 50, or 100 mg/m^2/day by 1 hr infusion to response or prohibitive toxicity. Includes all 1 and 4-hr infusion data, all schedules.
14	39	13 (2 CR)		3 to 5 mg/kg/day, "push" x $\geq$ 10 days. 51 patients treated. 39 had adequate trial. 9 patients had M_1 marrow. All refractory to "standard" chemotherapy. CCGA study.
18	–	–		Ara-C, 3 mg/kg/day x 10, IM, + Prednisone 2 mg/kg/day x 10, PO; then (if M_1 marrow), 6 mg/kg x 2/wk, Ara-C; if M_3, ↑ to 5 mg/kg/day x 10. See discussion.
19	34	4 (1 CR)	12 (3% CR)	150-200 mg/m^2/day as 24 hr continuous infusion x 5 days, q 2 wks. Children. 9 patients had inadequate trials.
	$\overline{122}$	$\overline{31}$ (9 CR)	25 (7% CR)	Total.

References

(1)   Chu, M., and Fischer, G. A proposed mechanism of action of
      1-β-D-arabinofuranosylcytosine as an inhibitor of the
      growth of leukemic cells. Biochem Pharmacol 11: 423, 1962.

(2)   Moore, E., and Cohen, S. Effects of arabinonucleotides on
      ribonucleotide reduction by an enzyme system from rat tumor.
      J Biol Chem 242: 2116, 1967.

(3)   Furth, J., and Cohen, S. Inhibition of mammalian DNA
      polymerase by the 5'-triphosphate of 1-β-D-arabinofuranosyl-
      cytosine and the 5'-triphosphate of 9-β-D-arabinofuranosyl-
      adenine. Cancer Res 28: 2061, 1968.

(4)   Skipper, H., Schabel, F., and Wilcox, W. Experimental
      evaluation of antitumor agents. XXI. Scheduling of
      arabinosylcytosine to take advantage of its S-phase
      specificity against leukemia cells. Cancer Chemother Rep
      51: 125, 1967.

(5)   Henderson, E., and Burke, P. Clinical experience with
      cytosine arabinoside. Proc Amer Assoc Cancer Res 6: #102,
      1965.

(6)   Carey, R., and Ellison, R. Continuous cytosine arabinoside
      infusions in patients with neoplastic disease. Clin Res
      13: 337, 1965.

(7)   Talley, R. Cytosine arabinoside: clinical pharmacology and
      human antineoplastic effects. Internat Cancer Congress
      (Tokyo), p. 441, 1966.

(8)   Yu, K., Howard, J., and Clarkson, B. Comparative studies of
      cytosine arabinoside (CA) and 5-fluoro-2'-deoxyuridine
      (FUdR) in leukemia in man. Proc Amer Assoc Cancer Res 7:
      78 (#310), 1966.

(9)   Bernard, J., Boiron, M., Jacquillat, C., et al. Un nouvel
      agent actif dans le traitement des leucemies aigues.
      Presse Med 74: 799, 1966.

(10) Howard, J., Cevik, N., and Murphy, M. Cytosine arabinoside
      (NSC 63878) in acute leukemia in children. Cancer Chemother
      Rep 50: 287, 1966.

(11) Henderson, E., Serpick, A., Leventhal, B., et al. Cytosine
      arabinoside infusions in adult and childhood acute myelocytic
      leukemia. Proc Amer Assoc Cancer Res 9: 29 (#113), 1968.

(12)   Brook, J., Scott, J., and Mass R. Intermittent cytosine
       arabinoside in the treatment of acute leukemia. Proc
       Amer Assoc Cancer Res 9: 9 (#32), 1968.

(13)   Ellison, R., Holland, J., Weil, M., et al. Arabinosyl
       cytosine: a useful agent in the treatment of acute
       leukemia in adults. Blood 32: 507, 1968.

(14)   Howard, J., Albo, V., and Newton, W. Cytosine arabinoside.
       Results of a cooperative study in acute childhood leukemia.
       Cancer 21: 341, 1968.

(15)   Bodey, G., Freireich, E., Monto, R., et al. Cytosine
       arabinoside (NSC 63878) therapy for acute leukemia in
       adults. Cancer Chemother Rep 53: 59, 1969.

(16)   Frei, E., Bickers, J., Hewlett, J., et al. Dose schedule
       and antitumor studies of arabinosyl cytosine (NSC 63878).
       Cancer Res 29: 1325, 1969.

(17)   Carey, R. Comparative study of cytosine arabinoside (CA)
       therapy alone and combined with thioguanine (TG),
       mercaptopurine (MP) or daunomycin (DN) in acute myelocytic
       leukemia (AML). Proc Amer Assoc Cancer Res 11: 15 (#55),
       1970.

(18)   Nesbit, M., and Hammond, D. Cytosine arabinoside (ara-C)
       and prednisone therapy of previously treated acute
       lymphoblastic and undifferentiated leukemia (ALL/AUL) of
       childhood. Proc Amer Assoc Cancer Res 11: 59, (#233), 1970.

(19)   Wang, J., Selawry, O., Vietti, T., et al. Prolonged infusion
       of arabinosyl cytosine in childhood leukemia. Cancer 25: 1,
       1970.

(20)   Wang, J., and Pratt, C. Intrathecal arabinosyl cytosine in
       meningeal leukemia. Cancer 25: 531, 1970.

(21)   Goodell, B., and Henderson, E. In press, Clin Pharm Ther.

(22)   Central Oncology Group. Unpublished results of protocol
       #550.

(23)   Central Oncology Group. Unpublished results of protocol
       #490.

Hydroxyurea

Synonyms: Hydrea

Structure:

$$NH_2 - \overset{\overset{\displaystyle O}{\|}}{C} - NH - OH$$

Dosage: 1. 80 mg/kg as a single dose, PO q 3 days, to
                 limiting toxicity or disease progression (~6 wks).
             2. 20-40 mg/kg/day, PO as a single dose or in two
                 divided daily doses, to limiting toxicity or
                 disease progression.
             (Neither schedule may be optimal – see discussion
             under "Role in Cancer Therapy")

Toxicity: I.   Hematological – usual dose-limiting toxicity
                  A. Leukopenia
                  B. Thrombocytopenia
                  C. Anemia

             II. Gastrointestinal – not usually severe
                  A. Anorexia
                  B. Nausea and vomiting
                  C. Diarrhea
                  D. Stomatitis – unusual

             III. Dermatological – rare
                  A. Maculopapular rash
                  B. Alopecia

Mechanism of Action: Hydroxyurea directly inhibits DNA synthesis,
             primarily through inhibition of ribonucleoside
             diphosphate reductase.[1,2,3,4] Its cytotoxic effect is,
             therefore, cell-cycle specific for the S phase. In
             this respect it resembles cytosine arabinoside, and,
             like that compound, hydroxyurea demonstrates marked
             schedule dependency in animal tumor models, in which
             treatments every 3 hours over a 24-hour period, with
             courses repeated every fourth day, are much more
             effective than a once-daily treatment schedule.[5,6]

Role in Cancer Therapy

    Hydroxyurea is currently recommended by the manufacturer
for use in malignant melanoma and in CML resistant to alkylating
agent therapy. In a total of 147 patients with malignant melanoma
reported in the literature, it produced a reported objective
response in 21% (in the largest series,[31] the criterion for tumor
regression was only $\geq$ 25% reduction in size; however, the same
series required a duration of response $\geq$ 30 days). Hydroxyurea
may be the most effective single agent now available for the
treatment of melanoma. The published data concerning the
usefulness of hydroxyurea in CML is scanty, but does indicate
activity. Fishbein et al[20] noted that "thrombocytopenia was less
frequent and marrow depression was more readily reversible with
hydroxyurea than with busulfan." Some clinicians feel, however,
that consistent, "smooth" control of the disease is more readily
obtained with 6 MP or busulfan.

The clinical pharmacology of this compound has been
extensively investigated. Davidson and Winter[7] found that
peak blood levels were obtained one hour after oral administration
at a variety of different doses, with rapid urinary clearance and
low serum levels at 4 to 6 hours. Krakoff et al[14] found that
peak blood levels were obtained two and one-half hours after oral
administration of a single dose of 60 mg/kg; half the administered
compound had been excreted in the urine within three and one-half
hours, and by five and one-half hours after oral administration,
no drug could be detected in the serum. These investigators
concluded: "Because hydroxyurea is excreted so rapidly it is
possible that frequent small doses may be more effective than
large doses given once daily; however, the influence of rate of
administration on the development of toxicity or the regression
of tumors has not yet been fully evaluated." Nevinny and Hall[29]
have made the same point: "Since inhibition of DNA synthesis
lasts only as long as effective concentrations of hydroxyurea
remain in circulation, the administration of hydroxyurea in
divided oral doses or by prolonged intravenous infusion may
produce an increase in antitumor effects because a greater
number of tumors cells might be destroyed as they go through
the supposedly most sensitive S phase of the mitotic cycle."
Such a dose schedule would be similar to that which is optimal
in mouse leukemias.[5,6] In spite of these theoretical
considerations, there have been no reported studies to date
of such a schedule in man. However, Lerner, Beckloff et al[24,33]
have utilized an intermittent, high single-dose schedule which
at least possesses many pharmacologic advantages over daily,
lower doses: they have shown that the mean peak serum
concentration obtained after a dose of 80 mg/kg is about six
times that obtained after a dose of 20 mg/kg, and that serum
levels of hydroxyurea 8 hours after administration of the 80
mg/kg dose are still higher than the maximum levels achieved
after a dose of 20 mg/kg. They offer the following rationale
for their approach:[33] "...it provides a cytotoxic concentration
of hydroxyurea to the tumor, but then allows the bone marrow
and other organs to recover during the intervening 2 days."

Bearing in mind that hydroxyurea may not have been used at
an optimal dose schedule, it has nonetheless shown some degree of
activity in tumor types other than CML and melanoma. The VA Lung
study[28] of hydroxyurea demonstrated an ability equivalent to CTX
to prolong life in the therapy of non-resectable bronchogenic
carcinoma. In this study, it was administered in a total amount per
day of approximately 9-14 mg/kg, usually in 3 or 4 divided daily
doses, for a relatively long period of time (ordinarily at least 42
days). The toxicity encountered was minimal, with only 17% of 153
patients having a fall in WBC to <4000/mm^3, and only 6 patients having

a reduction to <3000/mm^3. Nausea and vomiting and platelet count depression were even less common. Forty-seven percent of treated patients were alive at 90 days, vs 37% of controls; at 330 days from the start of therapy, 14% of the treated and 9% of the control patients were still alive. This apparent ability of hydroxyurea to influence survival time favorably in lung cancer is of interest, especially when one notes that the overall reported objective response rate is only 10% of 69 cases.

Hydroxyurea may be of value in the treatment of renal cell carcinoma (hypernephroma), a notoriously unresponsive tumor to chemotherapeutic agents in general. Seven of 25 patients treated were reported as having an objective response, including 5 of 14 in the series of Nevinny and Hall.[29]

Small numbers of cases, treated on a variety of regimens, indicate that hydroxyurea may also be of value in the treatment of bladder cancer (5 of 8 reported responses), liposarcoma, head and neck cancer (7 of 18 reported responses), and breast cancer (8 of 43 reported responses). Its reported trial in ALL-AUL and AML-AMoL has been inadequate for evaluation; the same is true for lymphomas.

Hydroxyurea has been used to some extent in combination with radiation therapy, in the hope that it may act as a radiopotentiator. Hreshchyshyn[32] reported encouraging preliminary results with this combination in patients with inoperable carcinoma of the cervix: 0/7 patients who received radiation therapy plus placebo and 3/8 patients who received radiation therapy plus hydroxyurea were alive and free of detectable tumor at 12 to 16 months after the start of treatment.

A common use of hydroxyurea, not alluded to in the accompanying tables, is as a preliminary adjunct to more definitive chemotherapy of acute leukemia, in patients presenting with WBC counts high enough to cause concern over thromboembolic complications. Hydroxyurea will cause a prompt lowering of the WBC count, usually within 24 to 48 hours after administration of a single large dose.

A recent paper by Ariel[34] summarized his experience with hydroxyurea in the treatment of 118 patients with advanced carcinoma. The criteria for objective response were more liberal than those in other series, so that these responses have not been included in our tables. However, it is worth noting that he observed some evidence of antitumor effect in 58% of patients with malignant melanoma, 30% of those with colorectal cancer, 50% of lymphomas, 37% of sarcomas, and 40% of head and neck tumors.

Tumor Type or Site

Melanoma

Ref #	# Pts Evaluated	# Pts Responding	% Response	Dose Schedule and Remarks
15	2	0		15–20 mg/kg/day, PO in single dose, as tolerated (up to 42 days).
17	15	10		40 mg/kg/day, PO in 2 divided daily doses, x 21 days (or to limiting toxicity). All responses PR, usually of short duration. First responses occurred between day 7 and 15 of treatment. SWCCG study.
21	2	0		50 mg/kg/day, PO in 2 divided daily doses (HU) — vs Testosterone, 400 mg x 3/wk for 4 wks, followed by HU (same dose) + Testosterone.
24	3	2		80 mg/kg, PO in single dose, q 3 days for 6 wks. (16/25 patients completed a course). Both PR.
26	15	0		25 to 37.5 mg/kg/day, PO in 2 divided daily doses, to median total dose of 740 mg/kg.
27	14	1		20 to 60 mg/kg/day, PO. Response was CR.
30	12	0		No regimen cited. South African data.
31	67	14	21	"Recommended dosage", apparently either 80 mg/kg q 3 days or 20–30 mg/kg/day, PO in single doses. Response defined as ≥ 25% regression of tumor, duration at least 30 days. Squibb data.

Melanoma (cont.)

Ref #	# Pts Evaluated	# Pts Responding	% Response	Dose Schedule and Remarks
33	5	3		80 mg/kg q 3 days, PO in single dose, for 6 wks. All responses $\geq$ 50% regression of tumor.
34	-	-		50 mg/kg/day, PO in 2 divided daily doses. See discussion.
35	12	1		40 mg/kg/day, PO, as 3 or 4 divided daily doses, for 21 days. Eastern CDEP study. PR.
	$\overline{147}$	$\overline{31}$	21	Total.

Breast

Ref #	# Pts Evaluated	# Pts Responding	% Response	Dose Schedule and Remarks
9	16	2		40 mg/kg/day, PO in 2 divided daily doses, x 28 days. SWCCG study. Both PR. Both patients may have had some antitumor effect from hormone administration.
20	3	1		25 to 75 mg/kg/day, PO "in single or divided doses", for 8 to 126 days. Response was >50% decrease in hepatomegaly.
24	2	1		80 mg/kg, PO in single doses, q 3 days for 6 wks. PR.
33	7	3		80 mg/kg, PO in single doses, q 3 days for 6 wks. All responses $\geq$ 50% regression of tumor.

Breast (cont.)

Ref #	# Pts Evaluated	# Pts Responding	% Response	Dose Schedule and Remarks
34	-	-		50 mg/kg/day, PO in 2 divided daily doses. See discussion.
35	15	1		40 mg/kg/day, PO, as 3 or 4 divided daily doses, for 21 days. PR. Eastern CDEP study.
	43	8	19	Total.
			Lung	
10	27	4		40 mg/kg/day, PO in 2 divided daily doses, x 10 to 29 days. Only 1/27 had ↓ in size of 1° tumor. Responses did not correspond with clinical benefit. SWCCG study.
15	2	0		20 mg/kg/day, PO in single daily dose, as tolerated (up to 42 days).
21	3	0		50 mg/kg/day, PO in 2 divided daily doses (HU) -- vs Testosterone, 400 mg x 3/wk for 4 wks, followed by HU + Testosterone.
24	4	0		80 mg/kg, PO in single dose, q 3 days for 6 wks.
28	-	-		1 capsule bid, tid, or qid to total daily dose of 9 to 14 mg/kg/day, as tolerated (usually for 42 days). Statistically significant prolongation of survival in VAL study. See discussion.

Lung (cont.)

Ref #	# Pts Evaluated	# Pts Responding	% Response	Dose Schedule and Remarks
33	6	0		80 mg/kg, PO in single dose, q 3 days for 6 wks.
35	27	3	11	40 mg/kg/day, PO, as 3 or 4 divided daily doses, for 21 days. All PR. Eastern CDEP study.
	69	7	10	Total.
Colorectal				
15	5	0		15 to 45 mg/kg/day, PO in single daily dose, as tolerated (up to 42 days).
17	14	0		40 mg/kg/day, PO in 2 divided daily doses, x 21 days (as tolerated).
20	3	0		25 to 75 mg/kg/day, PO "in single or divided doses", for 8 to 126 days.
21	2	0		50 mg/kg/day, PO in 2 divided daily doses (HU) -- vs Testosterone, 400 mg x 3/wk for 4 wks., then HU (same dose) + Testosterone.
22	23	0		50 to 100 mg/kg/day, IV in 8-hour infusion daily x 5. (Repeat course, if given, in 4 to 5 wks.)

Colorectal (cont.)

Ref #	# Pts Evaluated	# Pts Responding	% Response	Dose Schedule and Remarks
24	2	1		80 mg/kg, PO in single dose, q 3 days for 6 wks. Response = "100% reduction in ascitic-fluid production."
33	3	1		80 mg/kg, PO in single doses, q 3 days for 6 wks. Response = 100% reduction in ascites.
34	–	–		50 mg/kg/day, PO in 2 divided daily doses. See discussion.
35	28	4	14	40 mg/kg/day, PO, as 3 or 4 divided daily doses, for 21 days. All PR. Eastern CDEP study.
	$\overline{80}$	$\overline{6}$	7.5	Total.

Lymphoma

Ref #	# Pts Evaluated	# Pts Responding	% Response	Dose Schedule and Remarks
13	10	0		40 mg/kg/day, PO in 2 divided daily doses, x 4 to 38 days. 0/5 Hodgkin's. 0/5 reticulum-cell sarcoma.
14	1	1		40 to 80 mg/kg/day, PO or IV in single daily doses. Hodgkin's; "minor therapeutic effect."
16	1	0		2.5-120 mg/kg/day, PO or IV in single daily doses. "Optimum dose" = 40-80 mg/kg/day. Reticulum-cell sarcoma, child.

Lymphoma (cont.)

Ref #	# Pts Evaluated	# Pts Responding	% Response	Dose Schedule and Remarks
20	2	0		25 to 75 mg/kg/day, PO "in single or divided doses", for 8 to 126 days. Hodgkin's.
	$\overline{14}$	$\overline{1}$	7	Total.

ALL-AUL

Ref #	# Pts Evaluated	# Pts Responding	% Response	Dose Schedule and Remarks
12	1	0		40 mg/kg/day, PO in 2 divided daily doses, for 3 to 16 days.
16	10	1		2.5-120 mg/kg/day, PO or IV as single daily dose. "Optimum dose" = 40-80 mg/kg/day. PR No "significant" side effects seen in this study involving children.
19	6	1		40 mg/kg/day, PO in 2 divided daily doses, for 14 to 35 days. PR.
	$\overline{17}$	$\overline{2}$	12	Total.

"Acute Leukemia"

Ref #	# Pts Evaluated	# Pts Responding	% Response	Dose Schedule and Remarks
14	9	0		40 to 80 mg/kg/day, PO or IV as single daily dose. All adults.

"Acute Leukemia" (cont.)

Ref #	# Pts Evaluated	# Pts Responding	% Response	Dose Schedule and Remarks
20	13	1	5	25-75 mg/kg/day, PO "in single or divided doses", for 8 to 126 days. PR.
	22	1		Total.
			AML-AMoL	
12	7	0		40 mg/kg/day, PO in 2 divided daily doses, for 3 to 16 days.
	7	0		Total.
			Stomach	
15	2	0		30-40 mg/kg/day, PO in single daily dose, as tolerated.
17	7	1		40 mg/kg/day, PO in 2 divided daily doses, x 21 days (as tolerated).
21	2	0		50 mg/kg/day, PO in 2 divided daily doses (HU) -- vs Testosterone, 400 mg x 3/wk for 4 wks, then HU (same dose) + Testosterone.

Stomach (cont.)

Ref #	# Pts Evaluated	# Pts Responding	% Response	Dose Schedule and Remarks
22	6	1		50 to 100 mg/kg/day, IV in 8-hr infusion, x 5. (Repeat course, if given, in 4 to 5 wks.) Complete regression of abdominal mass.
24	2	1		80 mg/kg, PO in single dose, q 3 days for 6 wks.
33	3	1		80 mg/kg, PO in single dose, q 3 days for 6 wks.
35	9	2		40 mg/kg/day, PO, as 3 or 4 divided daily doses, x 21 days. Eastern CDEP study. Response PR.
	31	6	19	Total.
			Kidney	
11	1	1		40 mg/kg/day, PO in 2 divided daily doses, for 12 to 28 days.
20	2	0		25-75 mg/kg/day, PO "in single or divided doses", for 8 to 126 days.
21	5	0		50 mg/kg/day, PO in 2 divided daily doses (HU), -- vs Testosterone, 400 mg x 3/wk for 4 wks, then HU (same dose) + Testosterone.

Kidney (cont.)

Ref #	# Pts Evaluated	# Pts Responding	% Response	Dose Schedule and Remarks
24	1	0		80 mg/kg, PO in single dose, q 3 days x 6 wks.
29	14	5		10 to 50 (median, 25) mg/kg/day, PO as single daily dose (?) to median total dose of 120 gm over median of 100 days (treatment frequently interrupted, then restarted when toxicity abated). 18 patients treated, 14 received "adequate trial" of – 50 gm total dose. See discussion.
33	2	1		80 mg/kg, PO in single dose, q 3 days x 6 wks. Response = 35% regresson of pulmonary metastases for >3 mo.
	$\overline{25}$	$\overline{7}$	28	Total.

Cervix and Endometrium

Ref #	# Pts Evaluated	# Pts Responding	% Response	Dose Schedule and Remarks
11	11	1		40 mg/kg/day, PO in 2 divided daily doses, for 12 to 28 days. 0/10 cervix, 1/1 endometrium (minimal PR).
21	2	1		50 mg/kg/day, PO in 2 divided daily doses (HU), -- vs Testosterone, 400 mg x 3/wk for 4 wks, then HU (same dose) + Testosterone. Endometrial cancer. PR.

Cervix and Endometrium (cont.)

Ref #	# Pts Evaluated	# Pts Responding	% Response	Dose Schedule and Remarks
32	-	-		Radiation therapy + HU, 80 mg/kg q 3 days for 12 wks, -- vs radiation therapy + placebo, q 3 days for 12 wks. See discussion.
	$\overline{13}$	$\overline{2}$	15	Total.
			Bladder	
11	1	0		40 mg/kg/day, PO in 2 divided daily doses, for 12 to 28 days.
24	1	0		80 mg/kg, PO in single dose, q 3 days x 6 wks.
25	5	4		HU administered "either orally or by intra-arterial infusion." All patients had transitional cell carcinoma.
33	1	1		80 mg/kg, PO in single dose, q 3 days x 6 wks. 50% regression pulmonary metastasis.
	$\overline{8}$	$\overline{5}$	62.5	
			Multiple Myeloma	
13	11	0		40 mg/kg/day, PO in 2 divided daily doses, x 6-15.

Multiple Myeloma (cont.)

Ref #	# Pts Evaluated	# Pts Responding	% Response	Dose Schedule and Remarks
20	1	0		25-75 mg/kg/day, PO "in single or divided doses", for 8 to 126 days.
	$\overline{12}$	$\overline{0}$		Total.
			CML	
14	6	3		40-80 mg/kg/day, PO or IV in single daily dose.
20	12	-		25-75 mg/kg/day, PO "in single or divided doses", for 8 to 126 days. 8/9 had complete regression of splenomegaly, 3/6 had ↑ in Hb of 3 gm or more. Majority benefited from treatment.
			CLL	
14	2	0	0	40-80 mg/kg/day, PO or IV in single daily dose.
			Liposarcoma	
17	2	2	100	40 mg/kg/day, PO in 2 divided daily doses, for 21 days (as tolerated).

"Bone"

Ref #	# Pts Evaluated	# Pts Responding	% Response	Dose Schedule and Remarks
17	4	0		40 mg/kg/day, PO in 2 divided daily doses, for 21 days (as tolerated).
19	1	0		40 mg/kg/day, PO in 2 divided daily doses, for 14 to 35 days. Osteogenic sarcoma.
	5̅	0̅	0	Total.

Head and Neck

Ref #	# Pts Evaluated	# Pts Responding	% Response	Dose Schedule and Remarks
17	13	5		40 mg/kg/day, PO in 2 divided daily doses, for 21 days (as tolerated).
33	5	2		80 mg/kg, PO in single dose, q 3 days x 6 wks.
	1̅8̅	7̅	39	Total.

References

(1)   Young, C., and Hodas, S. Hydroxyurea: inhibitory effect
       on DNA metabolism. Science 146: 1172, 1964.

(2)   Turner, M., Abrams, R., and Lieberman, I. Meso-α, β-
       diphenylsuccinate and hydroxyurea as inhibitors of
       deoxycytidylate synthesis in extracts of Ehrlich ascites
       and L cells. J Biol Chem 241: 5777, 1966.

(3)   Elford, H. Effect of hydroxyurea on ribonucleotide
       reductase. Biochem Biophys Res Commun 33: 129, 1968.

(4)   Krakoff, I., Brown, N., and Reichard, P. Inhibition of
       ribonucleoside diphosphate reductase by hydroxyurea. Cancer
       Res 28: 1559, 1968.

(5)   Schabel, F. In vivo leukemic cell kill kinetics and
       "curability" in experimental systems. In "The
       Proliferation and Spread of Neoplastic Cells," (Twenty-
       first Annual Symposium on Fundamental Cancer Research,
       M.D. Anderson Hospital and Tumor Institute, University of
       Texas) Williams and Wilkins Co., Baltimore, pp 379-408, 1968.

(6)   Brockman, R., Shaddix, S., Laster, W., et al. Guanazole
       and hydroxyurea: inhibition of DNA synthesis,
       ribonucleotide reductase, and L1210 leukemia. Cancer Res
       (in press).

(7)   Davidson, J., and Winter, T. A method of analyzing for
       hydroxyurea in biological fluids. Cancer Chemother Rep 27:
       97, 1963.

(8)   Thurman, W., Bloedow, C., Howe, C., et al. A phase I study
       of hydroxyurea. Cancer Chemother Rep 29: 103, 1963.

(9)   Sears, M. Phase II studies of hydroxyurea (NSC 32065) in
       adults: cancer of the breast. Cancer Chemother Rep 40:
       43, 1964.

(10)   Bickers, J. Phase II study of hydroxyurea (NSC 32065) in
       adults: carcinoma of the lung. Cancer Chemother Rep 40:
       45, 1964.

(11)   Howe, C., and Samuels, M. Phase II studies of hydroxyurea
       (NSC 32065) in adults: urologic and gynecologic neoplasms.
       Cancer Chemother Rep 40: 47, 1964.

(12) Shullenberger, C. Phase II studies of hydroxyurea in adults:
      leukemia. Cancer Chemother Rep 40: 49, 1964.

(13) Davis, P. Phase II studies of hydroxyurea (NSC 32065) in
      adults: multiple myeloma and lymphoma. Cancer Chemother
      Rep 40: 51, 1964.

(14) Krakoff, I., Savel, H., and Murphy, M. Phase II studies of
      hydroxyurea (NSC 32065) in adults: clinical evaluation.
      Cancer Chemother Rep 40: 53, 1964.

(15) Bolton, B., Kaung, D., Lawton, R., et al. Hydroxyurea
      (NSC 32065) - a phase I study. Cancer Chemother Rep 39:
      47, 1964.

(16) Origenes, M., Beatly, E., Brubaker, C., et al. Trial of
      hydroxyurea (NSC 32065) in cancer in children. Cancer
      Chemother Rep 37: 41, 1964.

(17) Bloedow, C. Phase II studies of hydroxyurea (NSC 32065)
      in adults: miscellaneous tumors. Cancer Chemother Rep
      40: 39, 1964.

(18) Griffith, K. Hydroxyurea (NSC 32065): Results of a phase I
      study. Cancer Chemother Rep 40: 33, 1964.

(19) Fernbach, D. Pediatric clinical trials with hydroxyurea.
      Cancer Chemother Rep 40: 37, 1964.

(20) Fishbein, W., Carbone, P., Freireich, E., et al. Clinical
      trials of hydroxyurea in patients with cancer and leukemia.
      Clin Pharm Ther 5: 574, 1964.

(21) Kennedy, B., and Newton, K. Effect of androgenic hormone
      combined with hydroxyurea (NSC 32065) on hematopoietic
      system of patients with cancer. Cancer Chemother Rep 49:
      21, 1965.

(22) Moertel, C., Reitemeier, R., and Hahn, R. Evaluation of
      hydroxyurea (NSC 32065) by parenteral infusion. Cancer
      Chemother Rep 49: 27, 1965.

(23) Beckloff, G., Lerner, H., Frost, D., et al. Hydroxyurea
      (NSC 32065) in biologic fluids: dose-concentration
      relationship. Cancer Chemother Rep 48: 57, 1965.

(24) Lerner, H., and Beckloff, G. Hydroxyurea administered
      intermittently. JAMA 192: 1168, 1965.

(25) Beckloff, G., Lerner, H., Cole, R., et al. Hydroxyurea in
      bladder carcinoma. Invest Urol 3: 530, 1966.

(26) Nathanson, L., and Hall, T. Phase II study of hydroxyurea
      (NSC 32065) in malignant melanoma. Cancer Chemother Rep
      51: 503, 1967.

(27) Cassileth, P., and Hyman, G. Treatment of malignant melanoma
      with hydroxyurea. Cancer Res 27: 1843, 1967.

(28) Kaung, D., Walsh, W., Sbar, S., et al. Hydroxyurea (NSC
      32065) in therapy for nonresectable cancer of the lung.
      Cancer Chemother Rep 52: 271, 1968.

(29) Nevinny, H., and Hall, T. Chemotherapy with hydroxyurea
      (NSC 32065) in renal cell carcinoma. J Clin Pharm 8:
      352, 1968.

(30) Falkson, G., and van Dyke, J. The chemotherapy of
      malignant melanoma. South Africa Med J 42: 89, 1968.

(31) Squibb Institute for Medical Research. Clinical brochure,
      1968.

(32) Hreshchyshyn, M. Hydroxyurea (NSC 32065) with irradiation
      for cervical carcinoma - preliminary report. Cancer
      Chemother Rep 52: 601, 1968.

(33) Lerner, H., Beckloff, G., and Godwin, M. Hydroxyurea
      (NSC 32065) intermittent therapy in malignant diseases.
      Cancer Chemother Rep 53: 385, 1969.

(34) Ariel, I. Therapeutic effects of hydroxyurea. Experience
      with 118 patients with inoperable solid tumors. Cancer 25:
      705, 1970.

(35) Slack, N., and Jones, R. Single reversal trial of
      hydroxyurea (NSC 32065) in 91 patients with advanced cancer.
      Cancer Chemother Rep 54: 53, 1970.

Actinomycin D

Synonyms: Dactinomycin, Cosmegen

Structure:

Dosage: 10-15 mcg/kg/day x 5, IV; repeated at 2 to 4 week
               intervals as tolerated. (This dose schedule is most
               commonly employed; it may not be optimal).

Toxicity: I. Gastrointestinal
                   A. Anorexia, nausea, and vomiting
                       1. Usually begin within a few hours of
                           administration
                       2. May be ameliorated by phenothiazine
                           premedication
                   B. Diarrhea
                   C. Proctitis, glossitis, cheilitis, stomatitis -
                       common dose-limiting toxicities

              II. Hematological
                   A. Thrombocytopenia - often seen first
                   B. Leukopenia - may be dose-limiting
                   C. Anemia

             III. Dermatological
                   A. Alopecia
                   B. Erythema, desquamation, hyperpigmentation
                       of skin
                       1. Especially common in areas subjected to
                           x-irradiation
                   C. Acneiform eruption - reversible after
                       cessation of therapy

Mechanism of Action: Actinomycin D forms a stable complex with
          DNA which results in inhibition of DNA-dependent RNA
          synthesis. The formation of such a complex requires
          the presence of guanine, preferably in the minor groove
          of the DNA helix. At concentrations of the drug
          attainable in vivo, the synthesis of ribosomal RNA
          appears to be preferentially affected; somewhat higher
          concentrations result in inhibition of the synthesis of
          all species of RNA, and still higher concentrations
          (in vitro) can directly inhibit DNA synthesis. The
          synthesis of ribosomal RNA may be especially sensitive
          to actinomycin D because ribosomal RNA contains a greater
          proportion of guanine and cytosine than chromosomal DNA,
          which implies that the species of DNA governing synthesis
          of ribosomal RNA should have a relatively high guanine
          content. It would thus be preferentially impaired in its
          ability to code for RNA synthesis. There is some
          experimental data to support this hypothesis.[2]

          Cytotoxicity, seen primarily in proliferating cells,
          correlates better with prolonged tissue retention of
          actinomycin D then with the degree of acute inhibitory

effect on RNA synthesis.[3]   Resistance to actinomycin
D has been shown to correlate, in the DMBA murine
sarcoma[3] and in certain mouse leukemias,[4] with poor
uptake and retention of the drug. The factors which
determine cell uptake and retention or degradation of
the compound are, as yet, little understood.

Role in Cancer Therapy

A major role of actinomycin D to date has been in sequential
combination with radiation therapy, especially of Wilms' tumor.
Because it does represent a combined modality approach, the
results of such therapy are not included in our tables. However, it
should be noted that Wolff et al conclusively demonstrated that
long-term, "maintenance" administration of the drug adds
significantly to the salvage rate obtainable with either surgery
plus radiation therapy alone, or surgery and radiation plus short-
term, "adjuvant" actinomycin D, in this disease (New Eng J Med 279:
290, 1968).

Another use of actinomycin D which deserves mention, though
it does not fall strictly within the intent of this review, is in
regional perfusion, especially in the therapy of localized malignant
melanoma. The drug has been used usually as an adjuvant to surgery
or in combination with other agents in this fashion, and the results
obtained are difficult, if not impossible, to evaluate.

Used alone for the treatment of disseminated neoplasia,
actinomycin D has proven of value against testicular tumors,
trophoblastic malignancies, soft tissue sarcomas, and Wilms' tumor.
It may be the most effective agent available for testicular cancer,
as shown by the experience of Mackenzie,[17] who treated 12 patients
with only actinomycin D as initial chemotherapy, and obtained 3 CR
and 3 PR. Ten other patients in his series received actinomycin D
subsequent to other forms of chemotherapy, and one had a CR; in
addition, one who failed to respond initially responded with CR to
a second course at a different dose schedule. Of the 5 patients who
obtained CR, 4 were alive and clinically disease-free at 11+, 19+,
20+, and 21+ months, and one was alive with recurrence at 9+ months.
Two had embryonal cell and 3 had teratocarcinoma. Mackenzie
recommended 1 mg of actinomycin D daily x 4-5, by IV push at monthly
intervals for patients with metastatic testicular tumors other
than seminoma. It should be pointed out that only 2 patients in
his series received the drug on a low-dose, chronic schedule of
daily administration (0.25 mg/day x 22-32, by IV push), and one
obtained a CR. (In the B16 mouse melanoma, a relatively slow-
growing animal tumor model system, unpublished data indicates that
prolonged, chronic treatment at very low doses is optimal.[24]
Such a schedule has received insufficient trial in man for an
adequate evaluation).

Actinomycin D is probably as effective as MTX for the treatment of trophoblastic tumors, and there seems to be no clinical cross-resistance between the two agents.

The usefulness of this agent for treatment of patients with malignant melanoma is a subject of controversy. Reported response rates range from 0 of 23 (at a weekly, low dose)[18] to 16 of 24 (with a 5-6 day course, followed by weekly maintenance or none).[22] Controlled studies and, perhaps, further exploration of dose schedules, will be necessary before a statement can be made with confidence as to the role of actinomycin D in this disease.

Limited experience, usually with "loading-dose" type regimens, indicates little activity for actinomycin D as a single agent against breast, lung, or colorectal cancer. The scanty reported experience in lymphoma suggests that it has some activity, with 9 of 18 treated patients showing an objective response. This drug received a trial as an induction agent in ALL-AUL by Farber and others, reportedly with little or no effect, although the only published data in this regard is a report of two treatment failures by Tan et al.[11] Since the recent demonstration by Children's Group A of its effectiveness in remission maintenance (Leikin et al, Cancer, 24: 427, 1969), the question of the usefulness of actinomycin D in ALL-AUL has been reopened.

Finally, actinomycin D may be of value in the treatment of hypercalcemia associated with production of parathormone-like substances by tumors.[20] This area is currently receiving definitive investigation.

Tumor Type or Site

Breast

Ref #	# Pts Evaluated	# Pts Responding	% Response	Dose Schedule and Remarks
8	14	0		Total dose 100 mcg/kg over 21 days.
10	18	4		Usually total dose 75 mcg/kg, IV over 5 to 10 days. Short, partial responses.
11	7	0		15 mcg/kg/day x 5 (children). ~12 mcg/kg/day x 5 (to total dose ~ 60 mcg/kg) for adults.
13	1	0		(1) 75 mcg/kg over 5 days. (2) 65 mcg/kg over 5 days.
23	5	1		12 mcg/kg/day x 5, off one day, then 8 mcg/kg eod to toxicity or a maximum of four such doses. PR.
	$\overline{45}$	$\overline{5}$	11	Total.

Lung

Ref #	# Pts Evaluated	# Pts Responding	% Response	Dose Schedule and Remarks
10	8	0		Usually total dose 75 mcg/kg, IV over 5 to 10 days.
23	8	0		12 mcg/kg/day x 5, off one day, then 8 mcg/kg eod to toxicity or a maximum of four such doses.
	$\overline{16}$	$\overline{0}$		Total.

Melanoma

Ref #	# Pts Evaluated	# Pts Responding	% Response	Dose Schedule and Remarks
10	8	3		Usually total dose 75 mcg/kg, IV over 5 to 10 days. Short, partial responses.
13	1	0		(1) 75 mcg/kg over 5 days. (2) 65 mcg/kg over 5 days.
18	23	0		Not specified for IV route, but IV administration was apparently weekly. Cited doses varied from 400-1000 mcg/wk. (~5-15 mcg/kg/wk). Perfusion + subsequent weekly systemic therapy →remission in 5/10. Perfusion alone →0/5.
22	24	16		6-10 mcg/kg/day x 5-6, IV; then weekly maintenance therapy (in one-half of patients). Ceiteria of objective response unclear.
23	2	0		12 mcg/kg/day x 5, off one day, then 8 mcg/kg eod to toxicity or a maximum of four such doses.
	58	19	33	Total. See discussion.

Colon and Rectum

Ref #	# Pts Evaluated	# Pts Responding	% Response	Dose Schedule and Remarks
10	21	3		Usually total dose 75 mcg/kg, IV over 5 to 10 days. Transient PR.
13	6	0		(1) 75 mcg/kg over 5 days. (2) 65 mcg/kg over 5 days.

Colon and Rectum (cont.)

Ref #	# Pts Evaluated	# Pts Responding	% Response	Dose Schedule and Remarks
23	21	4		12 mcg/kg/day x 5, off one day, then 8 mcg/kg eod to toxicity or a maximum of four such doses. All PR.
	$\overline{48}$	$\overline{7}$	15	Total.

Lymphoma

Ref #	# Pts Evaluated	# Pts Responding	% Response	Dose Schedule and Remarks
5	3	0		Not given. Total dose up to 5 mg over 9-30 days, IV.
7	8	5		75 mcg/kg over 4-5 days (about 1.9 mg/m^2 over 5 days). 2/4 Hodgkin's, 1/2 reticulum-cell sarcoma, 2/2 lymphosarcoma. All PR.
10	6	3		Usually total dose 75 mcg/kg, IV over 5 to 10 days. All lymphosarcoma; 2 transient, 1 of 6 mo duration.
13	1	1		(1) 75 mcg/kg over 5 days. (2) 65 mcg/kg over 5 days. Hodgkin's. Objective response.
	$\overline{18}$	$\overline{9}$	50	Total.

Acute Leukemias

Ref #	# Pts Evaluated	# Pts Responding	% Response	Dose Schedule and Remarks
7	2	0		75 mcg/kg over 4-5 days (about 1.9 mg/m^2 over 5 days).
	$\overline{2}$	$\overline{0}$		Total. See discussion
			CLL	
19	14	5		Not given. "Shrinkage of nodes".
			Kidney	
10	4	0		Usually total dose 75 mcg/kg, IV over 5 to 10 days.
21	2	0		Not given.
23	1	0		12 mcg/kg/day x 5, off one day, then 8 mcg/kg eod to toxicity or a maximum of four such doses.
	$\overline{7}$	$\overline{0}$		Total.
			Wilms' Tumor	
6	3	1		2-3 mg/m^2 as 3-6 injections over 4-12 days.

Wilms' Tumor (cont.)

Ref #	# Pts Evaluated	# Pts Responding	% Response	Dose Schedule and Remarks
7	16	6		75 mcg/kg over 4-5 days (about 1.9 mg/m^2 over 5 days).
9	5	3		Varied. 24-250 mcg/kg total dose, given over 1-7 days. "Optimal" total dose = 75-100 mg/kg or 2.4 mg/m^2.
13	2	0		(1) 75 mcg/kg over 5 days. (2) 65 mcg/kg over 5 days. Adults.
	$\overline{26}$	$\overline{10}$	39	Total. See discussion.

Rhabdomyosarcoma

Ref #	# Pts Evaluated	# Pts Responding	% Response	Dose Schedule and Remarks
6	3	1		2-3 mg/m^2 as 3 to 6 injections over 4 to 12 days.
7	5	1		75 mcg/kg over 4-5 days (about 1.9 mg/m^2 over 5 days).
9	5	3		Varied. 24-250 mcg/kg total dose, given over 1-7 days. "Optimal" total dose = 75-100 mg/kg or 2.4 mg/m^2.
12	9	1		Total dose 2.4 mg/m^2 over 7 days.
	$\overline{21}$	$\overline{6}$	29	Total.

"Adult Sarcoma"

Ref #	# Pts Evaluated	# Pts Responding	% Response	Dose Schedule and Remarks
10	5	2		Usually total dose 75 mcg/kg, IV over 5 to 10 days. 1/1 liposarcoma; 1/3 leiomyosarcoma; 0/1 osteogenic sarcoma.
16	9	2		Not given. Mixed mesodermal (ovarian) sarcoma.
23	48	10		12 mcg/kg/day x 5, off one day, then 8 mcg/kg eod to toxicity or a maximum of four such doses. 1 CR. No further details.
	$\overline{62}$	$\overline{14}$	23	Total.

Trophoblastic Tumors

Ref #	# Pts Evaluated	# Pts Responding	% Response	Dose Schedule and Remarks
15	13	7		7-11 mcg/kg/day x 5; repeated as tolerated (actinomycin D); 10-30 mg/day, IM x 5; repeated as tolerated (MTX). Actinomycin D as initial therapy. MTX initially →45/87 CR. All CR. 3/7 choriocarcinoma, 4/6 others.
15	23	12		7-11 mcg/kg/day x 5; repeated as tolerated (actinomycin D); 10-30 mg/day, IM x 5; (methotrexate). All responses CR, 10/17 choriocarcinoma, 2/6 others. MTX in actinomycin D-resistant patients → 4/7 CR.
	$\overline{36}$	$\overline{19}$	53	Total. All CR. Actual response rate higher.

Testis

Ref #	# Pts Evaluated	# Pts Responding	% Response	Dose Schedule and Remarks
7	1	1		75 mcg/kg over 4-5 days (about 1.9 mg/m^2 over 5 days). Embryonal cell carcinoma.
11	2	0		15 mcg/kg/day x 5 (children). ~12 mcg/kg/day x 5 (to total dose ~ 60 mcg/kg) for adults.
17	12	6	50	(1) 1 mg/day x 5, IV rapid injection, at monthly intervals. (2) 1 mg/day x 4-5, continuous IV infusion. (3) 0.25 mg/day x 22-32, IV rapid injection. (4) 5 mg/day x 1 q 2 wks, IV rapid injection. 3 CR, 3 PR. Patients without previous chemotherapy.
17	10	1		(1) 1 mg/day x 5, IV rapid injection, at monthly intervals. (2) 1 mg/day x 4-5, continuous IV infusion. (3) 0.25 mg/day x 22-32, IV rapid injection. (4) 5 mg/day x 1 q 2 wks, IV rapid injection. Patients with previous chemotherapy.
	$\overline{25}$	$\overline{8}$	32	

Pancreas

Ref #	# Pts Evaluated	# Pts Responding	% Response	Dose Schedule and Remarks
10	3	0		Usually total dose 75 mcg/kg, IV over 5 to 10 days.
13	1	0		(1) 75 mcg/kg over 5 days. (2) 65 mcg/kg over 5 days.
	$\overline{4}$	$\overline{0}$		Total.

Head and Neck

Ref #	# Pts Evaluated	# Pts Responding	% Response	Dose Schedule and Remarks
13	5	0		(1) 75 mcg/kg over 5 days. (2) 65 mcg/kg over 5 days.
23	6	0		12 mcg/kg/day x 5, off one day, then 8 mcg/kg eod to toxicity or a maximum of four such doses.
	$\overline{11}$	$\overline{0}$		Total.

References

(1)   Young, C. Actinomycin and antitumor antibioties. Amer
       J Clin Path 52: 130, 1969.

(2)   Ro, T., Narayan, K., and Busch, H. Effects of actinomycin
       D on base composition and nearest neighbor frequency of
       nucleolar RNA of the Walker tumor and liver. Cancer Res
       26: 780, 1966.

(3)   Schwartz, H., Sodergren, J., and Ambaye, R. Actinomycin
       D: drug concentrations and actions in mouse tissues and
       tumors. Cancer Res 28: 192, 1968.

(4)   Kessel, D., and Wodinsky, I. Uptake _in vivo_ and _in vitro_
       of actinomycin D by mouse leukemias as a factor in survival.
       Biochem Pharmacol 17: 161, 1968.

(5)   Korst, D., and Meyer, O. Negative effect of actinomycin D
       treatment in three cases of Hodgkin's disease. Antibiot
       Med 1: 474, 1955.

(6)   Pinkel, D. Actinomycin D in childhood cancer. A
       preliminary report. Pediat 23: 342, 1959.

(7)   Tan, C., Dargeon, H., and Burchenal, J. The effect of
       actinomycin D on cancer in childhood. Pediat 24: 544, 1959.

(8)   Wright, J., Cobb, J., Golomb, F., et al. Chemotherapy of
       disseminated carcinoma of the breast. Ann Surg 150: 221, 1959.

(9)   Shaw, R., Moore, E., Mueller, P., et al. The effect of
       actinomycin D on childhood neoplasms. Am J Dis Child 99:
       628, 1960.

(10)   Watne, A., Badillo, J., Koike, A., et al. Clinical studies
       of actinomycin D. Ann N Y Acad Sci 89: 445, 1960.

(11)   Tan, C., Galbey, R., Yap, C., et al. Clinical experiences
       with actinomycin D, KS_2, and F_1 (KS_4). Ann N Y Acad Sci
       89: 426, 1960.

(12)   Pinkel, D., and Pickren, J. Rhabdomyosarcoma in children.
       JAMA 175: 293, 1961.

(13)   Humphrey, E., Hymes, A., Ausman, R., et al. An evaluation of
       actinomycin D and mitomycin C in patients with advanced cancer.
       Surgery 50: 881, 1961.

(14) Ross, G., Stolbach, L., and Hertz, R.   Actinomycin D in the
      treatment of methotrexate-resistant trophoblastic disease
      in women.   Proc Amer Assoc Cancer Res 3: 355, 1962, and
      Cancer Res 22: 1015, 1962.

(15) Hertz, R., Ross, G., and Lipsett, M.   Chemotherapy in women
      with trophoblastic disease: choriocarcinoma, chorioadenoma
      destruans, and complicated hydatidiform mole.   Ann N Y Acad
      Sci 114: 881, 1964.

(16) Hreshchyshyn, M.   Experiences with chemotherapy in
      gynecologic cancer.   N Y J Med 64: 2431, 1964.

(17) Mackenzie, A.   Chemotherapy of metastatic testis cancer:
      results in 154 patients.   Cancer 19: 1369, 1966.

(18) Golomb, F., Solowey, A., Postel, A., et al.   Induced
      remission of malignant melanoma with actinomycin D.
      Cancer 20: 656, 1967.

(19) Karnofsky, D.   The use of actinomycin in neoplastic disease
      in adults.   In "Actinomycin", (S. Waksman, ed), Interscience
      Publishers, New York, pp. 147-161, 1968.

(20) Muggia, F., Heinemann, H., Belanger, R., et al.
      Hyperparathyroid-like hypercalcemia in neoplastic disease -
      treatment with dactinomycin.   Clin Res 16: 558, 1968 (In
      Soc Proc).

(21) Talley, R., Moorhead, E., Tucker, W., et al.   Treatment of
      metastatic hypernephroma.   J Amer Med Assoc 207: 322, 1969.

(22) Molander, D., and Oropeza, R.   Management of metastatic
      malignant melanoma with actinomycin D.   Proc Amer Assoc
      Cancer Res 10: 60 (#237), 1969.

(23) Central Clinical Drug Evaluation Program.   Unpublished data,
      1965.

(24) Cancer Chemotherapy National Service Center, Drug Evaluation
      Branch.

Mithramycin

Synonyms: Mithracin

Structure:

Dosage: 1.   50 mcg/kg/dose on alternate days, IV by push or
                    infusion over several hours, for up to 8 doses per
                    course.
               2.   25 mcg/kg/day x 7, IV by push or infusion on
                    consecutive days. (May be more toxic.)

Toxicity, Mechanism of Action, and Role in Cancer Therapy

Mithramycin is an antibiotic with antitumor properties. Like
Actinomycin D, it appears to specifically inhibit DNA-directed
synthesis of RNA, without affecting the synthesis of DNA itself.
Unlike daunorubicin, which is felt to act by intercalating between
base pairs in the DNA helix, mithramycin is thought to stabilize
the secondary structure of DNA by forming bridges between
complementary strands of the helix.[10] The precise geometry of its
binding to DNA has not been determined.

It is a very toxic agent: an analysis of the clinical
brochure prepared by Pfizer (1966) reveals that, in a total of 900
cancer patients treated and evaluated for toxicity, 5.5% died of
hemorrhage associated with administration of the drug. Since that
time, other reports have appeared,[5,6,8] further confirming the
existence of a "hemorrhagic syndrome" associated with the
administration of mithramycin, and emphasizing that this may occur
in the absence of thrombocytopenia or abnormalities in the usual
measurements of clotting. The incidence of death directly
attributable to administration cf this drug has been reported to
be as high as 10% of the patients treated.[8] Recently, Kennedy[7]
has reported a sharp decrease in toxicity, and no mortality, in a
series of 28 patients treated with mithramycin on an every-other-
day schedule at 50 mcg/kg/dose. The antitumor effect was
preserved (7/28 patients with embryonal carcinoma of the testis
responded). This dose schedule was based on experimental evidence
of Yarbro and Kennedy (Cancer Research 27: 1779, 1967) which
demonstrated, in an in vitro test system, that normal liver cells
exposed to mithramycin recovered their capacity for RNA synthesis
more rapidly than tumor cells. Since Kennedy introduced it, two
cooperative groups have begun protocols which essentially utilize
Kennedy's dose schedule (SWCCG, WCCG). It is too early to know
whether they will confirm his results.

Mithramycin has received extensive clinical trials in the
therapy of patients with testicular cancer, mostly at a daily dose
schedule of 25 to 50 mcg/kg for 5 to 10 days. It has been
administered both as a rapid, single "push" injection and as an
infusion over 4 to 24 hours. Nausea and vomiting appear to be less
severe if the drug is given as an infusion, preferably over 24
hours.[4,6] Other toxic side effects, and therapeutic effects,
appear to be little influenced. Thirty-two percent of 346

reported patients with testicular cancer have shown an objective
response to therapy with this drug; about 9% have had CR, often for
sustained periods.   In general, patients seem to respond better to
mithramycin who have embryonal carcinoma as the predominant or
only histologic type, and those in the teratocarcinoma group have
the poorest chance of responding.[4,6]   The 32% response rate with
mithramycin compares to 32% for Actinomycin D alone (but in only
25 evaluable patients) in testicular cancer.   "Triple therapy"
(Actinomycin D + chlorambucil + MTX) has produced at least as
high a response rate, on the basis of published reports.   Since
mithramycin seems to be at least as toxic as triple therapy, and
probably more toxic than Actinomycin D used alone (at least on a
daily x 5-10 dose schedule), the drug probably should not be
recommended at present as first-line therapy in this group of
tumors.   The real and at times dramatic activity of mithramycin,
however, justifies continued evaluation of the every-other-day
dose schedule in controlled studies until definite conclusions
can be drawn as to the possibly greater value of this method of
administration.

As can be seen from examination of the tabulated results in
other solid tumor types, mithramycin received a minimal trial in a
wide variety, without demonstrating any significant antitumor
effect.   It has not received an evaluation in acute leukemia.
Should the alternate-day dose schedule (or some other schedule)
prove significantly more effective than daily administration in
testicular cancer therapy, the question of mithramycin's possible
usefulness in other tumors might be reopened.

Tumor Type or Site

Testicular

Ref #	# Pts Evaluated	# Pts Responding	% Response	Dose Schedule (IV) and Remarks
4	163	64	39	Usually 25-50 mcg/kg/day x 7-10, push or infusion. 17 CR = 10%. Death related to drug-induced bleeding in 5.5%.
5	8	3		25-50 mcg/kg/day x 3-10. 0 CR. Two patients had hemorrhage without thrombocytopenia. No response considered "worthwhile".
6	26	9		25 mcg/kg/day x 9-10 by constant infusion. 2 CR = 8%. All responses (9/20) in embryonal carcinoma with pulmonary metastases. One CR >32 mo, the other >12 mo at time of report. 8 patients had drug-associated bleeding, 5 without accompanying ↓ in platelets - 0 deaths. 0/6 teratocarcinoma responded.
7	28	7	25	50 mcg/kg every other day. "Elimination of hemorrhage and mortality" with new dose schedule.
8	48	19		(1) 0.8-1.2 mg/m^2/day x 10, by 8-hr infusion. (2) 1.5 mg/m^2 x 3/wk, by push to $\leq$ 10 doses. 3 CR, 14 PR of 34 embryonal carcinoma. 2 PR of 14 "others". 9/95 patients had drug-associated deaths (see discussion).

Testicular (cont.)

Ref #	# Pts Evaluated	# Pts Responding	% Response	Dose Schedule (IV) and Remarks
9	73	9	12	25 mcg/kg/day, by infusion of ? duration. 5 CR. 5 patients had "severe" drug-associated bleeding. 36% had "severe" effect on performance rating.
	346	111	32	Total. 27 CR of 295 = 9%.

Breast

Ref #	# Pts Evaluated	# Pts Responding	% Response	Dose Schedule (IV) and Remarks
1	1	0		50-80 mcg/kg/day x 10, "push".
2	3	1		50 mcg/kg/day x 5, "push" or 3-hr infusion. PR.
3	16	3		50 mcg/kg/day x 5, "push" (and other schedules). only one response >50%.
	20	4	20	Total.

Colorectal

Ref #	# Pts Evaluated	# Pts Responding	% Response	Dose Schedule (IV) and Remarks
1	1	0		50-80 mcg/kg/day x 10, "push".
3	2	0		50 mcg/kg/day x 5, "push" (and other schedules).
	3	0	0	Total.

Lung

Ref #	# Pts Evaluated	# Pts Responding	% Response	Dose Schedule (IV) and Remarks
1	2	0		50-80 mcg/kg/day x 10, "push".
	2	0		Total.

Melanoma

Ref #	# Pts Evaluated	# Pts Responding	% Response	Dose Schedule (IV) and Remarks
1	1	0		50-80 mcg/kg/day x 10, "push".
3	2	1		50 mcg/kg/day x 5, "push" (and other schedules). PR.
	3	1	33	Total.

Lymphoma

Ref #	# Pts Evaluated	# Pts Responding	% Response	Dose Schedule (IV) and Remarks
3	7	3		50 mcg/kg/day x 5, "push" (and other schedules). All PR, all <50%. 1/2 lymphosarcoma, 2/5 Hodgkin's.
	7	3		Total.

Prostate

Ref #	# Pts Evaluated	# Pts Responding	% Response	Dose Schedule (IV) and Remarks
3	5	1		50 mcg/kg/day x 5, "push" (and other schedules). 3 other patients had ↓ in acid phosphatase.

Prostate (cont.)

Ref #	# Pts Evaluated	# Pts Responding	% Response	Dose Schedule (IV) and Remarks
	$\overline{5}$	$\overline{1}$	20	Total.
Pancreas				
1	2	0		50-80 mcg/kg/day x 10, "push".
3	2	0		50 mcg/kg/day x 5, "push" (and other schedules).
	$\overline{4}$	$\overline{0}$	0	Total.

References

(1)   Parker, G., Wiltsie, D., and Jackson, C.   The clinical
        evaluation of PA-144 (mithramycin) in solid tumors of
        adults.   Cancer Chemother Rep 8: 23, 1960.

(2)   Curreri, A., and Ansfield, F.   Mithramycin – human
        toxicology and preliminary therapeutic investigation.
        Cancer Chemother Rep 8: 18, 1960.

(3)   Kofman, S., and Eisenstein, R.   Mithramycin in the
        treatment of disseminated cancer.   Cancer Chemother Rep 32:
        77, 1963.

(4)   Pfizer Laboratories.   Mithramycin: clinical studies and
        brochure, 1966.

(5)   Mackenzie, A., et al.   Mithramycin in metastatic urogenital
        cancer.   J Urol 98: 116, 1967.

(6)   Ream, N., et al.   Mithramycin therapy in disseminated
        germinal testicular cancer.   JAMA 204: 1030, 1968.

(7)   Kennedy, B.   Mithramycin treatment in testicular neoplasms.
        Am Soc Clin Oncol Abstracts (#20), 1969.

(8)   Talley, R.   (SWCCSG).   Unpublished results of protocol
        #221, 1969.   (Personal communication).

(9)   Johnson, R.   (COG).   Unpublished results of protocol #410,
        1969.   (Personal communication).

(10)   Kersten, W., Kersten, H., and Szybalski, W.   Physicochemical
        properties of complexes between deoxyribonucleic acid and
        antibiotics which affect ribonucleic acid synthesis
        (actinomycin, daunomycin, cinerubin, nogalomycin, chromomycin,
        mithramycin, and olivomycin).   Biochem 5: 236, 1966.

Vinblastine

Synonyms: Velban, VLB, vincaleukoblastine

Structure:

Dosage: Standard practice is to administer the drug initially
                 at a dose level of 0.1-0.15 mg/kg, IV once weekly.
                 Dosages can be then progressively increased, depending
                 on tumor response and individual patient tolerance,
                 to as high as 0.3 mg/kg once weekly. Vinblastine is
                 probably best given on a once weekly schedule.

Toxicity: I. Hematological
                 A. Leukopenia - usual dose-limiting side effect
                     1. Nadir of WBC usually 4-7 days after single
                         injection.
                 B. Thrombocytopenia
                 C. Anemia

            II. Gastrointestinal
                 A. Nausea, vomiting, anorexia - common
                 B. Stomatitis (usually associated with
                     leukopenia)
                 C. Weight loss
                 D. Constipation or diarrhea

           III. Neurological
                 A. All of complications associated with
                     vincristine can occur, but all are much less
                     common

            IV. Alopecia (uncommon)

Mechanism of Action: Current data are "consistent with the
                            existence of at least two separate sites
                            of action of vinca alkaloids: reversible
                            mitotic arrest through binding of drug to
                            a cytoplasmic precursor of the spindle,
                            and inhibition of RNA synthesis through
                            effects on the DNA-dependent RNA
                            polymerase system."[1] The binding of drug
                            to spindle precursor may take place in the
                            cell's S phase, when centriolar replication
                            occurs, with cellular spindle dis-
                            organization and consequent death not
                            becoming apparent until the next mitosis
                            is attempted.[2] On a molecular level, it
                            has been suggested that the vinca alkaloids
                            cause a rearrangement of binding sites in
                            the protein of the microtubular units which
                            comprise the mitotic spindle, permitting
                            polymerization of the tubule protein to
                            protofibrils.[3]

Role in Cancer Therapy

Vinblastine is one of the most active single agents against Hodgkin's disease. A summation of the data included in this review yields an overall response rate of 65%, with a complete response rate of 33% in the 145 patients for whom this could be analyzed. A study of Acute Leukemia Group B[32] in which cyclophosphamide, 15 mg/kg/wk IV, was compared with vinblastine, 0.1-0.3 mg/kg/wk IV, for remission induction of Hodgkin's disease, demonstrated that in the previously untreated **group** vinblastine gave a complete response rate of 27% (15/56) vs 18% for cyclophosphamide (10/54). The total response rate for vinblastine was significantly better than that for cyclophosphamide (P <0.05): 75% (42/56) vs 54% (29/54). In patients previously treated, the two drugs gave essentially the same results. In the authors' opinion, the sequence of vinblastine and then cyclophosphamide was superior to reversing the order.

In a similar comparative study reported by Stutzman and Ezdinli,[29] vinblastine gave 11/33 complete remissions and an 85% total response rate vs only 2/26 complete remissions and a 43% total response rate for cyclophosphamide, the latter given at 2 mg/kg/day x 6 weeks orally. In another study, however, the same authors compared vinblastine with nitrogen mustard (HN2) and obtained results which were the same for induction with either agent, although the sequence of HN2 followed by vinblastine gave an 89% response rate, vs 65% for vinblastine followed by nitrogen mustard.

Flatow, Ultmann, Hyman and Muggia studied both vinblastine and procarbazine (separately) in patients resistant to x-irradiation and alkylating agents. Objective improvement was achieved in 68% of the patients receiving vinblastine (13/19), and 100% (14/14) of those receiving procarbazine. The mean duration of vinblastine-induced remission was 10.5 months, vs 6 months for procarbazine. The differences were not statistically significant.[33]

Vinblastine may also be a useful agent in the treatment of reticulum-cell sarcoma and lymphosarcoma. About one-fourth of patients treated in these categories have reportedly obtained an objective response, but the complete response rate is quite low (only 3 of 54 cases analyzed). (Vincristine and cyclophosphamide each appear to be superior to vinblastine for the initial chemotherapy of these forms of lymphoma.)

In early clinical trials, vinblastine demonstrated activity against methotrexate-resistant choriocarcinoma in four of eight patients treated.[4] It has since been largely superseded, as a second-line drug after (or with) methotrexate in this disease, by actinomycin D.

Vinblastine has had a fairly extensive trial in the major solid tumors. The overall reported response rate in breast cancer is 20%, but marked variability exists among the results obtained by different investigators. Johnston and Novales[22] reported a response rate of 35% and Bleehen and Jelliffe[24] in England reported a response rate of 45%, but in both of these studies response criteria were not stated. Goldenberg,[17] on the other hand, reported no responses at all in 18 patients treated for at least 4 weeks on various schedules. The combined study of Acute Leukemia Group B and the Eastern Cooperative Oncology Group[25] reported 3 responses in 16 patients. The authors felt these were impressive responses.

In malignant melanoma, of a combined total of 54 patients reported, there have been 8 responses for a 15% response rate. The combined ALGB-ECOG Study[25] saw only one partial response out of 15 patients and represents the most extensive trial reported in this disease.

Against bronchogenic carcinoma the drug has shown only slight activity. The largest experience is again the combined ALGB-ECOG Study[25] in which 33 patients were treated, with three partial responses being seen. The best results reported are by Wright et al[18] of the Midwestern Cooperative Chemotherapy Group, who saw 5 partial responses in 21 cases.

In adenocarcinoma of the colon activity appears borderline at best, with two large studies[25,26] reporting no responses in 15 and 19 cases respectively.

The data on the use of vinblastine in acute leukemia are worthy of some comment. Although superficially this agent appears to have minimal effect against ALL, it has not received an extensive trial on a weekly basis, which is the most effective schedule in solid tumors and lymphomas, the most effective schedule for vincristine in ALL, and is a schedule which might be expected to produce dose-limiting toxicity less quickly. In the AML-AMoL category, the available data suggests that AMoL is particularly responsive to this agent, with a reported overall response >50% and one-eighth of patients treated achieving CR. In AML, on the other hand, only 4 PR and 0 CR were reported among 22 patients treated. On the basis of the available information, it would appear that vinblastine has some activity against acute leukemia. Its potential for remission induction at an optimal dose schedule remains to be definitively evaluated. Along these lines, the recent report by Massimo et al[5] of successful anti-leukemic treatment with the combination of vinblastine and vincristine in a group of children who were largely resistant to the latter drug is provocative, but as yet unconfirmed.

Current efforts to improve the therapeutic effectiveness of vinblastine are centered primarily on its use in combination with other active agents in the primary chemotherapy of Stage III and IV Hodgkin's disease (unpublished data, Acute Leukemia Group B).

Preliminary experiments in animals have shown (Smith and Wilson, 1967)[6] that the administration of either vinblastine or vincristine 2 days prior to irradiation resulted in a more rapid recovery of the cellular elements of the bone marrow from the effects of the radiation. No attempt has as yet been made to apply these findings in a clinical setting.

Tumor Type or Site

Breast

Ref #	# Pts Evaluated	# Pts Responding	% Response	Dose Schedule (IV) and Remarks
10	2	0		0.15 mg/kg x 2/wk to response or WBC <2000; then 0.1 mg/kg/wk maintenance.
12	4	0		0.2 mg/kg/wk as tolerated.
14	5	3		0.1→0.15→0.2→0.25→0.3 mg/kg/wk; weekly maintenance at dose one increment lower than that producing WBC of 3000. (Some patients received drug PO, in higher doses). PR, duration 3, 5, and 13 mo.
17	18	0		(a) 0.1 mg/kg/day x 3, off 10-14 days, then weekly. (b) 0.1→0.15→0.2 mg/kg/wk, etc. All evaluable patients received $\geq$ 4 wks treatment.
18	7	0		0.1-0.15 mg/kg/day x 1-3, then $\geq$ 0.1 mg/kg q 4-7 days, according to leukopenia.
21	9	0		0.1-0.3 mg/kg/wk.
22	23	8		10 mg/day to toxicity, then 10 mg/wk as tolerated. Response criteria not stated.
24	11	5		10-20 mg/dose (~0.15-0.3 mg/kg), usually weekly. British study. Response criteria not stated.

Breast (cont.)

Ref #	# Pts Evaluated	# Pts Responding	% Response	Dose Schedule (IV) and Remarks
25	16	3		$0.1 \rightarrow 0.2 \rightarrow 0.3$ mg/kg/wk, as tolerated x ≥ 8 wks. 1 CR, 2 PR. Cooperative study, ALGB-ECOG.
	$\overline{95}$	$\overline{19}$	20	Total.

Melanoma

7	1	0		0.15 mg/kg/day x 4, repeated as tolerated.
10	3	0		0.15 mg/kg x 2/wk to response or WBC <2000; then 0.1 mg/kg/wk maintenance.
11	9	0		(a) 0.1-0.4 mg/kg/wk. (b) .0025-.075 mg/kg/day. (c) 0.2-0.4 mg/kg x 1.
14	3	0		$0.1 \rightarrow 0.15 \rightarrow 0.2 \rightarrow 0.25 \rightarrow 0.3$ mg/kg/wk; weekly maintenance at dose one increment lower than that producing WBC of 3000. (Some patients received drug PO, in higher doses).
18	9	1		0.1-0.15 mg/kg/day x 1-3, then ≥ 0.1 mg/kg q 4-7 days, according to leukopenia.
24	3	1		10-20 mg/dose (~0.15-0.3 mg/kg), usually weekly. British study. Response criteria not stated.

Melanoma (cont.)

Ref #	# Pts Evaluated	# Pts Responding	% Response	Dose Schedule (IV) and Remarks
25	14	1		0.1→0.2→0.3 mg/kg/wk, as tolerated x $\geq$ 8 wks. PR. Cooperative study, ALGB-ECOG.
27	12	5		~.09 mg/kg/day, PO (mean dose). All PR. Daily dose oral study.
	$\overline{54}$	$\overline{8}$	15	Total.

Ovary

7	1	0		0.15 mg/kg/day x 4, repeated as tolerated.
12	2	1		0.2 mg/kg/wk as tolerated.
14	3	0		0.1→0.15→0.2→0.25→0.3 mg/kg/wk; weekly maintenance at dose one increment lower than that producing WBC of 3000. (Some patients received drug PO, in higher doses).
18	7	1		0.1→0.15 mg/kg/day x 1-3, then $\geq$ 0.1 mg/kg q 4-7 days according to leukopenia.
25	7	1		0.1→0.2→0.3 mg/kg/wk, as tolerated x $\geq$ 8 wks. PR. Cooperative study, ALGB-ECOG.
	$\overline{20}$	$\overline{3}$	15	Total.

Lung

Ref #	# Pts Evaluated	# Pts Responding	% Response	Dose Schedule (IV) and Remarks
11	9	0		(a) 0.1–0.4 mg/kg/wk. (b) .0025–.075 mg/kg/day. (c) 0.2–0.4 mg/kg x 1.
12	7	1		0.2 mg/kg/wk as tolerated. PR in adenocarcinoma.
14	6	1		0.1→0.15→0.2→0.25→0.3 mg/kg/wk; weekly maintenance at dose one increment lower than that producing WBC of 3000. (Some patients received drug PO, in higher doses). PR, duration 6 mo.
18	21	5		0.1–0.15 mg/kg/day x 1–3, then $\geq$ 0.1 mg/kg q 4–7 days according to leukopenia.
23	13	1		0.1–0.3 mg/kg/wk.
24	12	1		10–20 mg (~0.15–0.3 mg/kg) intermittently, usually weekly. British study.
25	33	3		0.1→0.2→0.3 mg/kg/wk, as tolerated x $\geq$ 8 wks. 3 PR. ALGB-ECOG cooperative study.
28	8	0		0.1→0.15→0.2 mg/kg/wk as tolerated. British study.
	$\overline{109}$	$\overline{12}$	11	Total.

Colorectal

Ref #	# Pts Evaluated	# Pts Responding	% Response	Dose Schedule (IV) and Remarks
7	1	1		0.15 mg/kg/day x 4 repeated as tolerated. PR, 4+ mo duration.
10	2	1		0.15 mg/kg x 2/wk (average) to response or WBC <2000; then 0.1 mg/kg/wk. "Marked" tumor response.
11	7	0		(a) 0.1-0.4 mg/kg/wk. (b) .0025-.075 mg/kg/day. (c) 0.2-0.4 mg/kg x 1.
12	4	1		0.2 mg/kg/wk as tolerated.
14	3	0		$0.1{\to}0.15{\to}0.2{\to}0.25{\to}0.3$ mg/kg/wk; weekly maintenance at dose one increment lower than that producing WBC of 3000. (Some patients received drug PO, in higher doses).
18	13	2		0.1-0.15 mg/kg/wk x 1-3, then $>$ 0.1 mg/kg q 4-7 days, according to leukopenia.
21	7	0		0.1-0.3 mg/kg/wk.
25	15	0		$0.1{\to}0.2{\to}0.3$ mg/kg/wk as tolerated x $\geq$ 8 wks. ALGB-ECOG cooperative study.
26	19	0		$0.15{\to}0.2{\to}0.3$ mg/kg/wk, then weekly maintenance at dose producing WBC of 3000.
	71	5	7	Total.

Hodgkin's Disease

Ref #	# Pts Evaluated	# Pts Responding	% Response	Dose Schedule (IV) and Remarks
7	1	1 (0 CR)		0.15 mg/kg/day x 4, repeated as tolerated. PR, 6 wks duration.
10	6	4 (0 CR)		0.15 mg/kg x 2/wk (average) to response or WBC <2000; then 0.1 mg/kg/wk.
11	8	5 (1 CR)		(a) 0.1-0.4 mg/kg/wk. (b) .0025-.075 mg/kg/day. (c) 0.2-0.4 mg/kg, single dose.
12	2	2		0.2 mg/kg/wk as tolerated.
13	14	9 (5 CR)		0.15-0.2 mg/kg/wk IV, or larger doses/wk, PO. Median duration CR = 3 mo.
14	10	10 (6 CR)		$0.1 \rightarrow 0.15 \rightarrow 0.2 \rightarrow 0.25 \rightarrow 0.3$ mg/kg/wk; weekly maintenance dose at one increment lower than that producing WBC of 3000. (Some patients received drug PO, in higher doses). Median duration CR = 6.5 mo.
15	22	8		(a) 0.3-0.6 mg/kg in 3 days. (b) 0.1-0.2 mg/kg q "week or two".
18	21	12		0.1-0.15 mg/kg/day x 1-3, then $\geq$ 0.1 mg/kg q 4-7 days, according to leukopenia.
21	6	6 (0 CR)		0.1-0.3 mg/kg/wk.
24	38	26		10-20 mg (~0.15-0.3 mg/kg) intermittently, usually weekly.

Hodgkin's Disease (cont.)

Ref #	# Pts Evaluated	# Pts Responding	% Response	Dose Schedule (IV) and Remarks
25	38	31 (7 CR)	82 (18% CR)	0.1→0.2→0.3 mg/kg/wk as tolerated x ≥ 7 wks. 75% of patients previously treated with both radiation therapy and alkylating agents. ALGB-ECOG cooperative study.
27	12	5 (0 CR)		~.09 mg/kg/day (average), PO as tolerated.
29	33	28 (11 CR)	85 (33% CR)	Vinblastine, 0.15 or 0.2 mg/kg/wk x ≥ 6 wks -- vs Cytoxan, 2 mg/kg/day to ≥ 6 wks, PO. Median remission duration = 7.5+ mo (for maintained patients - shorter for unmaintained). CTX →2 CR, 9 PR of 26.
30	27	20		Vinblastine 0.15 or 0.2 mg/kg/wk --- vs HN$_2$, 0.1 mg/kg/d x 4 or 0.2 mg/kg/day x 2. Comparison study with HN$_2$. HN$_2$ →22/27. Median duration unmaintained remission = 2.5 mo with either drug, HN$_2$ followed by VLB→ 89% response. VLB followed by HN$_2$ →65% response.
31	35	22		0.05-0.2 mg/kg/wk. 33/35 unresponsive to alkylating agents.
32	88	57 (18 CR)	65	Vinblastine, 0.1 mg/kg 1st wk, 0.2 mg/kg 2nd wk, 0.3 mg/kg 3rd wk, then 0.3 mg/kg/wk as tolerated. 75% response rate in patients without previous chemotherapy. Comparison study with CTX. CTX →54% response.

Hodgkin's Disease (cont.)

Ref #	# Pts Evaluated	# Pts Responding	% Response	Dose Schedule (IV) and Remarks
33	19	13	68	$0.15 \to 0.2 \to 0.25$ mg/kg, etc, "at weekly or biweekly intervals" to WBC 3000 or tumor regression; then weekly or biweekly maintenance. Median duration remission = 8 mo. Comparison study with procarbazine. Procarbazine$\to$14/14 responses, median duration 5 mo. Most patients refractory to both radiation therapy and alkylating agents.
	380	259	65	Total. CR = 48/145 analyzed, or 33%.

Reticulum-Cell Sarcoma + Lymphosarcoma

Ref #	# Pts Evaluated	# Pts Responding	% Response	Dose Schedule (IV) and Remarks
10	3	0		0.15 mg/kg x 2/wk (average) to response or WBC <2000; then 0.1 mg/kg/wk. All patients lymphosarcoma.
11	5	0		(a) 0.1-0.4 mg/kg/wk. (b) .0025-.075 mg/kg/day. (c) 0.2-0.4 mg/kg, single dose. All patients lymphosarcoma.
12	2	0 (0 CR)		0.2 mg/kg/wk as tolerated. All patients lymphosarcoma.
13	12	4 (0 CR)		0.15-0.2 mg/kg/wk, IV or large doses/wk, PO. 9 patients reticulum-cell sarcoma, 3 patients lymphosarcoma.

Reticulum-Cell Sarcoma + Lymphosarcoma (cont.)

Ref #	# Pts Evaluated	# Pts Responding	% Response	Dose Schedule (IV) and Remarks
14	1	1		$0.1\rightarrow0.15\rightarrow0.2\rightarrow0.25\rightarrow0.3$ mg/kg/wk; weekly maintenance dose at one increment lower than that producing WBC of 3000. (Some patients received drug PO, in higher doses). Response duration 16 mo.
18	13	4		$0.1-0.15$ mg/kg/day x 1-3 then ≥ 0.1 mg/kg q 4-7 days, according to leukopenia. 5 patients reticulum-cell sarcoma, 8 patients lymphosarcoma.
24	13	3		10-20 mg ($\sim$0.15-0.3 mg/kg) intermittently, usually weekly. British study.
25	19	3 (1 CR)		$0.1\rightarrow0.2\rightarrow0.3$ mg/kg/wk as tolerated x ≥ 7 wks. 3/13 responses in lymphosarcoma, 0.6 in reticulum cell sarcoma.
27	4	3 (1 CR)		$\sim$.09 mg/kg/day (average), PO. All patients reticulum-cell sarcoma.
29	17	6 (1 CR)		Vinblastine, 0.15 or 0.2 mg/kg/wk x ≥ 6 wks, -- vs CTX, 2 mg/kg/day, PO, for $\geq$ 6 wks. Median duration remission = 3+ mo. Comparison study with CTX. CTX $\rightarrow$3 CR, 7 PR of 15.
	$\overline{89}$	$\overline{24}$	27	Total. CR = 3/54 analyzed, or 5.5%.

ALL-AUL

Ref #	# Pts Evaluated	# Pts Responding	% Response	Dose Schedule (IV) and Remarks
7	2	0		0.15 mg/kg/day x 4, repeated as tolerated.
8	8	3		0.15 mg/kg/day x 3-4 or 0.2 mg/kg/wk (given as 10 injections of .02 mg/kg, hourly). All responses PR.
10	4	0		0.15 mg/kg x 2/wk (average) to response or WBC <2000; then 0.1 mg/kg/wk.
18	5	1		0.1-0.15 mg/kg/day x 1-3 then $\geq$ 0.1 mg/kg q 4-7 days, according to leukopenia. PR.
	$\overline{19}$	$\overline{4}$	21	Total.

AML-AMoL

Ref #	# Pts Evaluated	# Pts Responding	% Response	Dose Schedule (IV) and Remarks
7	13	3 (0 CR)		0.15 mg/kg/day x 4, repeated as tolerated. 3 PR of 12 with AMoL.
8	1	0		0.2 mg/kg/wk (given as 10 injections of .02 mg/kg, hourly).
9	18	3 (0 CR)		0.15 mg/kg/day x 4, repeated as tolerated. One PR of 6 mo duration in adult with AML.
10	6	0		0.15 mg/kg x 2/wk (average) to response or WBC <2000; then 0.1 mg/kg/wk.

AML–AMoL (cont.)

Ref #	# Pts Evaluated	# Pts Responding	% Response	Dose Schedule (IV) and Remarks
13	19	8 (2 CR)		0.15–0.2 mg/kg/wk, IV, or larger doses/wk, PO. CR of 4 and 8.5 mo duration, respectively.
14	2	2 (0 CR)		0.1→0.15→0.2→0.25→0.3 mg/kg/wk; weekly maintenance dose at one increment lower than that producing WBC of 3000. (Some patients received drug PO, in higher doses). Both PR: 3 and 4 mo duration, respectively.
15	2	0		(a) 0.3–0.6 mg/kg in 3 days -- vs (b) 0.1–0.2 mg/kg q "week or two".
18	18	3 (0 CR)		0.1–0.15 mg/kg/day x 1–3, then $\geq$ 0.1 mg/kg q 4–7 days, according to leukopenia.
20	12	1 (1 CR)		Not given.
27	7	5 (1 CR)		~.09 mg/kg/day (average), PO. All patients had "AMoL".
	$\overline{98}$	$\overline{25}$ (4 CR)	26 (4% CR)	Total.
				Head and Neck
21	35	10 (1 CR)	29	0.1–0.3 mg/kg/wk.
				Histiocytosis X
23	6	2	33	0.2–0.5 mg/kg/wk x 3 mo.

References

(1)   Creasey, W. Effect of the vinca alkaloids on RNA synthesis
      in relation to mitotic arrest. Fed Proc 27: 760 (Abstract
      #3053), 1968.

(2)   Madoc-Jones, H., and Mauro, F. Interphase action of
      vinblastine and vincristine: difference in their lethal
      action through the mitotic cycle of cultured mammalian
      cells. J Cell Physiol 72: 185, 1968.

(3)   Bensch, K., and Malawista, S. Microtubular crystals in
      mammalian cells. J Cell Biol 40: 95, 1969.

(4)   Hertz, R., Lipsett, M., and Moy, R. Effect of vinca-
      leukoblastine on metastatic choriocarcinoma and related
      trophoblastic tumors in women. Cancer Res 21: 1050, 1960.

(5)   Massimo, L. Vincristine plus vinblastine in acute childhood
      leukemia. Lancet 1: 469, 1969.

(6)   Smith, W., and Wilson, S. Post-irradiation recovery induced
      by vinblastine and vincristine. J Nat Cancer Inst 39:
      1055, 1967.

(7)   Hodes, M., Rohn, R., and Bond, W. Vincaleukoblastine I.
      Preliminary clinical studies. Cancer Res 20: 1041, 1960.

(8)   Warwick, O., Darte, J., and Brown, T. Some biological
      effects of vincaleukoblastine, an alkaloid in Vinca rosea
      Linn in patients with malignant disease. Cancer Res 20:
      1032, 1960.

(9)   Whitelaw, D., and Teasdale, J. Vincaleukoblastine in the
      treatment of malignant disease. Canad Med Assoc J 85:
      584, 1961.

(10) Hill, J., and Loeb, E. Treatment of leukemia, lymphoma and
      other malignant neoplasms with vinblastine. Cancer Chemother
      Rep 15: 41, 1961.

(11) Frei, E., III., Franzino, A., Shnider, B., et al. Clinical
      studies of vinblastine. Cancer Chemother Rep 12: 125, 1961.

(12) Vaitkevicius, V., Talley, R., Tucker, J., et al. Cytological
      and clinical observations during vincaleukoblastine
      therapy of disseminated cancer. Cancer 15: 294, 1962.

(13) Hodes, M., Rohn, R., Bond, W., et al. Vincaleukoblastine
      IV. A summary of two and one-half years' experience in the
      use of vinblastine. Cancer Chemother Rep 16: 401, 1962.

(14) Armstrong, J., Dyke, R., Fouts, P., et al. Hodgkin's
      disease, carcinoma of the breast, and other tumors treated
      with vinblastine sulfate. Cancer Chemother Rep 18: 49, 1962.

(15) Frost, J., Goldwein, M., and Bryan, J. Clinical experience
      with vincaleukoblastine in far-advanced Hodgkin's disease
      and various malignant states. Ann Intern Med 56: 854, 1962.

(16) Johnson, I., Armstrong, J., Gorman, M., et al. The vinca
      alkaloids: a new class of oncolytic agents. Cancer Res
      23: 1390, 1963.

(17) Goldenberg, I. Vinblastine sulfate therapy of women with
      advanced breast cancer. Cancer Chemother Rep 29: 111, 1963.

(18) Wright, T., Hurley, J., Korst, D., et al. (Midwest
      Cooperative Chemotherapy Group). Vinblastine in neoplastic
      disease. Cancer Res 23: 169, 1963.

(19) Costa, G., Carbone, P., Gold, G., et al. Clinical trials
      of vinblastine in multiple myeloma. Cancer Chemother Rep
      27: 87, 1963.

(20) Mathe, G. Some recent findings on the chemotherapy of
      leukemias and hematosarcomas. Proc 3rd Int Congr Chemother
      (Stuttgart) 1: 968, 1964.

(21) Smart, C., Rochlin, D., Nahum, A., et al. Clinical
      experience with vinblastine sulfate in squamous cell carcinoma
      and other malignancies. Cancer Chemother Rep 34: 31, 1964.

(22) Johnston, B., and Novales, E. The use of vinblastine sulfate
      (Velban) in advanced malignancies of the female reproductive
      tract. Proc Amer Assoc Cancer Res 5: 33 (Abstract #125),
      1964.

(23) Sharp, H., White, J., and Krivit, W. "Histiocytosis X"
      treated with vinblastine sulfate. Cancer Chemother Rep 39:
      53, 1964.

(24) Bleehen, N., and Jelliffe, A. Vinblastine sulfate in the
      treatment of malignant disease. Brit J Cancer 19: 268,
      1965.

(25) Cooperative study (Eastern Solid Tumor Group - Acute
      Leukemia Group B). Neoplastic disease-treatment with
      vinblastine. Arch Intern Med 116: 846, 1965.

(26) Ansfield, F. Clinical trial of vinblastine in colo-rectal
      cancer. Cancer Chemother Rep 47: 81, 1965.

(27) Bond, W., Rohn, R., Bates, L., et al. Treatment of
      neoplastic diseases with an improved oral preparation of
      vinblastine sulfate. Cancer 19: 213, 1966.

(28) Myles, A. A trial of vinblastine sulfate in the treatment
      of inoperable carcinoma of the lung. Brit J Cancer 20:
      264, 1966.

(29) Stutzman, L., and Ezdinli, E. Vinblastine sulfate vs
      cyclophosphamide in the therapy for lymphoma. JAMA 195:
      111, 1966.

(30) Ezdinli, E., and Stutzman, L. Nitrogen mustard vs
      vinblastine therapy of Hodgkin's disease. Proc Amer Assoc
      Cancer Res 9: 20 (Abstract #77), 1968.

(31) Sohier, W., Wong, R., and Aisenberg, A. Vinblastine in the
      treatment of advanced Hodgkin's disease. Cancer 22: 467,
      1968.

(32) Carbone, P., and Spurr, C. Management of patients with
      malignant lymphoma: a comparative study with cyclo-
      phosphamide and vinca alkaloids. Cancer Res 28: 811, 1968.

(33) Flatow, F., Ultmann, J., Hyman, G., et al. Treatment of
      advanced Hodgkin's disease with vinblastine (NSC 49842)
      or procarbazine (NSC 77213). Cancer Chemother Rep 53: 39,
      1969.

Vincristine

Synonyms: Oncovin, VCR, leurocristine

Structure:

Dosage: 1.5-2.0 mg/m^2/wk, IV. (Individual doses in adult
               patients should not exceed 2 mg, and older adults may
               require considerable dose reduction to avoid severe
               neurotoxicity).

Toxicity: I. Neurological
                   A. Loss of deep tendon reflexes, mild
                       paresthesias - usual side effects, not in
                       themselves dose-limiting
                   B. Severe paresthesias, peripheral neuropathy -
                       usual dose-limiting side effects
                   C. Constipation, abdominal pain - if severe, may
                       be dose-limiting
                   D. Hoarseness, ptosis, double vision - less
                       common dose-limiting side effects

               II. Alopecia - occurs in about 20% of patients

               III. Hematological - unusual
                    A. Leukopenia
                    B. Thrombocytopenia, anemia

Mechanism of Action: Current data are consistent with the
               existence of at least two separate sites of action of
               vinca alkaloids: reversible mitotic arrest through
               binding of drug to a cytoplasmic precursor of the
               spindle, and inhibition of RNA synthesis through
               effects on the DNA-dependent RNA polymerase system.[1]
               The binding of drug to spindle precursor may take place
               in the cell's S phase, when centriolar replication
               occurs, with cellular spindle disorganization and
               consequent death not becoming apparent until the next
               mitosis is attempted.[2] On a molecular level, it has
               been suggested that the vinca alkaloids cause a
               rearrangement of binding sites in the protein of the
               microtubular units which comprise the mitotic spindle,
               permitting polymerization of the tubule protein to
               protofibrils.[3]

                          Role in Cancer Therapy

     The principal role of vincristine to date has been in the
treatment of patients with acute leukemia, lymphomas, and solid tumors
of childhood.

     It is an extremely effective remission inducer in ALL-AUL, with
41% of 349 reported patients (nearly all of whom were previously
treated with other agents) obtaining an M_1 marrow from vincristine
used alone. It may be an agent of considerable value in the

treatment of AML-AMoL as well, with a 20% CR rate and 51% overall
response rate reported among 41 patients. However, almost all of
these were children. There is insufficient data available to state
whether vincristine by itself would demonstrate a similar degree of
activity in adults.

Vincristine is quite active in all forms of lymphoma, with
50-60% of treated patients obtaining tumor regression. Remissions
obtained with vincristine alone, however, tend to be quite short-
lived, so that now it is usually used (as in acute leukemia) in
combination with other drugs for remission induction.

As a single agent, vincristine appears to have considerable
effect against neuroblastoma, Wilms' tumor, rhabdomyosarcoma, and
possibly Ewing's sarcoma and retinoblastoma. Again, the remissions
obtained with vincristine alone are usually of short duration in
these tumor types, so that, when employed, it is now usually used in
concert with other agents.

Like vinblastine, vincristine appears to have some usefulness
in the treatment of disseminated breast cancer, with 20% of 164
reported patients responding. There may be a greater antitumor
effect at a relatively high weekly dose,[21] in contrast to the
situation with reticulum cell sarcoma, where low weekly doses appear
to be as effective as high ones.[39] The vinca alkaloids are probably
inferior to MTX, 5-FU, or CTX as single agents in the treatment
of breast cancer.

Scanty reported data suggest little or no activity for
vincristine against carcinoma of the colon and rectum, and only one
report[17] suggests that it has significant effects on malignant
melanoma, used alone. The numbers of patients with lung cancer
treated solely with vincristine and reported in the literature is
too small to make any statement about its effectiveness.

Vincristine may be a useful agent for the treatment of
primary brain tumors, with 57% of 56 patients having shown what was
described as an objective response, some, especially children with
medulloblastomas, for long periods of time.[28,30] The evalution of
antitumor effect is difficult in this type of tumor, but the results
reported for vincristine are distinctly superior to those reported
for other agents, with the possible exception of the investigational
drug, BCNU (unpublished data, Brain Tumor Study Group).

Vincristine has been reported to exert beneficial effects in
patients with choriocarcinoma, testicular tumors, and leiomyosarcoma,
in very small series. It appears, on the basis of the published
data, to be as effective as any other cytotoxic agent in the
treatment of carcinoma of the cervix, with 10/34 patients demonstrating

response. There are a number of tumor types in which vincristine
has essentially received no trial (multiple myeloma, CML, CLL,
pancreas, prostate, stomach) in the reported literature.

A final point worth emphasizing with respect to this agent
is that, because of its lack of significant overlapping toxicity
with other agents, vincristine lends itself well to combination
chemotherapy. In the future, it may be used much more widely in
such a role, even against tumor types where it demonstrates
relatively little activity used alone.

Tumor Type or Site

Breast

Ref #	# Pts Evaluated	# Pts Responding	% Response	Dose Schedule (always IV) and Remarks
6	2	1		.025–.075 mg/kg/wk.
7	6	1		.01–0.05 mg/kg/wk $\geq$ 4 wks. PR of 5 wks duration.
9	6	4		2–3 mg (.035–.12 mg/kg) twice weekly x 2, then weekly. All PR of ~50%.
12	43	11	26	(1) 75 mcg/kg/wk (most patients). (2) $<$ 50 mcg/kg/wk. ECOG study. Median time to onset of response = 4 wks.
14	2	0		25–75 mcg/kg/wk to $\geq$ 100–150 mcg/kg total dose.
15	15	3		.01–.05 mg/kg/wk x $\geq$ 4 wks. All were regressions of cutaneous lesions, of 2, 5, and 6 mo duration.
21	18	0		.0125 mg/kg/wk x $\geq$ 4 wks. (0.77 mg/kg mean dose).
21	25	3	12	.025 mg/kg/wk x $\geq$ 4 wks. (1.5 mg/kg mean dose). Responses of 3, 5, and 12 mo duration. No responses were in osseous lesions.
21	32	7	22	.035 mg/kg/wk x $\geq$ 4 wks.((2.1 mg/kg mean dose). Median duration response = 5.5 mo. 3 responses were regressions of osseous lesions. Toxicity severe in one patient.

Breast (cont.)

Ref #	# Pts Evaluated	# Pts Responding	% Response	Dose Schedule (always IV) and Remarks
23	10	1		Not given.
31	2	1		.04 mg/kg/wk or twice weekly.
39	3	0		.025-.05 mg/kg x $\geq$ 1, then .0075-.015 mg/kg/wk.
	164	32	20	Total.

Colorectal

4	1	0		~75 mcg/kg/wk.
14	3	0		25-75 mcg/kg/wk to $\geq$ 100-150 mcg/kg total dose.
17	9	0		1→1.5→→up to 6 mg/wk.
	13	0		Total.

Malignant Melanoma

4	5	0		~75 mcg/kg/wk.
7	2	0		.01-0.05 mg/kg/wk $\geq$ 4 wks.
14	10	3		25-75 mcg/kg/wk to $\geq$ 100-150 mcg/kg total dose. Included marked regression of pulmonary metastases.

Malignant Melanoma (cont.)

Ref #	# Pts Evaluated	# Pts Responding	% Response	Dose Schedule (always IV) and Remarks
17	3	0		1→1.5→→up to 6 mg/wk.
31	1	0		.04 mg/kg/wk or twice weekly.
38	7	0		Initially, .04→→.08 mg/kg/wk. Later, .015–.03 mg/kg/wk.
39	1	0		.025–.05 mg/kg x $\geq$ 1, then .0075–.015 mg/kg/wk.
	29	3	10	Total.

Lung

Ref #	# Pts Evaluated	# Pts Responding	% Response	Dose Schedule (always IV) and Remarks
14	4	2		25–75 mcg/kg/wk to $\geq$ 100–150 mcg/kg total dose. All patients had oat-cell; responses $\geq$ 50%.
17	1	0		1→1.5→→up to 6 mg/wk.
31	1	0		.04 mg/kg/wk or twice weekly.
39	3	0		.025–.05 mg/kg x $\geq$ 1, then .0075–.015 mg/kg/wk. One patient had oat-cell.
	9	2	22	Total.

AML-AMoL

Ref #	# Pts Evaluated	# Pts Responding	% Response	Dose Schedule (always IV) and Remarks
11	3	3		.01-.06 mg/kg/wk as tolerated. All AMoL. All PR.
14	1	0		25-75 mcg/kg/wk to $\geq$ 100-150 mcg/kg total dose.
24	12	5		.06 mg/kg/wk (mean dose). CCSGA study. 1 CR, 4 PR.
26	14	6		2 mg/m^2/wk. ALGB study. 5 CR, 1 PR.
29	7	6		1→1.5→2 mg/m^2/wk. 3 CR, 3 PR.
35	4	1		~2 mg/m^2/wk. Response was CR.
	$\overline{41}$	$\overline{21}$	51	Total. CR in 10/51 = 20%.

ALL-AUL

Ref #	# Pts Evaluated	# Pts Responding	% Response	Dose Schedule (always IV) and Remarks
14	8	6		25-75 mcg/kg/wk to $\geq$ 100-150 mcg/kg total dose. All PR.
24	109	48+		.06 mg/kg/wk (mean dose). 48 CR by M_1 marrow criterion. All patients resistant to previous therapy. CCSGA study.
26	103	76	74	2 mg/m^2/wk. 59 CR = 57%, by all criteria. All but 5 patients previously treated and refractory to previous treatment (usually 6 MP+ MTX). Study demonstrated no advantage for VCR over placebo in remission maintenance. ALGB study.

ALL-AUL (cont.)

Ref #	# Pts Evaluated	# Pts Responding	% Response	Dose Schedule (always IV) and Remarks
29	25	17	68	$1 \rightarrow 1.5 \rightarrow 2$ mg/m^2/wk. 5 CR. Figures are for first course only.
33	47	15	32	2 mg/m^2/wk. SWCCG study. Patients resistant to previous therapy. 7 CR by all criteria, 14 CR by M$_1$ criterion.
33	16	5		.075 mg/kg/wk. SWCCG study. Patients resistant to previous therapy. 0 CR, 1 M$_1$ marrow.
33	28	4		.02 mg/kg/day x 5, then .05 mg/kg/wk. SWCCG study. Patients resistant to previous therapy. 4 CR, 4 M$_1$ marrows.
35	21	12		$\sim$2 mg/m^2/wk. 12 CR. Patients previously treated.
35	13	10		$\sim$2 mg/m^2/wk. 10 CR. Patients previously untreated.
	$\overline{370}$	$\overline{193}$	52	Total. CR (by M$_1$ marrow criterion) in 142/349 previously treated patients = 41%.

Hodgkin's Disease

4	3	3		$\sim$75 mcg/kg/wk. All PR.
6	10	10		.025-.075 mg/kg/wk. 4 CR. Median response duration = 4 mo.

Hodgkin's Disease (cont.)

Ref #	# Pts Evaluated	# Pts Responding	% Response	Dose Schedule (always IV) and Remarks
7	1	0		.01-0.05 mg/kg/wk $\geq$ 4 wks.
9	8	5		2-3 mg (.035-.12 mg/kg) twice weekly x 2, then weekly.
10	23	9	39	.03-.05 mg/kg/wk. All responses >1 mo duration.
11	6	5		.01-.06 mg/kg/wk as tolerated. 2 CR.
12	21	10	48	(1) 75 mcg/kg/wk (most patients). (2) $\leq$ 50 mcg/kg/wk. ECOG study.
14	4	1		25-75 mcg/kg/wk to $\geq$ 100-150 mcg/kg total dose.
19	3	2		~1.5 mg/m^2/wk.
32	12	9		2.5 mg/m^2/wk (median dose) to dose-limiting neurotoxicity. 4 CR, 5 PR >50% regression. All children. Median response duration = 3 mo.
39	1	1		.025-.05 mg/kg x $\geq$ 1, then .0075-.015 mg/kg/wk.
	$\overline{92}$	$\overline{55}$	60	Total. 10 CR of 28 evaluated = 36%.

Lymphosarcoma

Ref #	# Pts Evaluated	# Pts Responding	% Response	Dose Schedule (always IV) and Remarks
4	1	1		~75 mcg/kg/wk. CR.
6	7	4		.025-.075 mg/kg/wk. Median response duration = 6 mo.

Lymphosarcoma (cont.)

Ref #	# Pts Evaluated	# Pts Responding	% Response	Dose Schedule (always IV) and Remarks
9	8	4		2-3 mg (.035-.12 mg/kg) twice weekly x 2, then weekly.
11	2	2		.01-.06 mg/kg/wk as tolerated. 2 CR.
12	16	11		(1) 75 mcg/kg/wk (most patients). (2) $<$ 50 mcg/kg/wk.
14	6	4		25-75 mcg/kg/wk to $\geq$ 100-150 mcg/kg total dose.
32	6	5		2.5 mg/m^2/wk (median dose) to dose-limiting neurotoxicity. 2 CR. Median response = 3 mo. Children.
37	35	16		.025 mg/kg/wk. 3 CR. No prior treatment. ALGB-ECOG study.
37	12	2		.025 mg/kg/wk. 0 CR. Prior treatment. ALGB-ECOG study.
	$\overline{93}$	$\overline{49}$	53	Total. 8/56 evaluated had CR = 14%.

Reticulum-cell Sarcoma

4	1	1		~75 mcg/kg/wk.
7	2	2		.01-0.05 mg/kg/wk $\geq$ 4 wks. 2 CR.

Reticulum-cell Sarcoma (cont.)

Ref #	# Pts Evaluated	# Pts Responding	% Response	Dose Schedule (always IV) and Remarks
9	9	8		2-3 mg (.035-.12 mg/kg) twice weekly x 2, then weekly. 4 CR. No prior treatment.
11	2	1		.01-.06 mg/kg/wk as tolerated. PR.
14	10	10		25-75 mcg/kg/wk to $\geq$ 100-150 mcg/kg total dose.
27	6	5		.0125 or .025 mg/kg/wk. 3 CR, 2 PR. Durations 4, 4, 7, 10, and 29 mo.
32	2	2		2.5 mg/m^2/wk (median dose) to dose-limiting neurotoxicity. 1 CR. Children.
37	27	10	37	.025 mg/kg/wk. 4 CR. No prior treatment. ECOG-ALGB study.
37	5	2		.025 mg/kg/wk. 0 CR. Patients had prior treatment. ECOG-ALGB study.
39	8	3		.025-.05 mg/kg x $\geq$ 1, then .0075-.015 mg/kg/wk. 2 CR.
	$\overline{72}$	$\overline{44}$	61	Total. 16 CR of 55 evaluated = 29%.

Primary Brain Tumors

Ref #	# Pts Evaluated	# Pts Responding	% Response	Dose Schedule (always IV) and Remarks
16	2	0		.02 mg/kg/day x 5, .05 mg/kg on day 7, then .05 mg/kg/wk.

Primary Brain Tumors (cont.)

Ref #	# Pts Evaluated	# Pts Responding	% Response	Dose Schedule (always IV) and Remarks
18	12	7		1-2 mg/day to total dose 20-30 mg, given by intra-arterial catheter perfusion. "Dramatic, though temporary" improvement seen.
22	12	6		~.05 mg/kg/wk. Adults. 1/1 medulloblastoma; 3/5 astrocytic glioma; 1/1 cerebral fibrosarcoma.
28	7	6		.05 mg/kg/wk. Children. 1/1 optic glioma, 17+ mo duration; 2/2 medulloblastoma, 8+ and 22+ mo; 1/1 cerebellar astrocytoma, 8+ mo; 2/3 cerebral astrocytoma.
30	1	1		.05→.075→.05 mg/kg/wk. Medulloblastoma. Response of 10+ mo duration.
31	6	4		.04 mg/kg/wk or twice weekly.
38	16	8		Initially, .04→→.08 mg/kg/wk. Later, .015-.03 mg/kg/wk. 4 responses rated as >50%.
	$\overline{56}$	$\overline{32}$	57	Total.

Neuroblastoma

Ref #	# Pts Evaluated	# Pts Responding	% Response	Dose Schedule (always IV) and Remarks
5	2	1		0.5 mg/kg x 1-3/wk to toxicity or response. Response <2 mo duration.

Neuroblastoma (cont.)

Ref #	# Pts Evaluated	# Pts Responding	% Response	Dose Schedule (always IV) and Remarks
19	7	3		~1.5 mg/m^2 wk.
25	16	3		.02 mg/kg/day x 5, then .03-.10 mg/kg/wk. SWCCG study. 1 CR, 3+ years' duration. 2 PR of 13 and 17 wks' duration.
32	33	18	55	2.5 mg/m^2/wk (median dose) to dose-limiting neurotoxicity. 4 CR. 5 PR >50%. Median response duration = 3.5 mo.
36	13	4		(1) .02 mg/kg/day x 5, then .05 mg/kg/wk. (2) .05 mg/kg/wk. (3) .075 mg/kg/wk, to total dose $\geq$ 0.2 mg/kg. (4) 2 mg/m^2/wk. 1 CR. SWCCG study.
	$\overline{71}$	$\overline{29}$	40	Total.

Wilms' Tumor

Ref #	# Pts Evaluated	# Pts Responding	% Response	Dose Schedule (always IV) and Remarks
5	4	1		0.5 mg/kg x 1-3/wk to toxicity or response.
8	13	8		.02 mg/kg/day x 5, then .05 mg/kg/wk. SWCCG study.
19	2	2		~1.5 mg/m^2/wk.
32	8	8		2.5 mg/m^2/wk (median dose) to dose-limiting neurotoxicity. 2 CR. 4 PR >50%. Median response duration = 2 mo.

Wilms' Tumor (cont.)

Ref #	# Pts Evaluated	# Pts Responding	% Response	Dose Schedule (always IV) and Remarks
34	4	4		.02 mg/kg/day x 5, then .05 mg/kg/wk x 11. 3 CR. Median response duration 6 mo. One possible cure. SWCCG study.
	$\overline{31}$	$\overline{23}$	74	Total.

Ewing's Sarcoma

19	1	1		~1.5 mg/m^2/wk.
32	2	2		2.5 mg/m^2/wk (median dose) to dose-limiting neurotoxicity. No CR. 1 PR >50%.
36	5	1		(1) .02 mg/kg/day x 5, then .05 mg/kg/wk. (2) .05 mg/kg/wk. (3) .075 mg/kg/wk, to total dose >0.2 mg/kg. (4) 2 mg/m^2/wk. PR of 4 wks duration.
	$\overline{8}$	$\overline{4}$	50	Total.

Cervix

4	1	1		~75 mcg/kg/wk. PR.

Cervix (cont.)

Ref #	# Pts Evaluated	# Pts Responding	% Response	Dose Schedule (always IV) and Remarks
13	31	9	29	(1) 75 mcg/kg/wk (20 patients). (2) 50 mcg/kg/wk (11 patients). 4/31 had both improved performance status and an objective response of >3 mo duration. 7/20 patients at 75 mcg/kg/wk and 2/11 patients at 50 mcg/kg/wk had objective responses.
17	2	0	29	1→1.5→up to 6 mg/wk.
	34	10	29	Total.

Choriocarcinoma

Ref #	# Pts Evaluated	# Pts Responding	% Response	Dose Schedule (always IV) and Remarks
4	1	1		~75 mcg/kg/wk. PR.
13	1	1		(1) 75 mcg/kg/wk (20 patients). (2) 50 mcg/kg/wk (11 patients). "Good" response.
	2	2	100	Total.

Leiomyosarcoma

Ref #	# Pts Evaluated	# Pts Responding	% Response	Dose Schedule (always IV) and Remarks
20	2	2		.03–.05 mg/kg/wk x 6–8, then q 3–4 wks, if response seen. Both CR, of 12+ and 14+ mo duration.

Leiomyosarcoma (cont.)

Ref #	# Pts Evaluated	# Pts Responding	% Response	Dose Schedule (always IV) and Remarks
39	5	0		.025–.05 mg/kg x $\geq$ 1, then .0075–.015 mg/kg/wk.
	$\overline{7}$	$\overline{2}$	29	Total.

Soft-tissue Sarcomas

Ref #	# Pts Evaluated	# Pts Responding	% Response	Dose Schedule (always IV) and Remarks
4	1	0		~75 mcg/kg/wk. Rhabdomyosarcoma.
5	3	2		0.5 mg/kg x 1–3/wk to toxicity or response. Rhabdomyosarcoma; responses <2 months' duration.
32	14	8		2.5 mg/m^2/wk (median dose) to dose-limiting neurotoxicity. 6/11 rhabdomyosarcoma; 1/2 neurofibrosarcoma; 1/1 liposarcoma had responses.
36	20	9	45	(1) .02 mg/kg/day x 5, then .05 mg/kg/wk. (2) .05 mg/kg/wk. (3) .075 mg/kg/wk, to total dose >0.2 mg/kg. (4) 2 mg/m^2/wk. 6 CR = 30%. SWCCG study.
	$\overline{38}$	$\overline{19}$	50	Total.

References

(1)   Creasey, W.   Effect of the vinca alkaloids on RNA
        synthesis in relation to mitotic arrest.   Fed Proc 27:
        760 (Abstract #3053), 1968.

(2)   Madoc-Jones, H., and Mauro, F.   Interphase action of vinblastine
        and vincristine: differences in their lethal action through
        the mitotic cycle of cultured mammalian cells.   J Cell
        Physiol 72: 185, 1968.

(3)   Bensch, K., and Malawista, S.   Microtubular crystals in
        mammalian cells.   J Cell Biol 40: 95, 1969.

(4)   Costa, G., Hreshchyshyn, M., and Holland, J.   Initial
        clinical studies with vincristine.   Cancer Chemother Rep
        24: 39, 1962.

(5)   Tan, C., and Aduna, N.   Preliminary clinical experience with
        leurocristine in children.   Proc Amer Assoc Cancer Res 3:
        367, 1962.

(6)   Carbone, P., Bono, V., Frei, E., et al.   Clinical studies
        with vincristine.   Blood 21: 640, 1963.

(7)   Gubisch, N., Norena, D., Perlia, C., et al.   Experience
        with vincristine in solid tumors.   Cancer Chemother Rep
        32: 19, 1963.

(8)   Sutow, W., Thurman, W., and Windmiller, J.   Vincristine
        (leurocristine) sulfate in the treatment of children with
        metastatic Wilms' tumor.   Pediatrics 32: 880, 1963.

(9)   Whitelaw, D., Cowan, D., Cassidy, F., and Patterson, T.
        Clinical experience with vincristine.   Cancer Chemother
        Rep 30: 13, 1963.

(10)   Bohannon, R., Miller, D., and Diamond, H.   Vincristine in
        the treatment of lymphomas and leukemias.   Cancer Res 23:
        613, 1963.

(11)   Martin, J.   Vincristine sulphate in the treatment of lymphoma
        and leukemia.   Lancet 2: 1080, 1963.

(12)   Gailani, S.   Phase II studies of vincristine (VCR) in human
        cancer.   Proc Amer Assoc Cancer Res 4: 21 (#82), 1963.

(13) Hreshchyshyn, M. Vincristine treatment of patients with
      carcinoma of the uterine cervix. Proc Amer Assoc Cancer Res
      4: 29 (#114), 1963.

(14) Shaw, R., and Bruner, J. Clinical evaluation of vincristine.
      Cancer Chemother Rep 42: 45, 1964.

(15) Goldenberg, I. Vincristine therapy of women with advanced
      breast cancer. Cancer Chemother Rep 41: 7, 1964.

(16) Haddy, T., Fernbach, D., Watkins, W., et al. Vincristine
      (NSC 67574) in uncommon malignant disease in children. Cancer
      Chemother Rep 41: 41, 1964.

(17) Reitemeier, R., Moertel, C., and Blackburn, C. Vincristine
      therapy of adult patients with solid tumors. Cancer Chemother
      Rep 34: 21, 1964.

(18) Owens, G. Chemotherapy of primary gliomas of the brain. N Y
      State J Med 64: 1933, 1964.

(19) James, D., and George, P. Vincristine in children with
      malignant solid tumors. J Pediat 64: 534, 1964.

(20) Godfrey, T., Good, J., Hall, B., et al. Experience with
      vincristine in the treatment of disseminated neoplastic
      disease. Proc Amer Assoc Cancer Res 5: 21 (#81), 1964.

 21) Grinberg, R., Nemoto, T., and Dao, T. Vincristine (NSC
      67574): dosage and response in advanced breast cancer.
      Cancer Chemother Rep 45: 57, 1965.

(22) Lassman, L., Pearce, G., and Gang, J. Sensitivity of
      intracranial gliomas to vincristine sulfate. Lancet 1:
      296, 1965.

(23) Silva, A., Smart, C., and Rochlin, D. Chemotherapy of breast
      cancer. Surg Gyn Obstet 121: 494, 1965.

(24) Heyn, R., Beatty, E., Hammond, D., et al. Vincristine in
      the treatment of acute leukemia in children. Pediatrics 38:
      82, 1966.

(25) Windmiller, J., Berry, D., Haddy, T., et al. Vincristine in
      the treatment of neuroblastoma of children. Amer J Dis Childh
      111: 75, 1966.

(26) Karon, M., Freireich, E., Frei, E., et al. The role of vincristine in the treatment of childhood acute leukemia. Clin Pharmacol Ther 7: 332, 1966.

(27) Yount, W., and Finkel, H. Treatment of refractory reticulum-cell sarcoma with low doses of vincristine sulfate. JAMA 197: 107, 1966.

(28) Lassman, L., Pearce, G., and Gang, J. Effect of vincristine sulphate on the intracranial gliomata of childhood. Brit J Surg 53: 774, 1966.

(29) Howard, J. Response of acute leukemia in children to repeated courses of vincristine. Cancer Chemother Rep 51: 465, 1967.

(30) Lampkin, B., Mauer, A., and McBride, B. Response of medulloblastoma to vincristine sulfate: a case report. Pediatrics 39: 761, 1967.

(31) Horn, Y., and Hochman, A. The alkaloids of Vinca rosea linn in malignant tumors. Oncology 21: 214, 1967.

(32) Selawry, O., Holland, J., and Wolman, I. Effect of vincristine on malignant solid tumors in children. Cancer Chemother Rep 52: 497, 1968.

(33) Haggard, M., Fernbach, D., Holcomb, T., et al. Vincristine in acute leukemia of childhood. Cancer 22: 438, 1968.

(34) Sullivan, M. Vincristine therapy for Wilms' tumor. Cancer Chemother Rep 52: 481, 1968.

(35) Evans, A. Vincristine in the treatment of children with acute leukemia. Cancer Chemother Rep 52: 469, 1968.

(36) Sutow, W. Vincristine therapy for malignant solid tumors in children (except Wilms' tumor). Cancer Chemother Rep 52: 485, 1968.

(37) Carbone, P., and Spurr, C. Management of patients with malignant lymphoma: a comparative study with cyclophosphamide and vinca alkaloids. Cancer Res 28: 811, 1968.

(38) Smart, C., Ottoman, R., Rochlin, D., et al. Clinical experience with vincristine in tumors of the central nervous system and other malignant diseases. Cancer Chemother Rep 52: 733, 1968.

(39) Korbitz, B., Davis, H., Ramirez, G., et al. Low doses of vincristine (NSC 67574) for malignant disease. Cancer Chemother Rep 53: 249, 1969.

Procarbazine

Synonyms: methylhydrazine (derivative), MIH, ibenzmethyl
             hydrazine, Natulan, Matulane

Structure:

$$CH_3-NH-NH-CH_2-\underset{}{\bigcirc}-\overset{\overset{O}{\|}}{C}-NH-\overset{\overset{CH_3}{|}}{CH}-CH_3$$

. HCl

Dosage: $50 \rightarrow 100$ mg/m^2/day, PO, for first week of therapy;
                 then 125-150 mg/m^2/day, PO as tolerated, until WBC
                 <4000, platelets <100,000, or maximum response obtained.
                 After recovery from hematologic toxicity, treatment
                 may be resumed at 50 or 100 mg/day, PO as tolerated.

Toxicity: I.   Hematological - usual dose-limiting toxicity
                      A. Leukopenia
                      B. Thrombocytopenia
                      C. Anemia

                 II. Gastrointestinal
                      A. Nausea and vomiting - frequent, may be dose-
                          limiting. Tolerance to this side effect
                          often develops with continued administration
                          of the drug, allowing the increase in dose
                          recommended after the first week.
                      B. Stomatitis, diarrhea - uncommon
                      C. Dry mouth, dysphagia - uncommon

                 III. Central nervous system
                      A. Pain - including myalgia and arthralgia
                      B. Lethargy and drowsiness
                      C. Paresthesias and neuropathies - uncommon
                      D. CNS hyperexcitability, including convulsions -
                          uncommon

                 IV. Dermatological
                      A. Occasional drug dermatitis or hyperpigmentation
                      B. Alopecia - uncommon

Note: Procarbazine is a monoamine oxidase inhibitor. As
                 such, it should not be administered in combination with
                 other drugs having monoamine oxidase inhibitory activity,
                 with sympathomimetic drugs, or with tricyclic antidepressants
                 (e.g., imipramine, amitryptyline). The patient should
                 avoid alcohol and foods with high tyramine content, such
                 as ripe cheese and bananas. Barbiturates, phenothiazines,
                 antihistamines, narcotics, and hypotensive agents may have
                 their effects potentiated by procarbazine.

Mechanism of Action: The mechanism of action of procarbazine is
                 uncertain. The agent has been shown to exert inhibitory
                 effects on the synthesis of protein, RNA, and DNA in cells
                 in vitro. It has been observed that cytotoxic derivatives
                 of methylhydrazine can degrade DNA in vitro, through a
                 mechanism involving the autoxidation of the methylhydrazine
                 derivative to hydrogen peroxide.[10] It has been suggested
                 that cytostatic methylhydrazine derivatives may, in vivo,

liberate formaldehyde, azomethine, and N-hydroxymethyl
derivatives, as well as hydrogen peroxide. Growth
inhibitory effects could thus cause both oxidation
and alkylation of cellular constituents.[2]

It was shown by Kreis and Yen[3] that N-demethylation of
procarbazine takes place in vivo. Subsequently, Kreis
reported a selective effect of the compound on the
methylation of transfer RNA, and suggested that this may
contribute to its carcinostatic activity.[4]

Role in Cancer Therapy

Procarbazine has been in clinical use against lymphomas,
especially Hodgkin's disease, for several years. Results in the
published English-language literature demonstrate a 69% objective
response rate in over 300 evaluable patients with Hodgkin's
disease. Of 119 patients evaluated for CR, 37% were reported to
have attained this status. These figures are even more impressive
when one considers that procarbazine has often been used as the
therapy of last resort, after the Hodgkin's patient has become
resistant to both standard alkylating agents and vinca alkaloids.
The number of patients with reticulum-cell sarcoma and lymphosarcoma
for whom results of treatment with procarbazine have been published
is still quite small. However, it does not appear to be as active
against these forms of lymphoma, and probably is inferior to
vincristine or CTX (but not to HN_2 or vinblastine) as single-drug
therapy for them.

Procarbazine appears to have some activity against malignant
melanoma. It deserves further trial in this disease. It has not
received an adequate trial in either breast or colon cancer.

In bronchogenic carcinoma, the data is confusing in spite of
the relatively large number of reported cases. The response rate
in series of reasonable size varies from 6% to 39%. As Samuels
points out,[25] this may be due to differences in the dose
administered or to differences in patient selection, especially
with respect to histologic type. Like CTX (and unlike HN_2),
procarbazine appears to be most effective against small cell
anaplastic ("oat cell") and least effective against squamous
cell bronchogenic cancer. Certainly procarbazine appears worthy
of further evaluation, especially in combination with other
agents of known activity (such as BCNU, CTX, imidazole carboxamide,
and HN_2) against this tumor group.

Procarbazine has not received an adequate trial in acute
leukemia. In addition to the two responses cited in the tabular
summary, it should be mentioned that Martz et al[5] reported

"objective regression" of disease in "one adult patient with acute leukemia resistant to corticosteroid treatment". No denominator was given.

Procarbazine has been reported to show clinical antitumor activity in embryonal cell carcinoma of the testis, ovarian carcinoma, bladder cancer, and neuroblastoma. The numbers are too small to draw conclusions as to its efficacy in these conditions relative to other agents. It received a trial alone against multiple myeloma, and demonstrated moderate activity. Currently, its use together with melphalan and prednisone in this entity is under evaluation by the Southwest Cancer Chemotherapy Group.

Current attempts to improve the effectiveness of procarbazine involve (1) its use in combination with other effective agents, especially in the treatment of Hodgkin's disease; and (2) higher-dose regimens with the drug alone in the more resistant tumor types, such as lung cancer.

Tumor Type or Site

Breast

Ref #	# Pts Evaluated	# Pts Responding	% Response	Dose Schedule and Remarks
7	1	0		50-100 mg →200 to 1000 mg/day, PO for 2-6 wks followed by 100 mg q 2-3 days as tolerated, PO.
8	7	1		300 mg/day PO or 250 mg/day IV = 4-8 mg/kg/day as tolerated. >50% regression.
9	1	0		50→450 mg/day, PO or IV, to limiting toxicity.
10	7	0		200 mg/day x 7, then 300 mg/day x 3-4 wks, PO. 4 had "slight" response.
15	2	0		(1) Day 1, 250 mg; day 2500 mg; days 3, 5, and 7, 1000 mg (IV). (2) Day 1, 250 mg; day 2, 500 mg; days 3, 5, 7, 9, etc., 1000 mg (IV). (3) 50→100→200→300 mg/day, PO as tolerated (usually to total dose of $\leq$ 8 gm).
16	1	0		250→500→then→1000 mg eod to 10 or 12 days, IV.
20	2	0		125-150 mg/m^2 or 250-300 mg/m^2/day, PO (30 patients). 300-1600 mg/m^2, IV (6 patients). 125-150 mg/m^2/day found to be oral MTD; 18 patients received median total dose of 11.7 gm over 42 day period.
	21	1	4.7	Total.

Melanoma

Ref #	# Pts Evaluated	# Pts Responding	% Response	Dose Schedule and Remarks
7	3	0		50-100 mg →200 to 1000 mg/day, PO for 2-6 wks, followed by 100 mg q 2-3 days as tolerated, PO.
9	1	0		50→450 mg/day, PO or IV, to limiting toxicity.
10	2	1		200 mg/day x 7, then 300 mg/day x 3-4 wks, PO.
11	13	3		Not given (daily oral). PR's of 3, 4, and 8 mo duration.
14	5	0		200-300 mg/day x 6-8 wks, PO.
15	1	0		(1) Day 1, 250 mg; day 2500 mg; days 3, 5, and 7, 1000 mg (IV). (2) Day 1, 250 mg; day 2, 500 mg; days 3, 5, 7, 9, etc., 1000 mg (IV). (3) 50→100→200→300 mg/day, PO as tolerated (usually to total dose of ~ 8 gm).
16	2	1		250→500→then→1000 mg eod to 10 or 12 days, IV. ? PR.
20	5	1		125-150 mg/m^2 or 250-300 mg/m^2/day, PO (30 patients). 300-1600 mg/m^2, IV (6 patients). 125-150 mg/m^2/day found to be oral MTD; 18 patients received median total dose of 11.7 gm over 42 day period.
	32̅	6̅	18.7	Total.

Colon

Ref #	# Pts Evaluated	# Pts Responding	% Response	Dose Schedule and Remarks
7	2	0		50–100 mg →200 to 1000 mg/day, PO for 2–6 wks, followed by 100 mg q 2–3 days as tolerated, PO.
9	2	0		50→450 mg/day, PO or IV, to limiting toxicity.
20	1	0		125–150 mg/m^2 or 250–300 mg/m^2/day, PO (30 patients). 300–1600 mg/m^2, IV (6 patients). 125–150 mg/m^2/day found to be oral MTD; 18 patients received median total dose of 11.7 gm over 42 day period.
	$\overline{5}$	$\overline{0}$		Total.

Lung

8	5	1		300 mg/day PO or 250 mg/day IV = 4–8 mg/kg/day as tolerated. 1/3 small cell. 0/1 anaplastic; 0/1 poorly differentiated.
14	40	3		200–300 mg/day x 6–8 wks, PO. All responses "poorly differentiated" group. Durations 2, 7, and 9 mo.
15	4	2		(1) Day 1, 250 mg; day 2500 mg; days 3, 5, and 7, 1000 mg (IV). (2) Day 1, 250 mg; day 2, 500 mg; days 3, 5, 7, 9, etc., 1000 mg (IV). (3) 50→100→200→300 mg/day, PO as tolerated (usually to total dose of ≤ 8 gm). Durations 5 and 11 mo.

Lung (cont.)

Ref #	# Pts Evaluated	# Pts Responding	% Response	Dose Schedule and Remarks
16	4	0		$250\rightarrow500\rightarrow$then$\rightarrow1000$ mg eod to 10 or 12 days, IV.
17	31	3		Varied, PO and IV, but in general escalating to daily dose of 300 mg/day, PO. Median duration of treatment, 34 days. All PR.
20	2	0		125-150 mg/m^2 or 250-300 mg/m^2/day, PO (30 patients). 300-1600 mg/m^2, IV (6 patients). 125-150 mg/m^2/day found to be oral MTD; 18 patients received median total dose of 11.7 gm over 42 day period.
24	50	3	6	200-300 mg/day, PO as tolerated. 1/25 squamous ("epidermoid") - 12 mo. 2/25 anaplastic - 5 and 6 mo.
25	36	14	39	100-150 mg/m^2/day, PO increased to maximum of 250 mg/m^2/day, x$\stackrel{>}{=}$ 21 days. Median dose = 180 mg/m^2/day x 28 (to response). Maintenance dose = 100 mg/day as tolerated. 7/9 small cell anaplastic. 3/9 adenocarcinoma. 3/13 squamous cell. 1/5 large cell anaplastic. MST responders = 26 wks. MST nonresponders = 18 wks (P = 0.15). MST overall = 21 wks for treated group.
	$\overline{172}$	$\overline{26}$	15.1	Total.

ALL

Ref #	# Pts Evaluated	# Pts Responding	% Response	Dose Schedule and Remarks
6	3	0		200–500 mg/day, IV or PO to mean total dose 9.75 gm.
22	3	0		125 mg/m^2/day, PO for $\geq$ 4 wks.
	$\overline{6}$	$\overline{0}$		Total.

AML-AMoL

Ref #	# Pts Evaluated	# Pts Responding	% Response	Dose Schedule and Remarks
7	2	1		50–100 mg →200 to 1000 mg/day, PO for 2–6 wks, followed by 100 mg q 2–3 days as tolerated, PO. CR – ? due to MIH.
20	2	0		125–150 mg/m^2 or 250–300 mg/m^2/day, PO (30 patients). 300–1600 mg/m^2, IV (6 patients). 125–150 mg/m^2/day found to be oral MTD; 18 patients received median total dose of 11.7 gm over 42 day period.
22	1	0		125 mg/m^2/day, PO for $\geq$ 4 wks.
	$\overline{5}$	$\overline{1}$	20	Total.

Hodgkin's

Ref #	# Pts Evaluated	# Pts Responding	% Response	Dose Schedule and Remarks
5	14	14		200–300 mg/day, PO or IV, x 3–5 wks, then 50–100 mg/day as tolerated. 10 CR.

Hodgkin's (cont.)

Ref #	# Pts Evaluated	# Pts Responding	% Response	Dose Schedule and Remarks
6	22	15		200-500 mg/day, IV or PO to mean total dose 9.75 gm. 7 CR.
7	20	12		50-100 mg →200 to 1000 mg/day, PO for 2-6 wks, followed by 100 mg q 2-3 days as tolerated, PO. All PR. 6/12 refractory to both vinca and alkylating agents had "useful response".
9	13	12		50→450 mg/day, PO or IV, to limiting toxicity. 8 remissions >1 mo.
10	16	15		200 mg/day x 7, then 300 mg/day x 3-4 wks, PO. Mean duration 4+ mo.
11	53	33		Not given (daily oral).
12	17	14		150 mg/day PO as tolerated.
13	27	15		100-300 mg/day, PO as tolerated. 12 CR, 3 PR. Mean duration 12 wks.
15	11	6		(1) Day 1, 250 mg; day 2500 mg; days 3, 5, and 7, 1000 mg (IV). (2) Day 1, 250 mg; day 2, 500 mg; days 3, 5, 7, 9, etc., 1000 mg (IV). (3) 50→100→200→300 mg/day, PO as tolerated (usually to total dose of ≤ 8 gm). 3 CR.
16	14	13		250→500→then→1000 mg eod to 10 or 12 days, IV. 9 CR.
18	21	16		50→→30° mg/day, PO.

Hodgkin's (cont.)

Ref #	# Pts Evaluated	# Pts Responding	% Response	Dose Schedule and Remarks
19	17	9		$50 \rightarrow 250$ mg/day, PO as tolerated. All patients refractory to CTX and to VLB.
20	10	5		125-150 mg/m^2 or 250-300 mg/m^2/day, PO (30 patients). 300-1600 mg/m^2, IV (6 patients). 125-150 mg/m^2/day found to be oral MTD; 18 patients received median total dose of 11.7 gm over 42 day period.
21	11	8		$50 \rightarrow 100 \rightarrow 150$ mg, then $\overset{>}{\sim} 150$ mg/m^2/day x 42 days, if tolerated, PO. 3 CR. Median duration 4 mo.
22	6	3		125 mg/m^2/day, PO for $\overset{>}{\sim}$ 4 wks. Durations 7, 13, 18 wks.
26	33	22		Up to 25-30 mg/kg/wk given in divided daily doses, PO. Median duration response = 98 days. All patients resistant to at least 2 other agents. WCCG study.
27	14	14		$50 \rightarrow 100 \rightarrow 150 \rightarrow 300$ mg/day, PO, as tolerated.
28	28	13		3-4 mg/kg/day x 30-40, then 1.5-2.5 mg/kg/day, PO as tolerated. Median duration 4 mo. All patients treated first with vinblastine.
	347	239	69	Total. 44 CR of 119 = 37%.

Reticulum-cell Sarcoma

Ref #	# Pts Evaluated	# Pts Responding	% Response	Dose Schedule and Remarks
6	2	2		200–500 mg/day, IV or PO to mean total dose 9.75 gm. 2 PR, 0 CR.
7	4	1		50–100 mg →200 to 1000 mg/day, PO for 2–6 wks, followed by 100 mg q 2–3 days as tolerated, PO. 5 wks' duration.
9	3	1		50→450 mg/day, PO or IV, to limiting toxicity. 3 mo duration. 1 PR.
11	2	0		Not given (daily oral).
13	3	2		100–300 mg/day, PO as tolerated. 2 PR, 0 CR. Remission durations 3 mo, 4 mo.
16	6	2		250→500→then→1000 mg eod to 10 or 12 days, IV. 2 PR, 0 CR.
18	5	2		50→→300 mg/day, PO.
21	5	1		50→100→150 mg, then $\geq$ 150 mg/m^2/day x 42 days, if tolerated, PO. PR.
26	3	1		Up to 25–30 mg/kg/wk given in divided daily doses, PO. WCGG study.
	$\overline{33}$	$\overline{12}$	36.4	Total.

Lymphosarcoma

Ref #	# Pts Evaluated	# Pts Responding	% Response	Dose Schedule and Remarks
5	1	1		200-300 mg/day, PO or IV, x 3-5 wks, then 50-100 mg/day as tolerated. 1 CR.
6	9	4		200-500 mg/day, IV or PO to mean total dose 9.75 gm. 4 PR, 0 CR.
7	2	1		50-100 mg →200 to 1000 mg/day, PO for 2-6 wks, followed by 100 mg q 2-3 days as tolerated, PO. Duration 5 wks.
9	1	0		50→450 mg/day, PO or IV, to limiting toxicity.
11	10	5		Not given (daily oral).
13	5	1		100-300 mg/day, PO as tolerated. CR, duration 13+ mo.
15	2	2		(1) Day 1, 250 mg; day 2500 mg; days 3, 5, and 7, 1000 mg (IV). (2) Day 1, 250 mg; day 2, 500 mg; days 3, 5, 7, 9, etc., 1000 mg (IV). (3) 50→100→200→300 mg/day, <PO as tolerated (usually to total dose of - 8 gm). 1 CR, 1 PR.
16	1	1		250→500→then→1000 mg eod to 10 or 12 days, IV.
18	1	0		50→→300 mg/day, PO.
20	5	0		125-150 mg/m^2 or 250-300 mg/m^2/day, PO (30 patients). 300-1600 mg/m^2, IV (6 patients). 125-150 mg/m^2/day found to be oral MTD; 18 patients received median total dose of 11.7 gm over 42 day period.

Lymphosarcoma (cont.)

Ref #	# Pts Evaluated	# Pts Responding	% Response	Dose Schedule and Remarks
22	1	0		125 mg/m^2/day, PO for $\geq$ 4 wks.
26	4	2		Up to 25-30 mg/kg/wk given in divided daily doses, PO. WCCG study.
	$\overline{42}$	$\overline{17}$	40.5	Total.

Head and Neck

Ref #	# Pts Evaluated	# Pts Responding	% Response	Dose Schedule and Remarks
17	31	3	10	Varied, PO and IV, but in general escalating to daily dose of 300 mg/day, PO. Median duration of treatment, 34 days.

Testicular

Ref #	# Pts Evaluated	# Pts Responding	% Response	Dose Schedule and Remarks
8	1	0		300 mg/day PO or 250 mg/day IV = 4-8 mg/kg/day as tolerated.
20	1	0		125-150 mg/m^2 or 250-300 mg/m^2/day, PO (30 patients). 300-1600 mg/m^2, IV (6 patients). 125-150 mg/m^2/day found to be oral MTD; 18 patients received median total dose of 11.7 gm over 42 day period.
21	1	1		50→100→150 mg, then $\geq$ 150 mg/m^2/day x 42 days, if tolerated, PO. PR; 3 mo duration.
	$\overline{3}$	$\overline{1}$	33	Total.

Ovary

Ref #	# Pts Evaluated	# Pts Responding	% Response	Dose Schedule and Remarks
9	1	0		50→450 mg/day, PO or IV, to limiting toxicity.
16	2	0		250→500→then→1000 mg eod to 10 or 12 days, IV.
17	4	1		Varied, PO and IV, but in general escalating to daily dose of 300 mg/day, PO. Median duration of treatment, 34 days.
	7	1	14.3	Total.

Bladder

21	3	1	33	50→100→150 mg, then $\geq$ 150 mg/m^2/day x 42 days, if tolerated, PO.

Multiple Myeloma

6	1	0		200-500 mg/day, IV or PO to mean total dose 9.75 gm.
9	1	0		50→450 mg/day, PO or IV, to limiting toxicity. Serum protein electrophoresis became normal.

Multiple Myeloma (cont.)

Ref #	# Pts Evaluated	# Pts Responding	% Response	Dose Schedule and Remarks
15	1	1		Day 1, 250 mg; day 2500 mg; days 3, 5, and 7, 1000 mg (IV). (2) Day 1, 250 mg; day 2, 500 mg; days 3, 5, 7, 9, etc., 1000 mg (IV). (3) 50→100→200→300 mg/day, PO as tolerated (usually to total dose of $\leq$ 8 gm). PR.
20	2	0		125-150 mg/m^2 or 250-300 mg/m^2/day, PO (30 patients). 300-1600 mg/m^2, IV (6 patients). 125-150 mg/m^2/day found to be oral MTD; 18 patients received median total dose of 11.7 gm over 42 day period.
21	8	1		50→100→150 mg, then $\geq$ 150 gm/m^2/day x 42 days, if tolerated, PO. PR.
23	20	3		300 mg/day, PO as tolerated. All PR.
	33	5	15	Total.

Hepatoma

Ref #	# Pts Evaluated	# Pts Responding	% Response	Dose Schedule and Remarks
9	14	0		50→450 mg/day, PO or IV, to limiting toxicity.

Neuroblastoma

Ref #	# Pts Evaluated	# Pts Responding	% Response	Dose Schedule and Remarks
10	1	1		200 mg/day x 7, then 300 mg/day x 3-4 wks, PO. PR; clearing of lung metastases.
22	2	0		125 mg/m^2/day, PO for $\geq$ 4 wks.
	3	1	33	Total.

References

(1)   Sartorelli, A., and Tsunamura, S. Studies on the biochemical
       mode of action of a cytotoxic methylhydrazine derivative,
       n-isopropyl-α-(2-methylhydrazino)-p-toluamide. Mol Pharmacol
       2: 275, 1966.

(2)   Berneis, K., Kofler, M., Bollag, W., et al. The degradation
       of deoxyribonucleic acid by new tumour inhibiting compounds:
       the intermediate formation of hydrogen peroxide. Experientia
       19: 132, 1963.

(3)   Kreis, W., and Yen, W. An antineoplastic ^{14}C-labeled
       methylhydrazine derivative in P815 mouse leukemia. A
       metabolic study. Experientia 21: 284, 1965.

(4)   Kreis, W. Metabolism of an antineoplastic methylhydrazine
       derivative in a P815 mouse neoplasm. Cancer Res 30: 82,
       1970.

(5)   Martz, G., D'Alessandri, A., Keel, H., et al. Preliminary
       clinical results with a new antitumor agent RO 4-6467
       (NSC 77213). Cancer Chemother Rep 33: 5, 1963.

(6)   Mathe, G., Berumen, L., Schweisguth, O., et al. Methyl-
       hydrazine in treatment of Hodgkin's disease and various forms
       of haematosarcoma and leukemia. Lancet 2: 1077, 1963.

(7)   Brunner, K., and Young, C. A methylhydrazine derivative in
       Hodgkin's disease and other malignant neoplasms. Ann Inter
       Med 63: 69, 1965.

(8)   Brule, G., Schlumberger, J., and Griscelli, C. N-isopropyl-
       α-(2-methylhydrazino)-p-toluamide, hydrochloride (NSC 77213)
       in treatment of solid tumors. Cancer Chemother Rep 44: 31,
       1965.

(9)   Falkson, G., Villiers, P., and Falkson, H. N-isopropyl-α-
       (2-methylhydrazino)-p-toluamide hydrochloride (NSC 77213) for
       treatment of cancer patients. Cancer Chemother Rep 46: 7,
       1965.

(10)   Hope-Stone, H. Ibenzmethyzin in the treatment of the
       reticuloses. In "Natulan (Ibenzmethyzin)", (Jelliffe, A.,
       and Marks, J., eds.), John Wright and Sons Ltd., pp 15-19,
       1965.

(11) Todd, I. Further experience with ibenzmethyzin. In
      "Natulan (Ibenzmethyzin)", (Jelliffe, A., and Marks, J.,
      eds.), John Wright and Sons Ltd., pp 20-25, 1965.

(12) Dawson, W. Ibenzmethyzin in the management of late Hodgkin's
      disease. In "Natulan (Ibenzmethyzin)", (Jelliffe, A., and
      Marks, J., eds.), John Wright and Sons Ltd., pp 31-34, 1965.

(13) Jelliffe, A., Bleehen, N., and Fenner, M. Short report.
      In "Natulan (Ibenzmethyzin)", (Jelliffe, A., and Marks, J.,
      eds.), John Wright and Sons Ltd., pp 35-39, 1965.

(14) Jelliffe, A., Bleehen, N., and Fenner, M. Ibenzmethyzin in
      the treatment of solid tumors. In "Natulan (Ibenzmethyzin),"
      (Jelliffe, A., and Marks, J., eds.), John Wright and Sons
      Ltd., pp 53-55, 1965.

(15) Backhouse, T., and Sicher, K. Initial experiences with
      methylhydrazine, a new cytotoxic agent. Clin Radiol 17:
      132, 1966.

(16) Hansen, M., Hertz, H., and Videback, A. Use of a methyl
      hydrazine derivative (Natulan), especially in Hodgkin's
      disease. Acta Med Scand 180: 211, 1966.

(17) Kenis, Y., DeSmedt, J., and Tagnon, H. Action de Natulan
      dans 94 cas de tumeurs solides. Europ J Cancer 2: 51, 1966.

(18) Spies, S., and Snyman, H. Procarbazine (Natulan) in the
      treatment of Hodgkin's disease and other lymphomas. S Afric
      Med J 40: 1061, 1966.

(19) Fairley, G., Patterson, M., and Scott, R. Chemotherapy of
      Hodgkin's disease with cyclophosphamide, vinblastine, and
      procarbazine. Brit Med J 2: 75, 1966.

(20) DeVita, V., Serpick, A., and Carbone, P. Preliminary clinical
      studies with ibenzmethyzin. Clin Pharm Ther 7: 542, 1966.

(21) Samuels, M., Leary, W., Alexanian, R., et al. Clinical trials
      with n-isopropyl-α-(2-methylhydrazino)-p-toluamide
      hydrochloride in malignant lymphoma and other disseminated
      neoplasia. Cancer 20: 1187, 1967.

(22) Holton, C., and Selawry, O. Clinical study of procarbazine
      hydrochloride in children with cancer. South Med J 60:
      1375, 1967.

(23)   Bousser, J. Essai de traitement du myelome multiple par
       une methylhydrazine. Europ J Cancer 3: 437, 1967.

(24)   Brouet, D., Flamant, R., and Hayat, M. Results of a trial of
       a methylhydrazine in the treatment of epidermoid and
       anaplastic lung cancer. European J Cancer 4: 129, 1968.

(25)   Samuels, M., Leary, W., and Howe, C. Procarbazine (NSC 77213)
       in the treatment of advanced bronchogenic carcinoma. Cancer
       Chemother Rep 53: 135, 1969.

(26)   Stolinsky, D., Solomon, J., Pugh, R., et al. Procarbazine
       HCL in Hodgkin's disease, reticulum-cell sarcoma and
       lymphosarcoma. Proc Amer Assoc Cancer Res 10: 88 (#350),
       1969.

(27)   Flatow, F., Ultmann, J., Hyman, G., et al. Treatment
       of advanced Hodgkin's disease with vinblastine (NSC 49842)
       or procarbazine (NSC 77213). Cancer Chemother Rep 53:
       39, 1969.

(28)   Bonadonna, G., Monfardini, S., and Oldini, C. Comparative
       effects of vinblastine and procarbazine in advanced Hodgkin's
       disease. Europ J Cancer 5: 393, 1969.

Prednisone and Prednisolone

Synonyms: deltacortisone (prednisone), deltahydrocortisone
             (prednisolone).   Numerous proprietary names

Structure:

$$CH_2-OH$$
$$C=O$$
$$----OH$$

Prednisone

$$CH_2O-\overset{O}{\overset{\|}{C}}-CH_2CH_2-\overset{O}{\overset{\|}{C}}-OH$$
$$C=O$$
$$-----OH$$

HO

. Na salt

Prednisolone

337

Dosage: 1. 2 mg/kg or 40 mg/m^2/day x $\geq$ 28 days, prednisone
                   (common induction regimens for ALL-AUL).
               2. Other schedules - see discussion and tables.

Toxicity: (see standard reference sources for more complete
            discussion)

                I.   Metabolic
                     A. Fluid and electrolyte disturbances
                         1. Sodium retention and potassium - wasting
                     B. Hyperglycemia and glycosuria

                II. Peptic ulceration - a common and dangerous
                     complication

                III. Increased susceptibility to infection

                IV. Myopathy

                V.   Psychoses and lesser psychiatric disturbances

                IV. Osteoporosis and vertebral compression
                     fractures

Mechanism of Action: Glucocorticoids have been known since 1944
                to exert profound effects on the volume, structure, and
                function of lymphoid tissue.[1,2] They possess, of
                course, a wide variety of other actions which are beyond
                the scope of discussion here, including anti-inflammatory
                effects and the related ability to suppress immune
                response.

                The ablative effect of pharmacologic doses of these
                compounds on lymphoid tissue, and specifically on
                abnormal lymphocytes or related cells, is not well
                understood at a molecular level. In vitro studies
                indicate that steroids can inhibit RNA and protein
                synthesis in such cells,[3,4] and it has been hypothesized
                that the inhibition of lymphocyte protein synthesis may
                ultimately result in the destruction of the cell.[4]
                Whatever the nature of the glucocorticoids' lympholytic
                effect, it does not seem to depend on the cell's being
                in a proliferating state, distinguishing the mechanism
                of action of the steroids from that of the "antimetabolites

                            Role in Cancer Therapy

    In this chapter, our survey of the literature has been confined
to the use of prednisone and prednisolone. A large body of earlier
data concerning the use of ACTH, cortisone, and hydrocortisone has

been omitted. The reasons for this are twofold: (1) prednisone and prednisolone have, in doses which are equally effective against sensitive tumors, fewer undesirable side effects than the other hormones, and might therefore be expected to produce somewhat better results; and (2) even if the steroids used were identical, the supportive aspects of care, especially in ALL-AUL, have changed so radically in the last 15 years that it becomes impossible to evaluate what the results of early steroid therapy might have been. (To some extent, of course, this caveat applies to a comparison of the use of prednisone and prednisolone even 10 years ago with that today). Prednisone and prednisolone have been considered essentially equivalent agents for the purposes of this report.

These compounds have not received a reported trial as single agents in the treatment of malignant melanoma or colorectal cancer. In lung cancer, an early trial of daily oral cortisone against inoperable disease produced a median survival time which was less than that of a control group treated with placebo.[19] (Along these lines, Berkheiser[33] subsequently showed that cortisone can cause pulmonary epithelial hyperplasia in rabbits, and found an increased incidence of alveolar epithelization and epidermal metaplasia in autopsied patients who had previously been on chronic steroid therapy). There has been no effort to examine the effects of the newer synthetic steroids on this disease.

Prednisone and prednisolone have, in contrast, proven to be extremely useful agents in the management of ALL-AUL and lymphomas, and to some extent disseminated breast cancer.

In ALL-AUL, the overall CR rate for a first course of daily therapy with one of these agents is 45% (391 of 863 patients evaluated).

Two additional facts seem worth emphasizing with reference to the effectiveness of predniso(lo)ne in ALL-AUL: (1) the antitumor effect is markedly reduced by therapy on an intermittent schedule, at least with equivalent doses per unit period of time;[47] and (2) the likelihood of remission is still substantial, though reduced, for patients receiving a first reinduction attempt.[25,39] Although it appears from the tabular summary that 40% of 90 patients evaluated for CR attained it on a second course of steroids, this per cent is derived from two reports in which very different criteria were used to define CR. In the first,[25] bone marrow examinations were not done routinely to establish remission status, and undoubtedly the "true" CR figure is <53%. In the second,[39] rigorous criteria were applied, and the CR figure drops to 25%. The important difference between a first and a second course of steroids is better illustrated by the change in proportion of patients achieving an M_1 marrow: from 52 to 29% in the Southwest Group's experience.

In summary, it appears that 50 to 60% of patients previously
unexposed to steroids will obtain an M_1 marrow on the initial
attempt, while only about half this number will do so on a second
attempt with the same agent alone.

The use of steroids in the treatment of patients with AML-AMoL
dates back to the 1940's. It was then, and remains, a controversial
topic. In 1954, Fessas, Wintrobe et al reviewed the treatment of
acute leukemia with cortisone and ACTH.[8] In all, 425 cases were
analyzed. They found the overall reported "complete" response rate
with these compounds to be 5.5% for patients with AML, 3.9% for
those with AMoL (acute monocytic), 27.3% for ALL, and 42.5% for
AUL (acute undifferentiated). The "complete" remission rate in AML
and AMoL did not seem significantly different from the 4%
spontaneous rate of CR reported for a large series of untreated
patients with acute leukemia of various types who received only
supportive care.[6] In a later review,[25] Boggs, Wintrobe, and
Cartwright reported their own experience with 50 consecutive cases
of AML who received steroid therapy: there were no remissions
seen, and only one patient was felt clinically to be improved. They
felt there was "no significant difference with ACTH, cortisone or
prednisone", and apparently treated all these patients with
"conventional" doses.

A number of other investigators have reported similar results.
The series of Rosenthal et al[5] and Shanbrom and Miller[26] showed no
response in a combined total of 33 patients with AML-AMoL. The
latter authors treated 15 patients with "massive" steroids (500 mg/
day x 10 of prednisolone) and felt that 7 were "made worse" by the
treatment. Bernard, using doses of prednisone that would now be
considered "conventional" (1-3 mg/kg/day) reported only 3 complete
responses in 47 patients treated between 1958 and 1962.[27]

Other investigators, however, have found steroids to be of
value against AML. Ranney and Gellhorn[11] treated 11 patients
classed as AML (or AMoL) and obtained 1 CR and 4 PR in this group,
using 1 gm/day x 10 of prednisone. However, 3 patients (of a total
of 18) had exacerbation of peptic ulcer disease on this dose, and one
had a perforated duodenal ulcer at necropsy. Three more patients
appeared to have the disease process accelerated while on steroid
therapy. "Finally, infection was an important and grave
complication of the massive steroid therapy." Granville et al[15]
from Dameshek's group used three dose schedules of predniso(lo)ne
in adults with AML: one gram/day, 250 mg/day, and 100 mg/day, for
14 days at each level. The dose was then tapered. At the highest
dose, there were 3 CR and 1 PR of 10 treated; however, only 3 of the
10 could tolerate a full 14-day course of therapy, and one patient
died of GI hemorrhage which may have been drug-related. At the
intermediate dose, there were 2 CR and 1 PR of 10 treated, and 9 of

the 10 were able to tolerate a full course, with no deaths felt to be drug-related. It should be noted that one of the CR in the high-dose group and one of the CR in the intermediate-dose group did not appear until the patients had received an additional "brief course" of 6 MP. At the low dose, there were 4 PR and no CR of 10 patients treated. The authors concluded that doses of steroids higher than "conventional" were capable of producing complete remissions in patients with AML, but that use of very high doses was associated with limiting toxicity. Unfortunately, their series was so small that there was no statistically significant difference (by chi-square), with regard to either CR or total response rate, among the 3 dose-level groups.

Bouroncle et al[16] reported favorable results in patients with AMoL, using high-dose prednisolone (500-1000 mg/day x 9-14): 2 of 5 patients with this diagnosis had "CR", with 0/1 AML patients responding.

The largest series of patients in the AML-AMoL group who were treated with steroid alone is that reported by the British investigators, Roath et al[35]. Using primarily "conventional" dosage, and usually prednisolone, they obtained 13/85 remissions in AML, and 1/34 in AMoL. "Remission" in their series was defined on the basis of improvement in the hemogram and physical condition rather than by marrow criteria; however, it was necessary to have an essentially normal differential and platelet count in order to qualify.

A final report worthy of mention is that of an MRC working party[42] which compared low-dose prednisone alone (40 mg/day) with 6 MP alone and with 6 MP + prednisone at the same doses of each in the treatment of a large number of patients, predominantly adults, with AML. With low-dose steroid alone, 6/39 "remissions" (criteria not defined) were reported. The median survival time with low-dose prednisone alone was 71.5 days; it was 61 days for 6 MP alone, and 40 days for 6 MP + prednisone. An earlier study had shown that high-dose prednisone + 6 MP gave the worst results of all, with MST = 21 days.

Overall, the results for the use of "massive" steroid therapy [$\geq$ 250 mg/day predniso(lo)ne] are as follows in AML-AMoL: 14/52 = 27% had a response, and 8/52 = 15% had a "CR" (based on varying criteria). For "conventional" steroid therapy [<250 mg/day predniso(lo)ne] these results are obtained: 30/297 = 10% had a response, and 3/57 = 5% had CR. Balanced against these data must be the reports which indicate that steroid therapy may accelerate the basic disease process in some patients, and those which show definitely greater toxic effects for patients who receive "high-dose" therapy with these agents. It is particularly

hard to evaluate the importance of steroids in increasing the
incidence of serious infections in this patient group, since the
disease itself predisposes them to sepsis.

In chronic lymphocytic leukemia, about two-thirds of patients
treated appear to have had a meaningful objective response. Such
an effect on the disease is not limited to patients with antiglobulin-
positive hemolytic anemias.[21] However, treated patients, at least
those on relatively prolonged continuous therapy, often have serious
side effects. In the study reported by Shaw et al[22] in 18
ambulatory patients, 12 had infections while on therapy, and these
were "generally more severe and more difficult to control when the
patients were receiving prednisone... Two fatal infections
occurred..." The same authors concluded that "corticosteroids
should not be used electively in patients with chronic lymphocytic
leukemia except in the presence of hemolytic anemia, significant
thrombocytopenia or in the presence of advanced disease associated
with bone marrow failure." Shaw et al also found that the
remissions obtained were of short duration, with loss of control
shortly after cessation of therapy. Other investigators have
reported prolonged responses, usually with low-dose prednisone
maintenance subsequent to a 1- to 5-week "induction" at higher
doses.[24,28,37] The paper of Burningham et al[37] describes the
results of weekly maintenance after such an induction period: these
authors obtained equivalent therapeutic effects and long-term
responses with "virtually no side effects". As such, their method
of using steroids may be optimal in this disease, although
confirmation of the superiority of their dose schedule remains to
be reported by others.

The activity of these agents against lymphomas, including
Hodgkin's disease, appears to be comparable to their activity against
chronic lymphocytic leukemia.[30,43] Current efforts to treat
lymphomas more effectively with drug combinations frequently involve
the use of predniso(lo)ne, since its toxicity does not significantly
overlap that of other active compounds.

The entire subject of hormonal therapy in breast cancer is
controversial, and the place of glucocorticoids in the therapy of
this disease is no exception. A review by Lemon of the literature
between 1954 and 1962 (quoted by Freckman et al[36]) reportedly
yielded a mean regression rate of 26% with either cortisone or
prednisone. The duration of objective regression, in this analysis,
varied from 1 to 6+ months, and most of the patients reported had not
undergone previous castration. The present review of predniso(lo)ne
data from the English-language literature totals an objective
response in 33 of 179 patients, or 18.5%. However, the reported
response rate ranges from 4% in an Eastern Solid Tumor Group Study[32]
to 48% in Lemon's own series.[17] This discrepancy is all the more
puzzling because all premenopausal women had undergone previous

castration in both series, so presumably this factor should not
have influenced the results. (Although predniso(lo)ne effectively
suppresses estrogen production by the adrenal via its effect on
ACTH secretion, it also stimulates FSH production, and thus could
augment estrogen production by functioning ovarian tissue)[17].

The activity of glucocorticoids in breast cancer is felt by
many clinicians to be entirely a function of their ability to
suppress adrenal estrogen production. As a result, they have been
"employed primarily in patients who reject the surgical ablative
procedure [adrenalectomy] or who are too ill to tolerate the
procedure. The rate of improvement has been less than that of the
surgical procedures, and the duration of such improvement is
shorter".[41] Another author states: "At present the greatest
usefulness of corticosteroids appears to reside in their availability
as an effective alternative to surgical adrenalectomy in patients
whose visceral encroachment contraindicates the operation".[46]
There appear to be at least two unanswered questions in this area
from a chemotherapist's point of view: (1) do glucocorticoids
have a specific antitumor effect in this disease, apart from their
ability to suppress estrogen production; and (2) would alternate-
day therapy offer any advantages, in terms of decreased long-term
steroid toxicity, over daily treatment, while still preserving
antitumor effect? To answer the first question, it would seem
to be necessary to randomize two comparable groups of previously
adrenalectomized women with recurrent disease to "replacement" vs
"pharmacologic" doses of prednisone, holding other therapeutic
modalities constant. In view of the difference between ALL on the
one hand and CLL and multiple myeloma on the other with regard to
the effectiveness of intermittent predniso(lo)ne therapy, the
second question would appear relevant, and might also be worth
answering.

Steroids appear to exert a real but modest antitumor effect
in multiple myeloma. Current efforts in investigative chemotherapy
involve the use of these agents in combination with others, such as
melphalan, or in patients refractory to alkylating agent therapy.

Finally, two useful actions of glucocorticoids in cancer therapy
which do not seem to be directly related to an antitumor effect
should be noted. The first is the ability of these agents to quickly
and often dramatically lessen cerebral edema; this has proven useful
both in the palliative treatment of primary brain tumors and of
cerebral metastases from other sites.[12,40] Secondly, these agents
will usually correct or alleviate the hypercalcemia associated with
breast cancer,[41] and sometimes that associated with other neoplastic
states. In this respect, they differ markedly from the sex steroids,
which can worsen or even induce the development of hypercalcemia
in these patients.

Tumor Type or Site

Breast

Ref #	# Pts Evaluated	# Pts Responding	% Response	Dose Schedule (PO in divided daily doses unless otherwise stated) and Remarks
14	45	8	18	Prednisolone, 50-100 mg/day. "Generalized tumor regression" in responders. Duration response >3 mo in 3/45 = 7%.
17	31	15	48	Prednisone, 30 mg/day. Longest response = 23 mo. All patients had undergone previous castration (see discussion).
32	23	1	4	Prednisolone, 40 mg/day. All premenopausal women had undergone previous castration. 0/32 patients treated with 9 α-bromo-11 β-ketoprogresterone ("BOP") responded.
34	80	9	11	Prednisolone, 30 mg/day. Patients did not as a rule undergo prior castration.
36	—	—		See discussion.
41	—	—		Prednisone, 60-80 mg/day, PO or methyl prednisolone, ~80 mg/day, IV. 32/40 treated patients with hypercalcemia had favorable response.
	179	33	18.5	Total.

Multiple Myeloma

Ref #	# Pts Evaluated	# Pts Responding	% Response	Dose Schedule (PO in divided daily doses unless otherwise stated) and Remarks
23	4	4		Prednisone, 60 →→→ 150 mg/day, then smaller daily maintenance. Response in each case in ≥ 2 objective parameters.
29	25	7		Prednisone, 40 mg/day -- vs Placebo. 7/25 had ↑ globulin of ~ 1.5 gm % from initial value of ~ 4.5 gm %. 1/22 placebo-treated patients had similar globulin ↓. 6/22 prednisone-treated patients had "significant" rise in Hb. MST 17 mo for both regimens.
45	10	8		Prednisone, 200 mg single dose PO, every other day x 8 wks; then 100 mg every other day x 4 wks; then 50 mg every other day. Response in each case in ≥ 2 objective parameters, by 8th wk. One patient had perforated gastric ulcer.
	$\overline{39}$	$\overline{19}$	49	Total.

ALL-AUL

| 10 | 21 | 16 (6 CR) | | 1.4-2.2 mg/kg/day, prednisone. Median duration remission (unmaintained) = 53 days. 4 children had previous exposure to cortisone. |
| 13 | 15 | 7 (5 CR) | | ~2 mg/kg/day, prednisone. |

ALL-AUL (cont.)

Ref #	# Pts Evaluated	# Pts Responding	% Response	Dose Schedule (PO in divided daily doses unless otherwise stated) and Remarks
16	24	8 (5 CR)		0.5-1.0 gm/day x 9-14, prednisone.
18	30	18 (16 CR)		2.2 mg/kg/day x 28 (induction) then no maintenance or 0.55 mg/kg/day, maintenance. All patients in relapse after 1st induction with 6 MP, 6 MP + azaserine, or 6 MP + DON. Continuous low-dose maintenance with prednisone after induction →79 days median remission duration; no maintenance →75 days.
25	100	91 (71 CR)	91 (71% CR)	~2 mg/kg/day, prednisone. First course steroids. (Bone marrow exams not done routinely to establish remission status.)
25	49	38 (26 CR)	78 (53% CR)	Second course steroids. (Bone marrow exams not done routinely to establish remission status.)
26	17	10 (6 CR)		500 mg/day x 10, prednisolone.
26	4	3 (3 CR)		50 mg/day x 10, prednisolone.
26	5	5 (2 CR)		50 mg/kg/day x 10, then 500 mg/kg/day prednisolone.
27	11	5 (5 CR)	(45% CR)	<1 mg/kg/day, prednisone. First course steroids.

ALL–AUL (cont.)

Ref #	# Pts Evaluated	# Pts Responding	% Response	Dose Schedule (PO in divided daily doses unless otherwise stated) and Remarks
27	45	29 (29 CR)	(64% CR)	1 to 3 mg/kg/day, prednisone. First course steroids.
27	62	45 (46 CR)	(74% CR)	> 3 mg/kg/day prednisone. First course steroids.
31	92	62 (56 CR)	67 (60% CR)	40 mg/m^2/day x > 28 days, prednisone. First course steroids. ALGB study. CR = M$_1$ marrow.
39	46	27 (12 CR)	59 (26% CR)	2.2 mg/kg/day x 4 to 6 wks, prednisone. First course steroids. 35 patients completed course. 24 patients = 52% achieved M$_1$ marrow. Median duration CR (unmaintained) = 57 days. SWCCSG study.
39	41	19 (10 CR)	(25% CR)	2.2 mg/kg/day x 4–6 wks, prednisone. Second course steroids. 38 patients completed course. 21 patients = 29% achieved M$_1$ marrow. Median duration CR (unmaintained) = 43 days. SWCCSG study.
44	391	244 (133 CR)	62 (34% CR)	2 mg/kg/day, prednisone. First course steroids. 330 patients had adequate trial.
47	77	59	77	2 mg/kg/day, prednisone. First course steroids. 59/77 = CR + GPR. (Children's Group A Study).
47	70	51	73	4 mg/kg/day, prednisone. First course steroids. 51/70 = CR + GPR. (Children's Group A Study).

ALL–AUL (cont.)

Ref #	# Pts Evaluated	# Pts Responding	% Response	Dose Schedule (PO in divided daily doses unless otherwise stated) and Remarks
47	24	6	25	8 mg/kg every other day, single dose, prednisone. First course steroids. 6/24 = CR + GPR. (Children's Group A Study).
47	16	3	19	16 mg/kg q 4 days, single dose, prednisone. First course steroids. 3/16 = CR + GPR. (Children's Group A Study).
	982	658	67	Total, overall response, daily treatment.
	892	601	67	Total, overall response to 1st course, daily treatment. Where information not given, data assumed to be for patients receiving a first course.
	90	57 (36 CR)	63 (40% CR)	Total, response to 2nd course, daily treatment. 40% "CR" is spuriously high by present standards (see discussion).
	863	391 (391 CR)	(45% CR)	Total, CR after 1st course, daily treatment.

AML–AMoL

Ref #	# Pts Evaluated	# Pts Responding	% Response	Dose Schedule (PO in divided daily doses unless otherwise stated) and Remarks
5	7	0		Varied (daily). 0/5 AML, 0/2 AMoL. Adults. Process felt to be accelerated in 4/7.
7	–	–		Cortisone, 1000 mg twice weekly for 4–6 wks. 2 CR, 10 PR of 18 adults with "acute leukemia" – no morphologic diagnosis.

AML-AMoL (cont.)

Ref #	# Pts Evaluated	# Pts Responding	% Response	Dose Schedule (PO in divided daily doses unless otherwise stated) and Remarks
8	-	-		Varied (daily). Review of literature. 5.5% CR in AML, 3.9% CR in AMoL reported overall.
9	-	-		250 mg/day. 2 CR, 1 PR in 6 patients over 30 on high-dose steroids. Questionable morphologic diagnosis.
11	11	5		1000 mg/day x 10, then tapered. (All patients also received KCl and antacids PO). 1 CR, 4 PR. High-dose prednisone. 3/18 had exacerbation of peptic ulcer disease, 1 had perforated ulcer. 3 patients appeared to have disease accelerated on steroid treatment.
15	10	4		1000 mg/day x 14, then tapered. 3 CR, 1 PR. One CR required 6 MP to obtain remission. Only 3 could tolerate full course. One patient on this high dose died of GI hemorrhage, possibly drug-related.
15	10	3		250 mg/day x 14, then tapered. "Medium" dose. One remission appeared only after "brief course" of 6 MP. 9/10 could tolerate full course. No clearly drug-related deaths. 2 CR, 1 PR.
15	10	4		100 mg/day x 14(?), then tapered. All PR.
16	6	2		500-1000 mg/day x 9-14. Both "CR". High-dose prednisolone.

AML–AMoL (cont.)

Ref #	# Pts Evaluated	# Pts Responding	% Response	Dose Schedule (PO in divided daily doses unless otherwise stated) and Remarks
25	50	0		"Conventional" daily low dose (?). 1 patient "improved". No discussion of dose regimen.
26	15	0		500 mg/day x 10. 0/12 AML, 0/3 AMoL. "Massive" steroids. 7/15 "made worse by treatment."
26	11	0		50 mg/day x 10. 0/5 AML, 0/6 AMoL. "Conventional" steroids.
27	47	3		1-3 mg/kg/day. 3 CR (PR not listed). "Conventional" steroids.
35	119	14	11.7	Varied, usually "conventional" low daily dose. 13/85 AML had hematologic remission. 1/34 AMoL responded. "Conventional" steroids.
42	39	6	15.3	(1) 40 mg/day; (2) 40 mg/day + 6 MP, 2.5 mg/kg/day; (3) 6 MP, 2.5 mg/kg/day.
47	14	3	21.4	(1) 2 mg/kg/day; (2) 4 mg/kg/day. Daily, low or moderate dose prednisone. Childhood AML. Response = CR or GPR.

CLL

Ref #	# Pts Evaluated	# Pts Responding	% Response	Dose Schedule (PO in divided daily doses unless otherwise stated) and Remarks
20	19	15		Prednisone, 40 mg/day or Cortisone, 200 mg/day; x ≥ 90 days.

CLL (cont.)

Ref #	# Pts Evaluated	# Pts Responding	% Response	Dose Schedule (PO in divided daily doses unless otherwise stated) and Remarks
22	18			Prednisone, 1 mg/kg/day x 4 wks, then 0.5 mg/kg/day x 4 wks, then 0.25 mg/kg/day x 4 wks, then discontinued. 10 CR, 2 PR of 14 with lymphadenopathy; 9 CR, 7 PR of 16 with hepatomegaly; 6 CR, 6 PR of 12 with splenomegaly. See discussion: responses short, infections frequent.
24	31	15		Prednisone 20-60 mg/day. 8 patients "benefit" (response >12 mo); 7 patients "some benefit."
28	20	20		Prednisone or prednisolone, 50-150 mg/day x 2-4 wks, then 5-25 mg/day maintenance. 7 "good", 13 "fair" responses. "Good" response = marked improvement for at least 6 mo (usually 6-12 mo).
37	12	7 (1 CR.)		Prednisone (or "equivalent") 60-145 mg/day x 1-5 wks, then 100-150 mg x 1 or 2 per wk, maintenance. Duration CR = 45+ mo. Range PR durations = 8+ to 36+ mo. See discussion.
	100	–	–	Total. 57/82 responses = 70%.

Lymphosarcoma

Ref #	# Pts Evaluated	# Pts Responding	% Response	Dose Schedule (PO in divided daily doses unless otherwise stated) and Remarks
28	20	17		Prednisone or prednisolone, 50–150 mg/day x 2–4 wks, then 5–25 mg/day maintenance. 10 "good", 7 "fair" responses. "Good" response = marked improvement for at least 6 mo (usually 6–12 mo).
30	22	15		(1) Prednisolone, 100–200 mg/day x 7–28. (2) Prednisolone, 1000 mg/day x 7, then 100–200 mg/day x 7–21. (3) Prednisolone, 30–60 mg/day. 1 regression >4 years duration.
37	2	1 (1 CR)		Prednisone (or "equivalent") 60–145 mg/day x 1–5 wks, then 100–150 mg x 1 or 2 per wk, maintenance. CR duration = 21+ mo. Other patient's condition "worse".
43	3	28	74	(1) Prednisone, 45–300 gm/day x $\geq$ 28 (25 patients). (2) Methylprednisolone or prednisolone, (7 patients), 60–600 mg/day x $\geq$ 28. (3) Cortisone, 100–200 mg/day x $\geq$ 28 (4 patients). [All patients received maintenance therapy if response occurred within 28 days]. 1 CR. Remissions of 4 wks and 7 mo duration. All patients refractory to radiation therapy and alkylating agents.
	$\overline{47}$	$\overline{35}$	74	Total.

Hodgkin's Disease

Ref #	# Pts Evaluated	# Pts Responding	% Response	Dose Schedule (PO in divided daily doses unless otherwise stated) and Remarks
30	22	9	41	(1) Prednisolone, 100–200 mg/day x 7–28. (2) Prednisolone, 1000 mg/day x 7, then 100–200 mg/day x 7–21. (3) Prednisolone, 30–60 mg/day. 4/53 in this series developed peptic ulcers on steroid treatment, one perforated. Adrenal insufficiency "not uncommon" in this series, treated successfully with cortisone or hydrocortisone.
43	24	16	67	(1) Prednisone, 45–300 mg/day x $\geq$ 28 (25 patients). (2) Methylprednisolone or prednisolone, 60–600 mg/day x $\geq$ 28 (7 patients). (3) Cortisone, 100–200 mg/day x $\geq$ 28 (4 patients). [All patients received maintenance therapy if response occurred within 28 days]. Median response = 10 wks; range, 3–104 wks. All patients refractory to radiation therapy and alkylating agents. Two responses >1 year's duration.
	$\overline{46}$	$\overline{25}$	54	Total.

Hodgkin's Disease (cont.)

Ref #	# Pts Evaluated	# Pts Responding	% Response	Dose Schedule (PO in divided daily doses unless otherwise stated) and Remarks
30	8	4		(1) Prednisolone, 100–200 mg/day x 7–28. (2) Prednisolone, 1000 mg/day x 7, then 100–200 mg/day x 7–21. (3) Prednisolone, 30–60 mg/day.
43	3	1		(1) Prednisone, 45–300 mg/day x $\geq$ 28 (25 patients). (2) Methylprednisolone or prednisolone, 60–600 mg/day x $\geq$ 28 (7 patients). (3) Cortisone, 100–200 mg/day x $\geq$ 28 (4 patients). [All patients received maintenance therapy if response occurred within 28 days]. Response duration 10 wks.

References

(1)   Dougherty, T., and White, A.   Influence of hormones on
        lymphoid tissue structure and function.   Role of pituitary
        adrenotrophic hromone in regulation of lymphocytes and other
        cellular elements of the blood.   Endocrinology 35: 1, 1944.

(2)   Dougherty, T., and White, A.   Evaluation of alterations
        produced in lymphoid tissue by pituitary adrenal cortical
        secretion.   J Lab Clin Med 32: 584, 1947.

(3)   Makman, M., Dvorkin, B., and White, A.   Influence of cortisol
        on the utilization of precursors of nucleic acids and protein
        by lymphoid cells in vitro.   J Biol Chem 243: 1485, 1968.

(4)   Werthamer, S., Hicks, C., and Arnaral, L.   Protein synthesis
        in human leukocytes and lymphocytes: 1.   Effect of steroid
        and sterols.   Blood 34: 348, 1969.

(5)   Rosenthal, M., Saunders, R., Schwartz, L., et al.   The use
        of adrenocorticotrophic hormone and cortisone in the treatment
        of leukemia and leukosarcoma.   Blood 6: 804, 1951.

(6)   Southam, C.   A study of the natural history of acute leukemia.
        Cancer 4: 39, 1951.

(7)   Bernard, J., and Deltour, G.   Les nouveaux traitements des
        leucoses: TEPA-GT 41 (Myleran)-6-mercaptopurine-mercapto-
        ethylamine: doses tres fortes de cortisone.   Sem hop de
        Paris 29: 3430, 1953.

(8)   Fessas, P., Wintrobe, M., Thompson, R., et al.   Treatment
        of acute leukemia with cortisone and corticotropin.   AMA
        Arch Intern Med 94: 384, 1954.

(9)   Hill, J., Marshall, G., and Falco, D.   Massive prednisone
        and prednisolone therapy in leukemia and lymphomas in adults.
        J Amer Geriat Soc 4: 627, 1956.

(10)   Hyman, C., and Sturgeon, P.   Prednisone therapy of acute
        lymphatic leukemia in children.   Cancer 9: 956, 1956.

(11)   Ranney, H., and Gellhorn, A.   The effect of massive prednisone
        and prednisolone therapy on acute leukemia and malignant
        lymphomas.   Amer J Med 22: 405, 1957.

(12)   Kofman, S., Garvin, J., Nagamani, D., et al.   Treatment
        of cerebral metastases from breast carcinoma with prednisolone.
        JAMA 163: 1473, 1957.

(13) Pierce, M. The acute leukemias of childhood. Pediat Clin N Amer 4: 497, 1957.

(14) Kofman, S., Nagamani, D., Buenger, R., et al. The use of prednisolone in the treatment of disseminated breast carcinoma. Cancer 11: 226, 1958.

(15) Granville, N., Rubio, F., Unugur, A., et al. Treatment of acute leukemia in adults with massive doses of prednisone and prednisolone. New Eng J Med 259: 207, 1958.

(16) Bouroncle, B., Doan, C., and Wiseman, B. Evaluation of the effect of massive prednisolone therapy in acute leukemia. Acta Haemat 22: 201, 1959.

(17) Lemon, H. Prednisone therapy of advanced mammary cancer. Cancer 12: 93, 1959.

(18) Hyman, C., Borda, E., Brubaker, C., et al. Prednisone in childhood leukemia. Comparison of interrupted with continuous therapy. Pediatrics 24: 1005, 1959.

(19) Wolf, J., Spear, P., Yessner, Y., et al. The sex hormones and cortisone in the treatment of inoperable bronchogenic carcinoma. In "Biological Activities of Steroids in Relation to Cancer", (Pincus, G., and Vollmer, E., eds.), Academic Press, New York, pp 413-426, 1960.

(20) Freymann, J., Vander, J., Burrell, S., et al. Corticosteroid therapy of chronic lymphocytic leukemia: a study of erythrocyte survival and leukocyte dynamics. Acta Un Int Cancr 16: 849, 1960.

(21) Freymann, J., Vander, J., Marler, E., et al. Corticosteroid therapy of chronic lymphocytic leukemia. Brit J Haemat 6: 303, 1960.

(22) Shaw, R., Boggs, D., Silberman, H., et al. A study of prednisone therapy in chronic lymphocytic leukemia. Blood 17: 182, 1961.

(23) Hume, R., Goldberg, A., and Garvic, D. Steroid therapy in multiple myeloma. Soct Med J 6: 189, 1961.

(24) Galton, D., Whiltshaw, E., Szur, L., et al. The use of chlorambucil and steroids in the treatment of chronic lymphocytic leukemia. Brit J Haemat 7: 73, 1961.

(25) Boggs, D., Wintrobe, M., and Cartwright, G. The acute
     leukemias. Medicine 41: 163, 1962.

(26) Shanbrom, E., and Miller, S. Critical evaluation of massive
     steroid therapy of acute leukemia. New Eng J Med 266: 1354,
     1962.

(27) Bernard, J., Boiron, M., Weil, M., et al. Etude de la remission
     complete des leucemies aigues. Nouv Rev France Hemat 2:
     195, 1962.

(28) Kyle, R., McParland, C., and Dameshek, W. Large doses of
     prednisone and prednisolone in the treatment of malignant
     lymphoproliferative disorders. Ann Intern Med 57: 717, 1962.

(29) Mass, R. A comparison of the effect of prednisone and a
     placebo in the treatment of multiple myeloma. Cancer Chemother
     Rep 16: 257, 1962.

(30) Kofman, S., Perlia, C., Boesen, E., et al. The role of
     corticosteroids in the treatment of malignant lymphomas. Cancer
     15: 338, 1962.

(31) Freireich, E., Gehan, E., Frei, E., et al. The effect of
     6-mercaptopurine on the duration of steroid-induced remissions
     in acute leukemia: a model for evaluation of other potentially
     useful therapy. Blood 21: 699, 1963.

(32) Colsky, J., Shnider, B., Jones, R., et al. A comparative
     study of 9α-bromo-11-β-ketoprogesterone and prednisolone in
     the treatment of advanced carcinoma of the female breast.
     Cancer 16: 502, 1963.

(33) Berkhirser, S. Epithelial proliferation of the lung associated
     with cortisone administration. Cancer 16: 1354, 1963.

(34) Stoll, B. Corticosteroids in therapy of advanced mammary cancer.
     Brit Med J 5351: 210, 1963.

(35) Roath, S., Israels, M., and Wilkinson, J. The acute leukemias:
     a study of 580 patients. Quarterly J Med 33: 257, 1964.

(36) Freckman, H., Fry, H., Mendez, F., et al. Chlorambucil-
     prednisolone therapy for disseminated breast carcinoma. JAMA
     189: 23, 1964.

(37) Burningham, R., Restrepo, A., Pugh, R., et al. Weekly high-dose
     glucocorticosteroid treatment of lymphocytic leukemias and
     lymphomas. New Eng J Med 270: 1160, 1964.

(38) Nissen-Meyer, R.   Endocrine treatment of breast cancer.
      Acta Un Int Cancr 20: 531, 1964.

(39) Vietti, T., Sullivan, M., Berry, D., et al.   The
      response of acute childhood leukemia to an initial and a
      second course of prednisone.   J Pediat 66: 18, 1965.

(40) Ruderman, N., and Hall, T.   Use of glucocorticoids in the
      palliative treatment of metastatic brain tumors.   Cancer 18:
      298, 1965.

(41) Mannheimer, I.   Hypercalcemia of breast cancer.   Management
      with corticosteroids.   Cancer 18: 679, 1965.

(42) Berlin, N., Andervont, H., Shimkin, M., et al.   Breast cancer.
      Combined clinical staff conference at the National Institutes
      of Health.   Ann Intern Med 63: 321, 1965.

(43) Working party on the evaluation of different methods of
      therapy in leukemia.   Brit Med J 1: 1383, 1966.

(44) Hall, T., Choi, O., Abadi, A., et al.   High-dose corticoid
      therapy in Hodgkin's disease and other lymphomas.   Ann Intern
      Med 66: 1144, 1967.

(45) Wolff, J., Brubaker, C., Murphy, M., et al.   Prednisone
      therapy of acute childhood leukemia: prognosis and duration
      of response in 330 treated patients.   J Pediat 70: 626, 1967.

(46) Salmon, S., Shadduck, R., and Schilling, A.   Intermittent
      high-dose prednisone (NSC 10023) therapy for multiple myeloma.
      Cancer Chemother Rep 51: 179, 1967.

(47) Moore, F., Woodrow, S., Aliapoulions, M., et al.   Medical
      progress.   Carcinoma of the breast.   A decade of new results
      with old concepts.   New Eng J Med 277: 460, 1967.

(48) Leikin, S., Brubaker, C., Hartmann, J., et al.   Varying
      prednisone dosage in remission induction of previously
      untreated childhood leukemia.   Cancer 21: 346, 1968.

Investigational Agents

1. 1,3-Bis(2-chloroethyl)-1-nitrosourea (BCNU)
2. Daunorubicin (Daunomycin, rubidomycin)
3. Dimethyl triazeno imidazole carboxamide
4. Streptozotocin
5. Dibromomannitol
6. Methyl-GAG
7. Mitomycin C
8. Streptonigrin
9. L-asparaginase

Investigational agents are drugs which are not commercially available to physicians through the use of prescriptions. The chemotherapy program of the National Cancer Institute has developed a series of compounds which are in various stages of clinical trial. Some of these have shown definite activity against some types of human cancer. This chapter will briefly review what information is currently available in the published literature about nine agents which fall into the category of clinically active.

1,3-Bis(2-chloroethyl)-1-nitrosourea (BCNU)

1,3-Bis(2-chloroethyl)-1-nitrosourea is a synthetic chemical agent with a wide range of effectiveness against experimental tumors.[1,2] The biochemical effects of BCNU have been studied in three experimental systems:[3] L1210 ascites cells in vitro; L1210 solid tumors and host livers in vivo; and plasmacytoma-1 and plasmacytoma-1/cyclophosphamide in vivo in hamsters. Formate-^{14}C and adenine-8-^{14}C were used as substrates in each of these systems, and DL-leucine-4,5-^{3}H was also used as a substrate for the L1210 solid tumors in vivo. The results show the incorporation of ^{14}C from formate-^{14}C into purines of both RNA and DNA inhibited by BCNU, with the inhibition of DNA synthesis being greater than that of RNA in the ascites cells and L1210 solid tumors. At high doses BCNU inhibits the synthesis of purine nucleotides. When the substrate is adenine-8-^{14}C, inhibition of DNA incorporation occurs in the absence of inhibition of incorporation into the RNA. These results are consistent with interference with the de novo synthesis of purine ribonucleotides to components of DNA. The inhibition of synthesis of DNA occurs in the absence of inhibition of protein as measured by the extent of fixation of ^{3}H from DL-leucine-4,5-[3]H.

The suggested loci of inhibition for BCNU are precisely the same as those considered in a study of the mode of action of nitrogen mustard, cyclophosphamide, triethylenemelamine, and triethyleneiminothiophosphoramide.[4] This similarity of inhibitory effects and the observed cross resistance of the hamster plasmocytoma-1/cyclophosphamide to BCNU and the above agents suggest strongly that BCNU functions as an alkylating agent, which has been suggested in other studies.[5]

It has been shown that certain N-alkyl-N-nitroso compounds serve as aklylating agents, such as N-methyl-N-nitrosourethan and N-methyl-N-nitroso-N-nitroguanidine.[6,7] Studies have shown that after the in vivo administration of N-nitrosodimethylamine, N-nitrosodiethylamine, and N-methyl-N-nitrosobutylamine, there is alkylation of the 7-position of guanine in the nucleic acids.[8,10]

The inhibition of the synthesis of DNA in vivo is a delayed one.[3] Since the biologic half-life of BCNU is probably less than one hour, the delayed inhibition is probably due to some phenomenon other than the progressive reaction of the agent with cellular constituents. It is reasonable to suggest that the delay results from the gradual disappearance of metabolically active materials whose further formation has been prevented by the drug.

BCNU has been compared with nitrogen mustard as to effects on the metabolism of protein, DNA and RNA (soluble and insoluble), glycolysis, the inhibitory action of sulfhydryl groups on the chemical agent's activity, and measurement of carbon-to-chlorine bonds.[11] There is no conclusive evidence to show that the mechanism of action of BCNU differs from that of HN_2 although some differences in response in the test system are seen. The alkylating nature of BCNU (as determined from the low order of reactivity of its carbon-to-chlorine bonds) is due to the **stability** of the carbon-to-chlorine bond, and it is felt that this may account, in part, for the drug's effectiveness, in that therapeutically effective long-term blood levels of the compound can be maintained.

In BCNU-treated Ehrlich ascites tumor cells investigated in vitro by measuring rates of incorporation of radioactive precursors into the acid-insoluble fraction of cells, there was a marked reduction in the rate of DNA synthesis, accompanied by an increase in the rate of RNA synthesis,[12] at concentrations compatible with those obtainable in vivo. Protein synthesis was affected only slightly at lower drug concentrations. At higher concentrations all three parameters are inhibited. The concentration of DNA in the cells is increased at low drug concentrations and depressed at higher levels.

The dose response curve of Saccharomyces cerevisiae to BCNU when compared to nitrogen mustard shows marked differences indicating different mechanisms of action.[11] Further suggestions of differences between the two regard antagonism by sulfhydryl groups of the inhibition mediated by each compound. The action of BCNU is overcome by sulfhydryl compounds to a much greater degree than that of HN_2.

BCNU is a potent inhibitor of nonproliferating microorganisms.[13] Comparative studies with 1-methyl-1-nitrosourea (NSC 23909) and 1-methyl-3-nitro-1-nitrosoguanidine show a similar mechanism of action. A strain of E. coli resistant to BCNU is cross-resistant to mitomycin C, porfiromycin, several alkylating agents, azaserine, DON, a terephthalanilide (NSC 60339), and ionizing and ultraviolet irradiation, but not to 6-mercaptopurine or methotrexate. Strains of E. coli resistant to mitomycin C, porfiromycin, nitrogen mustard, or azaserine were cross-resistant to BCNU.

BCNU has shown significant activity against advanced Hodgkin's disease. In DeVita's original study,[14] two partial responses were seen. This was followed by Lessner's study:[15] of 34 patients with Hodgkin's disease treated, 28 had Stage IVB disease and the remaining six had Stage IIIB disease. Of the 31 evaluable patients, there were four complete remissions, twelve partial remissions and one fair response. Objective improvement usually occurred within two to three weeks. The duration of remissions achieved varied from 38 days to more than a year. The dose used in most patients was 100 mg/m^2/day x 2, IV, with maintenance being repeat courses at 4-6 week intervals. The remissions achieved in Lessner's study are particularly striking since most patients were resistant to standard chemotherapeutic agents, including alkylating agents.

The toxicity seen included leukopenia and thrombocytopenia, noteworthy for its delayed onset, which is characteristic of the drug. The nadir of platelet and WBC counts may not be reached for 4-6 weeks after treatment. Other toxicity seen included nausea and vomiting, usually occurring about two hours after drug administration, transient local venous pain relieved by slowing the rate of administration, and a possibly drug-related maculopapular skin eruption in one patient.

Some activity has been seen in other lymphomas[8,9] but the number treated is small, and the degree of response does not seem equivalent to that seen in Hodgkin's disease.

Moertel et al[16] from the Mayo Clinic have used BCNU in 72 cases of advanced gastrointestinal cancer. Most patients were given a total dose of 300 mg/m^2 over three to five days and most patients had received prior chemotherapy with fluorinated pyrimidines. Nine of the 72 treated showed an objective response (12.5%) with the mean duration of response being 19 weeks and the range 8-32 weeks. No difference in response rates among specific tumor types was noted. Leukopenia below 4000 was seen in 66% of the patients receiving 300 mg/m^2 total dose, with a mean day of nadir of 38, and a range of 18-56 days. Thrombocytopenia was seen in 56%, with mean nadir on day 29 and the range 14-56 days. Nausea was seen in 57%, vomiting in 33% and jaundice was observed in 6%.

The authors compared their results to their own results with fluorinated pyrimidine therapy. In 290 patients treated with 5-FU, they obtained an objective regression rate of 17% with a mean duration of regression of 8 months, and in 150 patients treated with FUDR, a regression rate of 21% was seen with a mean duration of nine months. They did not state that fraction of patients treated with these agents had received previous chemotherapy; 60% of the BCNU-treated group had already received fluorinated pyrimidine therapy.

It is known that a relationship exists between relative water-lipoid solubility, degree of ionization, and the capacity of administered antileukemia agents to affect meningeal (intracerebrally inoculated) L1210 leukemia, as first elucidated by Rall and Zubrod. Only those agents which have a high degree of lipoid solubility and which are essentially not ionized have this ability, or the ability to cross the so-called "blood-brain barrier" in man. BCNU has shown this activity to an encouraging degree.[3,18,19]

In 1963 Rall reported giving BCNU to nine patients with ALL, five of whom had meningeal leukemia.[18] The dose range was 15-150 mg/m^2. No remissions were observed in the leukemic patients, but meningeal leukemia was controlled in all five patients. The predominant toxic effect was severe, prolonged bone marrow depression.

Some increase in BUN and SGOT was seen. Pulmonary edema and pleural effusion occurred in three patients. Other toxic signs included dysphagia, esophagitis, anorexia and diarrhea. It was felt that the drug was uniquely effective when given orally in clearing meningeal leukemia.

Iriarte et al reported on the use of BCNU in six children with central nervous system leukemia and eight children with solid tumors.[19] The dose was 150 mg/m^2 IV daily for three days. Three of the six children treated for CNS leukemia had a remission of their CNS manifestations. All three were experiencing their first episode of CNS involvement by acute lymphoblastic leukemia and their marrows were in remission when BCNU was given. One child had a clinical and marrow relapse shortly after his CNS leukemia improved. The three whose treatment failed had all had previous therapy for CNS involvement with either methotrexate intrathecally or radiation. This raises the question of cross resistance between BCNU and methotrexate and of previous radiation altering the effectiveness of BCNU.

Antitumor response was noted in three of the eight children with solid tumors. One was a Ewing's sarcoma, and there were two responses in neuroblastoma. Toxicity included immediate reactions such as nausea, vomiting, and flushing of the face in all patients. Diuresis was seen in one child. These immediate reactions were benign and self-limited. Thrombocytopenia was a constant feature in this series with onset at 14-23 days after therapy. Bone marrow examinations revealed a decrease in all of the cellular elements. The thrombocytopenia was a potentially reversible process with recovery 2-7 weeks after onset, but two children died from uncontrolled gastrointestinal hemorrhage. Peripheral white counts showed depressions of granulocytes and lymphocytes. Interestingly, no note was made in this series of delayed onset of toxicity.

BCNU has been shown to have exciting activity in preliminary studies in brain tumors. Walker and Hurwitz[20] have reported on 27 patients with primary or secondary brain tumors treated with 100-125 mg/m^2 for three successive days. Patients received from 300-975 mg/m^2 total dose. Treatment could be repeated at two to three month intervals dependent upon bone marrow depression. Significant initial clinical improvement was seen in 10 of 16 patients with intensive intermittent therapy, including dramatic improvement in hemiplegia and reversal of semi-coma in patients who failed to respond to high dose corticosteroid therapy.

Wilson and Boldrey[21] have reported on 36 primary brain tumors treated with BCNU. The majority of tumors had recurred after conventional surgery and irradiation, and without exception the tumors were large and readily demonstrated. Objective responses were seen in 7 of 18 glioblastomas, 4 of 6 astrocytomas and 4 of 8 miscellaneous tumors.

The Brain Tumor Study Group of the National Cancer Institute is currently evaluating the drug in a controlled fashion in glioblastomas.

References

(1)   Skipper, H.E., Schabel, F.M., Trader, M.W., and Thomson,
        J.R. Experimental evaluation of potential anticancer
        agents. VI. Anatomical distribution of leukemic cells and
        failure of chemotherapy. Cancer Res 21: 1154, 1964.

(2)   Skinner, W.W., Gren, H.F., Greene, M.O., Greenberg, J., and
        Baker, B.R. Potential anticancer agents. XXXI. The
        relationship of chemical structure to antileukemia activity
        with analogs of 1-methyl-1-nitro-1-nitrosoguanidine. J Med
        Pharm Chem 2: 299, 1960.

(3)   Wheeler, G.P., and Bowdon, B.J. Some of effects of BCNU on
        the synthesis of protein and nucleic acids. Cancer Res 25:
        1770, 1965.

(4)   Wheeler, G.P., and Alexander, J.A. Studies with mustards.
        VI. Effects of alkylating agents upon nucleic acid synthesis.
        Cancer Res 24: 1338, 1964.

(5)   Schabel, F.M., Johnston, T.P., McCaleb, G.S., Montgomery, J.A.,
        and Skipper, H.E. Experimental evaluation of potential
        anticancer agents. VIII. Effects of certain nitrosoureas on
        intracerebral L1210. Cancer Res 23: 725, 1963.

(6)   Henry, R.A. The reaction of amines with N-methyl-N-nitroso-
        N-nitroguanidine. J Amer Chem Soc 72: 3287, 1950.

(7)   Schoental, R., and Rive, D.J. The interaction of carcinogen-
        N-methyl-N-nitrosourethane with cystine in vitro. Biochem J
        87: 228, 1963.

(8)   Lee, K.Y., Lijinsky, W., and Magee, P.N. Methylation of
        ribonucleic acids of liver and other organs in different
        species treated with C^{14} and H^3 dimethylnitrosamines in vivo.
        J Natl Cancer Inst 32: 65, 1964.

(9)   Magee, P.N., and Farber, E. Toxic liver injury and
        carcinogenesis--methylation of rat liver nucleic acids by
        dimethylnitrosamine in vivo. Biochem J 83: 114, 1962.

(10)   Magee, P.N., and Lee, K.Y. Cellular injury and carcinogens--
        alkylation of ribonucleic acid of rat liver by diethylnitrosamine
        and N-butylmethylnitrosamine in vivo. Biochem J 91: 35, 1964.

(11)   Gale, G.R. Effect of BCNU on saccharomyces cerevisiae. Proc
        Soc Exp Biol Med 119(4): 1004, 1965.

(12) Gale, G.R. Effect of BCNU on Ehrlich ascites tumor cells.
      Biochem Pharmacol 15: 1707, 1965.

(13) Pittillo, R.F., Narkates, A.J., and Burns, J. Microbiological
      evaluation of BCNU. Cancer Res 24(7): 1222, 1964.

(14) DeVita, V., Carbone, P., Owens, A., et al. Clinical trials
      with BCNU. Cancer Res 25: 1876, 1965.

(15) Lessner, H. BCNU - Effects on advanced Hodgkin's disease
      and other neoplasia. Cancer 22: 2, 1968.

(16) Moertel, C., Reitemeier, R., and Hahn, G. Therapy of advanced
      gastrointestinal cancer with BCNU. Clin Pharm and Ther 9:
      652, 1968.

(17) Rall, D.P., and Zubrod, C.G. Mechanisms of drug absorption and
      excretion. Passage of drugs in and out of the CNS. Ann Rev
      Pharmacol 2: 109, 1962.

(18) Rall, D.P., Ben, M., and McCarthy, D.M. BCNU toxicity and
      initial clinical trial. Proc Amer Assoc Cancer Res 4(1): 55,
      1963.

(19) Iriarte, P.V., Hananian, J., and Cortner, J.A. CNS leukemia
      and solid tumors of childhood: treatment with BCNU. Cancer
      19: 1187, 1966.

(20) Walker, M.D., and Hurwitz, B.S. BCNU in the treatment of
      malignant brain tumor. In press, Cancer Chemother Rep 54,
      1970.

(21) Wilson, C.B., Boldrey, E.B., and Enot, K. BCNU in the
      treatment of brain tumors, In press, Cancer Chemother Rep
      54, 1970.

Daunorubicin (Daunomycin, rubidomycin)

Daunorubicin (DNR) is an antitumor antibiotic of the anthracycline group which was isolated from cultures of <u>Streptomyces peucetius</u> by Grein et al in 1963.[1] The structure of DNR consists of a pigmented aglycone (daunomycinone) in glycoside linkage with an amino sugar (daunosamine). The drug is classified as an anthracycline and is in the same group with rhodomycins, cinerubins, pyrromycins and rutilantins.[2]

The drug's mechanism of action involves the formation of complexes with DNA, thereby inhibiting both DNA replication and DNA-dependent synthesis of RNA. It is believed to bind to DNA by intercalation between base pairs.[3] The compound appears to have a greater effect on DNA than on RNA synthesis in mammalian cells [3,4] in contrast to actinomycin D which seems to be specific for DNA-directed RNA synthesis. In addition, DNR has the unique ability to delay the onset of mitosis in cells which have already synthesized DNA,[4] an observation which may be relevant to the scheduling of this agent when used in combination with others.

The most important toxicity associated with the use of DNR is suppression of the bone marrow. Such suppression is nearly always severe at therapeutically effective levels of the drug, and irreversible aplasia can occur, especially in leukemic patients. The frequency of this lethal complication ranges between 20 and 30% when a dose of 60 mg/m^2/day for three to five days is employed.[5]

The second major side effect which accompanies the use of DNR is cardiac damage, often lethal when it occurs. It was initially felt that the development of cardiac toxicity was related to the cumulative total dose given, and that doses <20 mg/kg were relatively "safe". Although this observation may still have some validity when dealing with children, it is important to note that a number of cases of cardiac toxicity have been seen in adults, especially patients over the age of 50, at total doses as low as 2 mg/kg (in other words, at any biologically effective dose of the drug).[6,8]

DNR has established activity against acute leukemia. Most of the published results are from the French literature, but studies soon to be published in the American literature will basically confirm the European experience.

The results against acute myelogenous leukemia from the French literature are quite impressive.[5,9,10,11] A total of 135 patients have been treated with regimens such as 2 mg/kg/day x 3-5,[5] or 2 mg/kg on day 1, repeat dose on day 4 at 1-2 mg/kg, depending on WBC count, with the remainder of the schedule being intermittent.[9] The results were 53 patients achieving complete remission (32%) and 19 achieving PR for a total response rate of 53%.

In acute lymphocytic leukemia the results are not quite as impressive because of the availability of many other agents with comparable or better activity and greater therapeutic indices. The published results in ALL are outlined on the following page.

Investigator	Schedule	# Pts Evaluated	# Pts CR	# Pts PR	# CR + PR
Holton et al (12)	25 mg/m²/day x 3, off 4 days; then 25 mg/m²/day x 3, off 4 days; then weekly, 25 mg/m²	23	0	3	3
Tan et al (13)	1 mg/kg/day x 4-5, off 3 days; then 1.5 mg/kg x 1, off 3 days; then 1-2 mg/kg/wk	28	2	13	15
Mathe (14)	30 mg/m²/day x 3-5, off 5 days and repeat course as tolerated, up to a total of 2-3 courses	13	3	2	5
Jones (15)	45 mg/m²/day x 5	18	7	-	7
Total		82	12 (15%)	18 (22%)	30 (37%)

Current studies include utilizing DNR in combination with vincristine and prednisone.

DNR has some activity in childhood solid tumors. Tan et al[13] reported 6 PR in 18 children treated, the median duration of remission being 3 months.

Slight activity has also been reported in lymphoma. Mathe[14] has reported 1 CR and 4 PR in 20 patients with Hodgkin's disease treated at a dosage of 30 mg/m^2/day x 3-5, then off 5 days, repeating the course as tolerated. The CR lasted 2 months and 10/20 developed marrow aplasia.

The use of DNR against adult solid tumors has been minimal.

References

(1)   Grein, A., Spalla, C., Di Marco, A. Descrizione e
       classificazione di un attimomicete (Streptomyces peucetius
       sp nova) produttoce di una sostaviza ad attivata
       antitumorale--la daunomicina. Giorn Microbiol 11: 109, 1963.

(2)   Di Marco, A., Gaetani, M., Dorigotti, L., et al. Daunomycin,
       a new antibiotic of the rhodomycin group. Nature 201: 706,
       1964.

(3)   Calendi, E., Di Marco, A., Reggiani, B., et al. On physico-
       chemical interactions between daunomycin and nucleic acids.
       Biochim Biophys Acta 103: 25, 1965.

(4)   Whang-Pang, J., Leventhal, B., Adamson, J., et al. The effect
       of daunomycin on human cells in vivo and in vitro. Cancer
       23: 113, 1969.

(5)   Boiron, M., Jacquillat, C., Weil, M., et al. Daunorubicin
       in the treatment of acute myelocytic leukemia. Lancet 1:
       330, 1969.

(6)   Bonadonna, G., and Monfardini, S. Cardiac toxicity of
       daunorubicin. Lancet 1: 837, 1969.

(7)   Malpas, J.S., and Bodley Scott, A. Rubidomycin in acute
       leukemia in adults. Brit Med J 3: 227, 1968.

(8)   Malpos, J.S., and Bodley Scott, A. Daunorubicin in acute
       myelocytic leukemia. Lancet 1: 469, 1969.

(9)   Organisation Europienne de Recherche sur le traitement du
       Cancer. (OERTC). Essai de traitement des leucemies aigues
       granulocytaires par la daunomycine. Europ J Cancer 5: 339, 1969.

(10)   Bernard, J., et al. Experimental treatment of acute
       lymphoblastic and myeloblastic leukemias with a new antibiotic
       --rubidomycin. Presse Med 75: 951, 1967.

(11)   Bernard, J. Acute leukemia treatment. Cancer Res 26: 2565,
       1967.

(12)   Mathe, G., Schwartzenberg, L., Schneider, M., et al. Acute
       lymphoblastic leukemia treated with a combination of prednisone,
       vincristine, and rubidomycin. Value of pathogen-free rooms.
       Lancet 2: 380, 1967.

(13)   Holton, C., Lonsdale, D., Nora, A., et al. Clinical study
        of daunomycin (NSC 82151) in children with acute leukemia.
        Cancer 22: 1014, 1968.

(14)   Tan, C., Tasaka, H., Yu, K., et al. Daunomycin, an antitumor
        antibiotic, in the treatment of neoplastic disease. Cancer
        20: 333, 1967.

(15)   Mathe, G. Essai de traitement des leucemies aigues et de la
        maladie de Hodgkin par la rubidomycine seule ou en
        association. Sem Hop Paris 43: 2108, 1967.

(16)   Jones, B. Daunorubicin vs daunorubicin and prednisone vs
        daunorubicin and vincristine and prednisone in resistant
        childhood leukemia. Proc Am Assoc Cancer Res 11: 41, 1970.

Dimethyl triazeno imidazole carboxamide

5-(3,3-dimethyl-1-triazeno)-imidazole-4-carboxamide (DTIC, DIC, imidazole carboxamide) is a structural analogue of 5-aminoimidazole-4-carboxamide, which is a precursor in de novo purine biosynthesis. Its mechanism of action is unknown but speculation has centered around possible roles as either an alkylating agent or a purine antimetabolite.[1,5]

Clinical studies have shown this drug to have significant activity against malignant melanoma. Luce et al reported on the treatment of 110 patients with melanoma with DTIC.[6] Most patients were treated at doses of 250 mg/m^2/day x 5, IV, with repeat courses given at 3 week intervals, and a minimum of 2 treatment courses constituting an adequate trial. Sixteen partial and 5 complete responses occurred in the 110 patients.

Toxicity seen included nausea and vomiting which usually began 1-3 hours after drug administration and was most severe after the first dose, and myelosuppression which included leukopenia and thrombocytopenia. Other side effects seen less frequently were pain along the injection vein, a "flu"-like syndrome and hepatotoxicity.

Nathanson has reported treating melanoma at dosages of 2.0 and 4.5 mg/kg/day x 10 intravenously.[7] Four of 11 patients given the low dose (2.0 mg/kg) and four of 18 patients on the high dose (4.5 mg/kg) were observed to undergo partial objective responses persisting for one month or more.

Skibba et al have reported 5 of 15 patients with disseminated or recurrent malignant melanoma having objective responses to DTIC therapy at a dosage of 4.5 mg/kg/day x 10 intravenously.[8] Three of these responding patients had complete disappearance of all radiographic and visible or palpable evidence of disease for 9.9 and 19+ months. Toxicity was manifested by nausea and vomiting, leukopenia and thrombocytopenia.

The overall response rate in melanoma in the reported literature is 22% (34/154) and compares favorably with that of any other agent used against this disease.

Reported studies in other diseases have been meager. Luce[6] et al reported five of 23 patients (22%) with various sarcomas responding to drug. One of 3 patients who had squamous cell carcinoma of the lung and the one patient with oat cell carcinoma of the lung responded to DTIC in Luce's series.

References

(1)   Shealy, Y.F., and Krauth, C.A. Complete inhibition of
       mouse leukemia L1210 by 5-[3,3-bis(2-chloroethyl)-1-
       triazeno] imidazole-4-carboxamide (NSC 82196). Nature 210:
       208, 1966.

(2)   Shealy, Y.F., Krauth, C.A., Holum, L.B., et al. Synthesis
       and properties of the antileukemic agent 5-[3,3-bis(2-
       chloroethyl)-1-triazeno] imidazole-4-carboxamide. J Pharm
       Sci 57: 83, 1968.

(3)   Shealy, Y.F., Montgomery, J.A., and Laster, W.R., Jr.
       Antitumor activity of triazeno-imidazoles. Biochem
       Pharmacol 11: 674, 1962.

(4)   Hano, K., Alsashi, A., Yamamoto, J., et al. Further
       investigation on the carcinostatic activity of 4-amino-
       imidazole-5-carboxamide derivatives: structure activity
       relationship. GANN 59: 207, 1968.

(5)   Hano, K., Alsashi, A., Suzuki, Y., et al. Pharmacologic
       studies on 4(or 5)-aminoimidazole-5 (or 4)-carboxamide (AICA)
       derivatives. Jap J Pharmacol 17: 668, 1967.

(6)   Luce, J.K., Thurman, W.G., Isaacs, B.L., et al. Clinical
       trials with the antitumor agent 5-(3,3-dimethyl-1-triazeno)-
       imidazole-4-carboxamide (NSC 45388). Cancer Chemother Rep
       54(2): 119, 1970.

(7)   Nathanson, L. The effectiveness of 5(or 4)-(3,3-dimethyl-1-
       triazeno)-imidazole-(4 or 5)-carboxamide (DTIC, NSC 45388).
       Internat Malignant Melanoma Proc 6th Internat Congress of
       Chemother, Tokyo, p 348, 1969.

(8)   Skibba, J.L., Ramirez, G., Beal, D.D., et al. Preliminary
       clinical trial and the physiologic disposition of 4(5)-
       (3,3-dimethyl-1-triazeno) imidazole-5(4)-carboxamide in man.
       Cancer Res 29: 1944, 1969.

Streptozotocin

Streptozotocin is an antibiotic derived from Streptomyces acromogenes.[1] It has been shown to inhibit synthesis of DNA in Escherichia coli without markedly inhibiting synthesis of RNA or protein.[2] Its mechanism of action is not yet defined.

Streptozotocin is diabetogenic in animals but does not appear to be so in man. In the rat pancreas, the drug causes dilatation of the endoplasmic reticulum, swollen mitochondria and degranulation in the beta cells. In animals it has been shown that nicotinamide can protect against the diabetogenic effect.[3]

Recently, clinical activity has been shown against functional malignant pancreatic islet cell tumors.

Murray-Lyon[4] et al have reported on the treatment of a patient who had a malignant pancreatic islet cell tumor, was suffering from recurrent episodes of hypoglycemia and was unable to tolerate therapy with diazoxide. She was initially given 1.5 gm of streptozotocin IV, felt nauseated for some hours, and had a drop in blood sugar to 45 mg/100 ml 2 hours after the injection. Her condition then began to improve, however, and no more episodes of hypoglycemia occurred. Three weeks later a dose of 3 gm streptozotocin was given, followed by 4 gm after 3 more weeks: "no new side effects were encountered. After the second dose it was possible to leave the patient 8 hours overnight without giving her carbohydrate. At this time the liver [which had been involved by metastases] was considerably smaller and this was confirmed by a repeat liver scan which also showed considerable improvement in the uptake of colloid with diminution in the size of the filling defects." The patient remained asymptomatic and had gained 11 kg when seen for follow-up examination 4 months after starting streptozotocin therapy. The total dose of streptozotocin given in the 3 injections over 6 weeks was 8.5 gm (about 170 mg/kg). The patient's islet cell tumor appeared to be responsible for elevated blood levels of glucagon and gastrin, in addition to insulin. The levels of all of these dropped with streptozotocin therapy.

More recently, Sadoff[5] has studied the effects of streptozotocin in another patient with islet cell carcinoma. This patient had had initial surgical resection and had received 5-FU, nitrogen mustard, hydroxyurea, and a combination of methotrexate and actinomycin D. There was no objective response to these agents. The patient then was given tubercidin (another investigational agent) for 3 months to a total dose of 165 mg, and responded initially by a transient decrease in serum insulin and hypoglycemic episodes. During the last month of tubercidin therapy serum insulin levels rose rapidly and hepatic angiography demonstrated increasing metastases. She was given diazoxide, 100 mg twice daily, but was unable to tolerate it because of severe vomiting. At the time of admission for streptozotocin therapy, her blood sugar was 45 mg/100 ml and her serum insulin level was 170 microunits/ml. She was given 1 gm of streptozotocin daily by rapid push through an indwelling arterial catheter just above the celiac axis, for 10 consecutive days (total dose 10 gm). Treatment was stopped on day 10 because of progressive vomiting. From day 5 of treatment to day 8 the patient had marked lessening of hypoglycemic symptoms. Three days after the end of treatment, however, her hypoglycemic symptoms returned, the blood sugar was 45 mg/100 ml, and serum insulin was 300 microunits/ml. At the same time, she had glycosuria, and further investigation of the patient for renal tubular defects revealed marked aminoaciduria. She also had acidosis, with a serum bicarbonate level of 12 mEq/liter, chloride 113, and strongly alkaline urine pH. The renal tubular acidosis persisted, but was controlled with 120 gm of supplemental sodium bicarbonate daily. Meanwhile, the hypoglycemic symptoms diminished gradually, while vomiting continued for 3 weeks after therapy. The patient became dehydrated and required IV fluid therapy, but recovered, although the renal tubular defect persisted.

Six weeks after the completion of the 10-day course of streptozotocin, the patient's blood sugar level was 83 mg/100 ml and the serum insulin had fallen to 37 microunits/ml. Two months after treatment she had no hypoglycemic symptoms or vomiting, and had a diabetic-appearing glucose tolerance test. She had returned to full-time employment by 4 months after streptozotocin therapy. Clinical diabetes did not develop.

A liver scan showed regression of tumor metastases. Determinations of gastrin and glycagon serum activity were not done. The serum insulin level 2 months after treatment was 15 microunits/ml (normal = 4.25 microunits/ml).

In addition to the persistent renal tubular acidosis, aminoaciduria, and glycosuria, which were apparently induced in this patient by streptozotocin, Sadoff noted persistent elevation of the serum alkaline phosphatase and SGOT levels and reversal of the ablumin/globulin ratio, suggesting a hepatotoxic effect of the drug. Sadoff also commented on the similarity between the streptozotocin-induced renal changes and the changes seen in type I glycogen storage disease (de Toni-Fanconi syndrome): in both states, there is glycosuria ketonuria, aminoaciduria, and acidosis. Glycogen deposits are present in the proximal tubules in the glycogen storage disease and in rats treated with streptozotocin. Glucose 6-phosphatase activity is usually absent in the renal tubules of affected children. This poses the question of whether streptozotocin affects the metabolism of glucose 6-phosphatase, which is as yet unanswered.

Additional cases have been reported confirming the activity of streptozotocin in this rare tumor. Evaluation of this drug in other more common tumor types is currently ongoing.

References

(1)   Herr, R.R., Jahnke, H.K., and Argoudelis, A.D. Structure of
       streptozotocin. J Amer Chem Soc 89: 4808, 1967.

(2)   Heinemann, B., and Howard, A.J. Effect of compounds with
       both antitumor and bacteriophage-inducing activities on
       E. coli nucleic acid synthesis. Antimicrob Agents Chemother
       5: 488, 1965.

(3)   Schein, P.S., Cooney, D.A., and Varnon, M.L. The use of
       nicotinamide to modify the toxicity of streptozotocin diabetes
       without loss of antitumor activity. Cancer Res 27: 2324,
       1967.

(4)   Murray-Lyon, I.M., Eddlesten, A.L., Williams, R., et al.
       Treatment of multiple-hormone-producing malignant islet-cell
       tumor with streptozotocin. Lancet 895, 1968.

(5)   Sadoff, L. Effects of streptozotocin in a patient with
       islet-cell sarcinoma. Diabetes 18: 675, 1969.

Dibromomannitol

Dibromomannitol (DBM) is an alpha, omega-substituted hexitol chosen for clinical trial on the basis of its activity against the Walker 256 carcinosarcoma in rats and its record of clinical effectiveness against chronic myelogenous leukemia, in European studies.[1,8]

The mechanism of action of DBM is a subject of controversy in the literature. It probably functions as a non-classial alkylating agent. Csanyi and Halasz[9] developed a DBM-resistant line of Yoshida sarcoma and found it resistant to various alkylating agents. Institoris[10,12] has pointed out that the picture of clinical resistance in cells appears to resemble those of the antimetabolites, and not that of busulfan. He has also shown a difference in drug distribution and excretion between DBM and busulfan. The bromide group of DBM is slowly detected by a reaction taking place in the tissues and appears subsequently in the urine covalently bonded to biotransformation products rather than as an anion. Busulfan, on the other hand, behaves as a classical alkylating agent, as its functional group (methane sulfonate) is rapidly detached as an anion by the alkylating reaction with nucleophilic reactive groups in the tissues resulting in an early peak in, and rapid disappearance from, the blood.

DBM is an agent of proven clinical usefulness in the treatment of chronic myelogenous leukemia. The largest available series is that of Eckhardt from the State Oncological Institute at Budapest.[1] He induced remissions with a daily dose of 5 mg/kg to a total dose of 10-15 grams and then used a maintenance dose of 5-10 mg/kg/wk. In 29 previously untreated patients, complete remission was obtained in 22 (76%) and partial remissions in the remaining seven. Of 21 patients previously treated with busulfan, mannitol myleran and/or radiation, CR was obtained in 14 (67%) and PR in 5 with 2 failures.

The only clinical report in the literature from this country is by Casazza, Cahn and Carbone[13] who treated 15 patients with the stable form of CML at an initial dosage of DBM of 250 mg/day orally, decreasing to 250 mg every 2 or 3 days after the WBC dropped to 20,000. Ten of the 15 patients had received prior therapy. At the end of 12 weeks of treatment, 12/15 patients (80%) were in remission, 2 in complete remission and 10 in partial remission. The only toxic effects were leukopenia and thrombocytopenia.

The question as to whether DBM has any superiority to busulfan is currently being investigated. DBM has not received a trial in any diseases except CML in this country. The Hungarians have reported some activity in polycythemia vera.[14]

References

(1)   Eckhardt, S. Chronic myelogenous leukemia and its
        treatment with dibromomannitol. 5th Internat Congress of
        Chemother, Vienna, Austria, 3: 259, 1967.

(2)   Bohnel, J., and Stacher, A. The effect of a new cytosatic
        (myelobromol) in chronic myeloid leukemia. Wien Med Wschr
        117: 535, 1967.

(3)   Mathe, G., Schneider, M., Cottan, A., et al. Experiment
        of treating chronic myeloid leukemia with dibromomannitol.
        Presse Med 72: 2135, 1964.

(4)   Petranyi, G., and Bobory, J. Treatment of chronic myeloid
        leukemia with myelobromol. Ther Hung 14: 136, 1966.

(5)   Csomor, G. Experiences with myelobromol/DBM in chronic
        myelocytic leukemia. Gyoyrpzereink 16: 261, 1965.

(6)   Cerny, V., Ujhazy, V., Sander, L., et al. Clinical
        application of myelobromol in chronic myeloses. Neoplasma
        13: 177, 1966.

(7)   Kassirskii, I.A., and Volkova, M.A. Myelosan treatment of
        chronic myeloid leukemia. Ter Arkh 39: 1967.

(8)   Cherntsova, T.A., and Susoeva, V.M. Clinical experience
        with myelobromol in the treatment of chronic myeloid leukemia.
        Hematologia (Budapest) 1: 61, 1967.

(9)   Csanyi, E., and Halasz, M. Cross-resistance studies on 1,6-
        dibromo-dideoxy-D-mannitol (DBM)-resistant Yoshida S.C.
        sarcoma. Brit J Cancer 21: 353, 1967.

(10)   Institoris, L., et al. Comparative data on the action mechanism
        of 1,6-dibromo-1,6-dideoxy-D-mannitol and 1,4-dimethanesulfonyl-
        oxy-butane. Arzneimittelforschung 16: 45, 1966.

(11)   Institoris, L., Horuath, I.P., Pethes, G., et al. Metabolic
        pathway of cytostatic dibromohexitols. Cancer Chemother Rep
        51: 261, 1967.

(12)   Institoris, L., Horvath, I.P., Csanyl, E., et al. Study on
        the distribution and metabolism of Br^{82}-labelled DBM in
        normal and tumor-bearing rats. Neoplasma 11: 245, 1964.

(13)   Casazza, A.R., Cahn, E.L., and Carbone, P.P. Preliminary
        studies with dibromomannitol (NSC 94100) in patients with

chronic myelogenous leukemia. Cancer Chemother Rep 51: 91, 1967.

(14)   Szentklaray, J., and Hartman, E. Treatment of polycythemia vera with myelobromol. Ther Hung 14: 143, 1966.

Methyl-GAG

Methylglyoxal-bis-guanylhydrazone (methyl-GAG) is a synthetic compound whose mechanism of action is uncertain; a variety of effects and possible sites of action in tissue have been described. These include inhibition of DNA synthesis through binding to nucleic acids[1] and uncoupling of the phosphorylation of mitochondria. Methyl-GAG selectively inhibits the incorporation of acetate into lipid via this effect on the mitochondria, and inhibition of lipid synthesis may be a factor in its antitumor effect.[2] The drug inhibits anaerobic glycolysis partially in both normal and leukemic bone marrow cells with no differential inhibition being observed.[3] Adamson has shown that L1210 tumors resistant to methyl-GAG had a diminished capacity to bind the drug and in one case, also diminished permeability to it.[4]

The toxicity associated with the clinical use of methyl-GAG has been dramatic, severe, and sometimes catastrophic. When administered on a daily schedule at a high enough dose to be effective, the drug often produces diffuse mucositis of the GI tract (manifesting as stomatitis, laryngitis, diarrhea, etc). Later side effects include myelosuppression which may be severe and irreversible, and the development of extremely painful skin manifestations, especially furunculosis and desquamation of the feet; the latter may not appear until after the course of therapy is completed. The incidence of toxicity is strikingly related to the length of continued drug administration.

Methyl-GAG has received extensive clinical evaluation in only one type of human malignancy: acute myelocytic leukemia. A summary of the published results in this disease is given on the following page.

Investigator	Schedule	# Pts Evaluated	# CR	# PR	% CR	% Response
Mathe[5]	1.5-2.5 mg/kg/day to a mean total dose of 1.6 gm IV	12	4	-	33	-
Regelson & Holland[6]	5 mg/kg/day to response or limiting toxicity (mean duration treatment = 10 days)	15	0	4	0	27
Shaw & Creger[7]	150 mg/m^2/day to response or limiting toxicity	15	1	3	7	27
Levin, Henderson & Karon[8]	<100 mg/m^2/day	4	0	1	0	25
	100-125 mg/m^2/day	22	4	6	18	45
	126-160 mg/m^2/day	31	14	3	45	55
	>160 mg/m^2/day	11	1	3	9	36
Schwartzenberg[9]	30-400 mg/day IV	15	4	1	27	33
Total		125	28	21	22	39

The current feeling about this compound is that the toxicity outweighs most of the potential therapeutic value.

References

(1)   Sartorelli, A.   Complex formation with DNA and inhibition
       of nucleic acid synthesis by methyl-GAG.   Biochim Biophys Acta
       103: 174, 1965.

(2)   Pine, M., and De Paolo, J.   The antimitochondrial action of
       2-chloro-4',4-bis (2-imidazolin-2-yl) terephthalanilide and
       methylglyoxal bis (guanylhydrazone).   Cancer Res 26: 18, 1966.

(3)   Kolmeier, K.   Anaerobic glycolysis in normal and leukemic
       bone marrow leukocytes.   Effect of methyl-GAG.   Cancer 19:
       1195, 1966.

(4)   Adamson, B.   Studies of resistance to methyl-GAG and its
       metabolic fate in rodents.   (Abstract).   Excerpta Medica
       1642, 1967.

(5)   Mathe, G., et al.   Essai de traitement des leucemies aigues
       par la methylglyoxal-bis (guanylhydrazone).   Rev Franc Etud
       Clin Biol 8: 1035, 1963.

(6)   Regelson, W., and Holland, J.   Clinical experience with
       methylglyoxal bis (guanylhydrazone) dihydrochloride:
       a new agent with clinical activity in acute myelocytic
       leukemia and the lymphomas.   Cancer Chemother Rep 27: 15,
       1963.

(7)   Shaw, R., and Greger, W.   Methylglyoxal bis (guanylhydrazone),
       NSC 32946, in the treatment of acute myeloblastic and
       monoblastic leukemia in adults.   Cancer Chemother Rep 36:
       63, 1964.

(8)   Levin, R., Henderson, E., Karon, M., et al.   Treatment of
       acute leukemia with methylglyoxal-bis-guanylhydrazone
       (methyl-GAG).   Clin Pharm Ther 6: 31, 1965.

(9)   Schwarzenberg, L.   Treatment of acute leukemia by methyl-GAG
       and its combination with 2-hydroxystilbamidine.   Sem Hop Paris
       42: 2955, 1966.

Mitomycin C

Mitomycin C is an antibiotic isolated from the broth of
Streptomyces caespitosus.[1] It selectively inhibits the synthesis
of DNA in susceptible organisms and leads to extensive breakdown
of the DNA in some, but not in all.[2] At high levels of antibiotic,
cellular RNA and protein synthesis are also suppressed. The
biologic effects of Mitomycin C and the presence of an aziridine
ring in its structure suggest that its mechanism of action is
similar to that of the alkylating agents. The drug may be inert
until activated in vivo by a reductive step which unmasks the
alkylating aziridine ring. The lethal effects are presumably due
to changes in the structure of DNA preventing its replication and
induced by the activated alkylating agent.

Mitomycin C has been in clinical trial in the United States
since 1959 when reported of activity from Japan excited interest.
In 1960, Frank and Osterberg evaluated the Japanese reports.[3]
They found that in only 351 patients was it possible to determine
whether the patient did or did not present objective evidence of
chemotherapeutic effect. The usual dose given was 1-2 mg daily for
20-40 days. By established criteria 130/351 (37%) patients showed
objective evidence of response. The greatest response rate occurred
in patients with chronic myelogenous leukemia (10/11), certain
epithelial tumors, chorioepithelioma, reticulum cell sarcoma (11/25)
and seminoma. Responses of other tumors were 11/26 in breast
cancer and 9/24 in lung tumors.

Clinically in this country there is an extensive experience
reported in the literature and this is outlined on the following
page.

Study	Dose Regimen	# Evaluable Pts	# Pts Responded	%
Bross[4]	0.05 mg/kg/day IV x 6	134	28	21
Reitmeier[5]	0.05 mg/kg every other day to 50 mg or toxicity	39	6	15.4
	0.05 mg/kg/day over 40 days (50 mg total)	13	2	15
Watne[6]	0.125-0.175 mg/kg/day x 5	24	8	33
Ausman[7]	50 mg total	201	50	25
Jones[8]	50 mg total in no more than 60 days	120	21	17.5
	10-250 µg/kg/day till toxicity			
Ferguson & Humphrey[9]	50 µg/kg/day x 6 then 50 µg/kg/day every other day till toxicity	21	1	5
Evans[10]	0.4-1.0 mg/kg IV over 2-10 days	57	8	14
Bergsagel[11,12]	0.5 mg/kg IV x 10 0.02 mg/kg/day x 25	13	0	0
Miller[13]	24 hour infusion 1.1-2.1 mg/kg 3-12 days	30	17	56
Manheimer[14]	50-100 µg/kg/day IV till toxicity	46	14	30

The toxicity with mitomycin C includes severe bone marrow depression and gastrointestinal disturbances. Its narrow therapeutic index, a high degree of toxicity being associated with effectiveness, has made it a difficult compound to handle.

Activity of some sort has been seen in almost all the tumors in which it has been adequately tried. The study of Reitemeier and Moertel[5] was entirely in gastrointestinal cancer and showed activity in the range of 15% but at a prohibitively high cost in toxicity. Manheimer saw responses in 7/28 gastrointestinal tumors and Miller and Sullivan in 8/52.

A breakdown of responses seen in 14 tumor types from the literature, including Frank and Osterberg's review of the Japanese literature, is given below:

	Total Evaluable	Total Response	% Responses
	1,040	285	28%
Colon	58	16	27
Breast	70	29	41
Lung	56	16	29
Stomach	143	46	32
Pancreas	18	6	33
Osteogenic sarcoma	22	6	28
Hodgkin's disease	19	8	42
Lymphoma	32	15	47
Rhabdomyosarcoma	11	4	36
Melanoma	8	1	12
Myeloma	15	0	0
Head and neck	11	2	18
Liver	8	3	37
Chronic myelogenous leukemia	16	15	93

Despite this activity, Mitomycin C is infrequently used today due to its severe toxic potential.

References

(1)   Wakaki et al. Isolation of new fractions of antitumor
        Mitomycins. Antibiot Chemother 8: 228, 1958.

(2)   Goldberg, I.H. Mode of action of antibiotics. II. Drugs
        affecting nucleic acid and protein synthesis. Amer J Med
        39: 722, 1965.

(3)   Frank, W., and Osterberg, A.E. Mitomycin C--an evaluation
        of the Japanese reports. Cancer Chemother Rep 9: 114, 1960

(4)   Bross, I.D., Rimm, A.A., Sleek, N.H., Ausman, R.K., and
        Jones, R. Is toxicity really necessary? Cancer 19: 1785,
        1966.

(5)   Reitemeier, R.J., Moertel, C.G., and Hahn, R.G. Mitomycin
        C therapy of advanced gastrointestinal adenocarcinoma.
        Comparison of short and long term schedules. Proc Amer
        Assoc Cancer Res 8: 56 (# 220), 1967.

(6)   Watne, A.L., Moore, D., and Gorgun, B. Solid tumor
        chemotherapy with Mitomycin C. Proc Amer Assoc Cancer Res
        8: 71 (# 279), 1967.

(7)   Ausman, R.K. Mitomycin C--Phase II broad spectrum trial.
        Proc Amer Assoc Cancer Res 6: 30 (# 7), 1965.

(8)   Jones, R., Jr. Mitomycin C: A preliminary report of
        studies of human pharmacology and initial therapeutic trial.
        Cancer Chemother Rep 2: 3, 1959.

(9)   Ferguson, D., and Humphrey, E. Mitomycin C. Cancer Chemother
        Rep 8: 154, 1960.

(10)   Evans, A.E. Mitomycin C. Cancer Chemother Rep 14: 1, 1961.

(11)   Bergsagel, D.E., Ross, S.W., and Davis, P. Evaluation of
        new chemotherapeutic agents in the treatment of multiple
        myeloma. II. Mitomycin C. Cancer Chemother Rep 21: 75, 1962.

(12)   Bergsagel, D.E. Phase II trials of Mitomycin C, AB-100
        NSC 1026, L-sarcolysin, and meta-sarcolysin in the treatment
        of multiple myeloma. Cancer Chemother Rep 16: 261, 1962.

(13)   Miller, E., Sullivan, R.D., and Chryssochoos, T. The clinical
        effects of Mitomycin C by continuous intravenous administration.
        Cancer Chemother Rep 21: 129, 1962.

(14)   Manheimer, L.H., and Vital, J. Mitomycin C in the therapy of
        far advanced malignant tumors. Cancer 19: 207, 1966.

Streptonigrin

Streptonigrin is an antitumor antibiotic derived from
Streptomyces flocaulus.[1] Its clinical studies date back to 1961.
Levine and Borthwick have shown that the drug has a preferential
deleterious action on bacterial DNA synthesis with net DNA
synthesis practically ceasing in the presence of appropriate
concentrations while synthesis of protein and RNA proceeds.[2,3]
When used in extreme dilutions, it inhibits the mitosis of cultured
human leukocytes and causes extensive chromosomal breakage and
rearrangements.[4] In primary tissue cultures of human neoplasms it
produces cytomorphological changes consistent with inhibition of
RNA synthesis[5] which appears to differ from that seen in bacteria.
Another study in cell free preparations has shown streptonigrin
inhibiting DNA-dependent RNA synthesis with inhibition of DNA
synthesis approximately parallel to that of DNA-dependent RNA
synthesis.[6]

Biochemical studies have shown that streptonigrin causes
a non-stoichiometric disappearance of reduced glutathione from
erythrocytes incubated without glucose.[7] In leukemic white cells,
anaerobic glycolysis was inhibited strongly and cellular ATP levels
decreased markedly.

Streptonigrin has moderate activity against leukemia L1210
and marked activity against Walker carcinosarcoma 256 as well as
activity against a host of experimental tumors and Hela cells in
culture.[8,10]

A summary of the published clinical usage with this drug
is shown in the table on the following page.

Study	Tumor Types	# Evaluable Pts	# Objective Response	%	Dosage
Wilson[11]	Far advanced solid tumors some almost terminal	42	4	10	4-10 μg/kg/day x 4-5 IV
Hacken, Thal, Tan et al[12]	Mixed solid & Hodgkin's	27	5	26	10 μg/kg/day x 4 IV
Humphrey[13]	Advanced mixed solid tumors	23	3	16	6-7 μg/kg/day x 5 IV
Sullivan and Miller[14]	Mixed solid tumors and lymphoma	39	16	41	7 μg/kg/day x 7 by continuous IV infusion
McCracken and Aboody[15]	Bronchogenic carcinoma	20	0	0	7 μg/kg/day x 6-7 by continuous IV infusion
Nora et al[16]	Far advanced mixed tumors without evidence of metastasis	10	2	20	7 μg/kg/day x 7 by intraarterial continuous infusion
Harris, Medrek, Golomb, Gumport and Wright[17]	Mixed solid tumors and lymphoma	(A) 49	17	34	0.2-0.4 mg/day till toxicity PO
		(B) 24	7	34	5-7 μg/kg/day x 6 by continuous IV infusion
		(C) 9	2	22	7 μg/kg/day x 5 by IA infusion
		(D) 3	2	66	35 μg/kg by isolation perfusion

Study	Tumor Types	# Evaluable Pts	# Objective Response	%	Dosage
Hurley[18]	Mixed pelvic neoplasms (cervix, bladder, colon)	15	3	20	8-20 µg/kg by pelvic perfusion
Moertel and Reitmeier[19]	Advanced gastrointestinal malignances	47	2	43	5-7 µg/kg/day x 7 by continuous IV infusion
Totals		308	63	20.4	

A total of 308 treated cases of lymphoma and solid tumors have been reported; many of these were far advanced and resistant to other forms of therapy. The dose regimens used have been almost exclusively 7 mcg/kg/day x 4-7 IV, either by pulse dose or by continuous infusion. A somewhat better response is seen with the continuous infusion regimens. Daily oral dosage to toxicity has been attempted with success as has isolated perfusion and intra-arterial infusion. The drug appears to have definite activity against lymphoma and little activity against the usual range of solid tumors.

The toxicity encountered with streptonigrin includes severe bone marrow depression, nausea, vomiting, diarrhea and alopecia.

References

(1) Rao, K.V., Bieman, K., and Woodard, R.B. The structure of streptonigrin. J Amer Chem Soc 85: 2532, 1963.

(2) Levine, M., and Borthwick, M. The action of streptonigrin on bacterial DNA metabolism and on induction of phage production in lyncogenic bacteria. Virology 21: 568, 1963.

(3) Levine, M., and Borthwick, M. Induction of phage production in lysogenic bacteria with streptonigrin. Bacteriol Proc, Abstract, p 153, 1963.

(4) Cohen, M.M., Shaw, M.W., and Craig, A.P. The effects of streptonigrin on cultured human leukocytes. Proc Nat Acad Sci 50: 16, 1963.

(5) Walker, D.G., Lyons, M.M., Medrek, T.J., and Wright, T.C. Autoradiographic studies on the effect of mithramycin and streptonigrin in primary tissue cultures of human neoplasms. Internat Cancer Cong, Abstract, p 357, 1967.

(6) Koschel, K. Effect of chromomycins and several anthracycline antibiotics on DNA dependent nucleic acid synthesis. Biochem Z 344: 76, 1966.

(7) Kremer, W.B., and Laszol, J. Biochemical effects of streptonigrin and its methyl ester. Biochem Pharmacol 15: 111, 1966.

(8) Oleson, J.J., Caiderella, L.A., Mjos, K.J., et al. I. The effects of streptonigrin on experimental tumors. Antibiot Chemother 11: 158, 1961.

(9) Teller, M.N., Wagshul, S.F., and Wooley, G.W. Transplantable human tumors in experimental chemotherapy: Effects of SN on HS #1 and HEp #3 in the rat. Antibiot Chemother 11: 165, 1961.

(10) Reilly, C.H., and Sugivra, K. An antitumor spectrum of streptonigrin. Antibiot Chemother 11: 174, 1961.

(11) Wilson, W.L., Labra, C., and Barrist, E. Preliminary observations on the use of streptonigrin as an antitumor agent in human beings. Antibiot Chemother 11: 147, 1961.

(12) Hackethal, C.A., Golbey, R.B., Tan, T.C., et al. Clinical observations on the effect of streptonigrin in patients with neoplastic disease. Antibiot Chemother 11: 178, 1961.

(13) Humphrey, E.W., and Blank, N. Clinical experience with
      streptonigrin. Cancer Chemother Rep 12: 99, 1961.

(14) Sullivan, R.D., Miller, E., Zurek, W.Z., et al. Clinical
      effects of prolonged continuous infusion of streptonigrin in
      advanced cancer. Cancer Chemother Rep 33: 27, 1963.

(15) McCracken, S., and Aboody, A. Continuous IV. Infusion of
      streptonigrin in patients with bronchogenic carcinoma.
      Cancer Chemother Rep 46: 23, 1965.

(16) Nora, P.F., Kukral, J.C., Soper, T., et al. Intra-arterial
      infusion of streptonigrin in advanced cancer. Cancer Chemother
      Rep 48: 41, 1965.

(17) Harris, M.N., Medrek, T.J., Golomb, F.M., et al. Chemotherapy
      with streptonigrin in advanced cancer. Cancer 18: 49, 1965.

(18) Hurley, J.D. Perfusion therapy with streptonigrin. Proc
      Amer Assoc Cancer Res 5: 29, 1964.

(19) Moertel, C.G., and Reitemeier, R.J. Evaluation of strep-
      tonigrin by continuous IV infusion in advanced gastrointestinal
      cancer. Cancer Chemother Rep 51: 73, 1967.

L-asparaginase

L-asparaginase is an enzyme which catalyzes the hydrolysis of L-asparagine to L-aspartic acid and ammonia. It has been partially purified from several sources: guinea pig serum,[1] yeast, Pseudomonas spp, E. coli[2] and Erwinia carotovora.[3] From E. coli, two different L-asparaginases have been isolated: EC-1 and EC-2.[4] These may be separated from each other by means of DEAE-cellulose column chromatography and have differential activities at different pH levels. Both of the E. coli enzymes have a limited ability to hydrolyze L-glutamine,[5] while the form of L-asparaginase found in guinea pig serum catalyzes only the hydrolysis of L-asparagine. EC-2 is the only form of the enzyme of E. coli origin with antitumor activity, and is the enzyme that has been used exclusively for clinical trials in this country.

In 1953, Kidd noted that the growth of certain lymphomas of mice and rats was inhibited by guinea pig serum, but not by rabbit or horse sera.[6] Ten years later, Broome was the first to show that the L-asparaginase of guinea pig serum was responsible for its antilymphoma effects.[7] It has since been demonstrated that the antitumor action of L-asparaginase is dependent on its ability to catalyze hydrolysis of asparagine; tumor cells which are sensitive to L-asparaginase are, in general, those which require exogenous L-asparagine for optimal growth when grown in tissue culture,[8,9] while neoplastic cells which are able to synthesize sufficient endogenous asparagine for optimal growth are not sensitive to L-asparaginase in vitro. Normal tissues in man and other mammals are able to synthesize asparagine, thus providing the biochemical basis for the differential ability of L-asparaginase to kill sensitive tumor cells.

In what fashion asparagine deprivation acts within the cell to cause its death is still uncertain. The only known metabolic pathways of asparagine in animal tissues are its conversion to aspartate by hydrolysis and to α-ketosuccinamic acid by transamination, and its utilization in protein synthesis.[10] Sobin and Kidd have demonstrated that in 6C3HED-OG cells (from a murine lymphoma), which are sensitive to L-asparaginase, protein synthesis in vivo is inhibited by 25 to 50% (as measured by the rate of incorporation of ^{14}C-labeled L-valine) within 15 minutes of injection of heated guinea pig serum. In the same setting, DNA synthesis proceeded undiminished for 60 minutes or more, and was curtailed only after 120 minutes of exposure to the guinea pig serum in vivo. RNA synthesis was not inhibited until 240 minutes after injection.

Broome also feels that inhibition of protein synthesis is likely to be the primary mechanism of action of L-asparaginase. He studied the fate of ^{14}C-labeled asparagine in 6C3HED lymphoma cells, and found no incorporation of the label for any purpose other than

protein synthesis.[11] He noted further that labeled asparagine,
once incorporated, remained within the cell, and that it was not
converted to aspartate in cell proteins. Of special interest was
his observation that, in solid tumors in vivo, protein synthesis in
sensitive cells is strongly inhibited by L-asparaginase at levels
of total cell asparagine which are adequate for normal synthesis
in resistant cells. He speculated that this might be due to
linkage between sites of asparagine synthesis and sites of
utilization in asparaginase-resistant cells, which would allow
synthesized asparagine to be used preferentially for protein
formation before equilibration with the whole cell pool. In this
way, essential proteins, such as enzymes, might be selectively
spared in cells capable of endogenous asparagine synthesis, even
though the total cell pool of asparagine was depleted by L-
asparaginase treatment. To support such a hypothesis, there is
evidence of preferential utilization of endogenous over exogenous
L-asparagine in protein formation by HeLa and other L-asparagine-
independent lines.[12]

     Mashburn and Wriston have shown that within an hour after L-
asparaginase treatment there is activation of alkaline ribonuclease
in sensitive tumor cells, and within two hours after L-asparaginase
administration, alkaline ribonuclease in sensitive cells had
increased by 80%, while the increase in a resistant subline of
tumor cells was only 18%.[13] Broome feels this increase in
ribonuclease activity may be a manifestation of metabolic control
mechanisms, activated by the primary inhibition of protein
synthesis.[11]

     The hydrolysis of asparagine results, of course, not only in
asparagine depletion but in aspartic acid accumulation, to levels
twelve times normal in 6C3HED lymphoma cells.[11] Such high
intracellular levels of aspartate may exert a growth-inhibitory
effect per se, but it has not been feasible so far to test this
possibility; no comparable rise in intracellular levels occurs
when cells are incubated in high concentrations of aspartic acid
(up to 3×10^{-3}M).[11]

     A final possibility with regard to the role of asparagine in
sensitive tumor systems is that asparagine may furnish its amido
group for nucleic acid biosynthesis, as glutamine is known to do in
normal cells. The only biological system in which this has so far
been shown to occur, however, is the wheat germ.[14]

     The ability of L-asparaginase to block incorporation of
valine-^{3}H and uridine-^{3}H into protein and RNA, respectively, of
sensitive tumor tissues has been exploited in an in vitro test of
L-asparaginase sensitivity aimed at predicting which specific
tumors, both in animals and in man, might respond to treatment with

the enzyme. This test consists of measuring the synthesis of
protein and RNA by cells in vitro, using labeled valine and labeled
uridine in the presence and absence of L-asparagine and L-
asparaginase.[15] If a patient's tumor cells do not incorporate
either valine or uridine in the absence of L-asparagine or in the
presence of L-asparaginase, the test would predict a favorable
response to L-asparaginase therapy. This test has proven of very
limited usefulness in clinical trials of L-asparaginase. Its
predictive value has so far proven disappointing. A number of
other in vitro predictive tests have been used in animal tumors,
with varying success.[16] Among them are measurements of (1) amount
of L-asparagine synthetase activity in the tumor; (2) growth of
tumor cells in tissue culture in the presence and the absence of
L-asparagine; and (3) the effect of L-asparaginase on the
viability of tumor cells in tissue culture. So far, technical
difficulties have prevented these tests from having clinical
application.

L-asparaginase has proven to have definite activity in ALL-
AUL and an outline of published results in this disease is given
below:

Investigator	Regimen (all IV)	# Evaluable Pts	# CR	# PR
Leventhal, Skeel, Yankee & Henderson[17]	6000 IU/m^2, 3 of 4 days x 28	11	5	2
Pratt & Holton[18]	500 IU/m^2 twice weekly x 4	11	5	1
	10,000 IU/m^2/wk x 2	10	4	1
	Totals	32	14	4

Investigator	Regimen (all IV)	# Evaluable Pts	# CR & PR
Rausen & Glidewell[19]	5000 IU/kg/wk x 3	15	10
	1000 IU/kg/day x 15	15	6
Tallal, Tan et al[20]	10 IU/kg/day x 28	12	6
	200 IU/kg/day x 28	23	16
	400 IU/kg/day x 28	5	2
	100 IU/kg/day x 28	22	14
	5000 IU/kg/day x 28	11	7
	Totals	103	61

Most of these cases were children with far advanced disease who had received most, if not all, of the standard agents. The duration of remissions was, unfortunately, only a few months in almost all the cases. It is clear, however, that L-asparaginase has a definite role to play in the therapy of ALL-AUL.

Clarkson et al[21] have administered L-asparaginase to 163 adults with different forms of leukemia, lymphoma and solid tumors. Six of 11 patients with ALL and 4 of 32 with AML-AMoL or AUL had complete or good partial remissions. Doses of 10 to 5000 IU/kg/day were used, but there was no clear correlation between dose and therapeutic response. Partial hematologic responses occurred in one patient with untreated CML, in 4 of 5 in the blastic phase of CML, and in 2 of 3 with CLL, but in none of these patients was the response of substantial clinical benefit. Two patients with disseminated lymphosarcoma or reticulum-cell sarcoma had excellent therapeutic responses and 4 others showed some improvement, while 14 had no detectable response. Of 30 patients with melanoma, only one responded and no responses were seen in 45 other patients with various types of solid tumors.

Whitecar et al[22] have reported treating 33 adult patients with acute leukemia and 15 with various solid tumors. Dosage levels ranged from 600-400,000 IU/m^2 in 30 of 33 patients with acute leukemia. There was a rapid fall in the white-cell count and

diminution in the blast population of the peripheral blood, but
further therapy with other agents was required in all but 5
patients who responded. Three of 17 patients with AML responded
with two patients achieving good partial remissions. One of
nine patients with ALL and one of 5 with AUL achieved partial
remissions. No responses were seen in any of the patients with
solid tumors.

The toxicity of L-asparaginase has proven to be extensive
and has been exhaustively reviewed by Oettgen et al,[23] by Haskell,
Canellos et al,[24,25] and by Whitecar et al.[22] The toxicity includes
fever, anorexia, nausea, vomiting, weight loss, lethargy,
somnolence, confusion, hemorrhage, hypolipidemia and occasionally
hyperlipidemia, hypoproteinemia, hypocalcemia, abnormal liver
function tests, azotemia, hyperglycemia, allergic reactions,
anaphylactic shock and hemorrhagic pancreatitis. This is an
impressive list of systems liable to damage from a single drug
and several, such as anaphylaxis and pancreatitis, are
potentially fatal. It is possible, but unproven, that the
utilization of lower doses may make it possible to treat the
majority of patients without serious side effects.

References

(1)   Tower, D., Peters, E., and Curtis, W. Guinea pig serum L-asparaginase. J Biol Chem 238: 983, 1963.

(2)   Mashburn, L., and Wriston, J. Tumor inhibitory effect of L-asparaginase from Escherichia coli. Arch Biochem Biophys 105: 450, 1964.

(3)   Wade, H. A new L-asparaginase with antitumor activity. Lancet 757: 776, 1968.

(4)   Campbell, H., Mashburn, L., Boyse, E., et al. Two L-asparaginases from Escherichia coli B. Their separation, purification, and antitumor activity. Biochem 6: 721, 1967.

(5)   Adamson, R., and Fabro, S. Antitumor activity and other biologic properties of L-asparaginase -- a review. Cancer Chemother Rep 52: 6, 1968.

(6)   Kidd, J. Regression of transplanted lymphomas induced in vivo by means of normal guinea pig serum. I. Course of trans-planted cancers of various kinds in mice and rats given guinea pig serum, horse serum, or rat serum. J Exp Med 98: 565, 1953.

(7)   Broome, J. Evidence that the L-asparaginase of guinea pig serum is responsible for its antilymphoma effects. I. Properties of the L-asparaginase of guinea pig serum in relation to those of the antilymphoma substance. J Exp Med 118: 99, 1963.

(8)   Boyse, E., Old, L., Campbell, H., et al. Suppression of murine leukemias by L-asparaginase. Incidence of sensitivity among leukemias of various types: comparative inhibitory activities of guinea pig serum L-asparaginase and E. coli L-asparaginase. J Exp Med 125: 17, 1967.

(9)   Broome, J. Evidence that the L-asparaginase activity of guinea pig serum is responsible for its antilymphoma effects. Nature 191: 1114, 1961.

(10)   Broome, J. Evidence that the L-asparaginase of guinea pig serum is responsible for its antilymphoma effects. II. Lymphoma 63HED cells cultured in a medium devoid of L-asparagine lose their susceptibility to the effects of guinea pig serum in vivo. J Exp Med 118: 121, 1963.

(11)   Broome, J. Studies on the mechanism of tumor inhibition by L-asparaginase. Effects of the enzyme on asparagine levels in the blood, normal tissues, and 6C3HED lymphomas of mice:

differences in asparagine formation and utilization in
asparaginase-sensitive and -resistant lymphoma cells.
J Exp Med 127: 1055, 1968.

(12) Eagle, H., Washington, C., Levy, M., et al. The population-
      dependent requirement by cultured mammalian cells for
      metabolites which they can synthesize. II. Glutamic acid
      and glutamine; aspartic acid and asparagine. J Biol Chem 241:
      4994, 1966.

(13) Mashburn, L., and Wriston, J. Change in ribonuclease
      concentrations in L-asparaginase-treated lymphosarcoma.
      Nature 211: 1403, 1966.

(14) Kapoor, M., and Waygood, E. Initial steps of purine biosynthesis
      in wheat germ. Biochem and Biophys Res Comm 1: 7, 1962.

(15) Oettgen, H. Inhibition of leukemias in man by L-asparaginase.
      Cancer Res 27: 2619, 1967.

(16) Old, L. Treatment of lymphosarcoma in the dog with L-asparaginase.
      Cancer 20: 1066, 1967.

(17) Leventhal, B., Skeel, R., Yankee, R. L-asparaginase plus
      azaserine in acute lymphatic leukemia. Cancer Chemother Rep
      54 1: 47, 1970.

(18) Pratt, C., and Holton, C. Comparison of weekly and twice
      weekly L-asparaginase in the treatment of childhood lymphocytic
      leukemia. Proc Amer Assoc Cancer Res 11: 64, 1970.

(19) Rausen, A., and Glidewell, O. L-asparaginase in advanced
      childhood leukemia: comparative trial of drug schedules
      singly and in combination. Proc Amer Assoc Cancer Res 11:
      66, 1970.

(20) Tallal, L., Tan, C., Oettgen, H., et al. E. coli L-
      asparaginase in the treatment of leukemia and solid tumors in
      131 children. Cancer 25: 306, 1970.

(21) Clarkson, B., Krakoff, I., Burchenal, J., et al. Clinical
      results of treatment with E. coli L-asparaginase in adults
      with leukemia, lymphoma and solid tumors. Cancer 25: 279,
      1970.

(22) Whitecar, J.P., Bodey, G., Harris, J., et al. Current concepts:
      L-asparaginase. New Eng J Med 282: 732, 1970.

(23) Oettgen, H., Stephenson, P., Schwartz, M., et al. Toxicity
      of E. coli L-asparaginase in man. Cancer 25: 253, 1970.

(24) Canellos, G.P., Haskell, C.M., Arseneau, J., et al.
      Hypoalbuminemia and hypocholesterolemic effect of L-
      asparaginase treatment in man -- a preliminary report. Cancer
      Chemother Rep 53: 67, 1969.

(25) Haskell, C., Canellos, G., Leventhal, B., et al. L-
      asparaginase toxicity. Cancer Res 29: 974, 1969.

Index

ACTH, 340
Actinomycin D, 257-270,273,282,367
"Acute leukemia", 11,102,198,209,210,241,247,248,264,273,282,299,
                  300,320,367
ALL-AUL, 29,30,50-53,83,86,105,117,132-135,145-148,229,234,235,241,
                  247,260,282,299,305,306,326,338,339,343,345-348,362,363,
                  368,369,397,398,399
AML-AMoL, 30,53,54,83,86,117,118,135,149,150,228,232,233,241,248,
                  282,293,294,300,305,326,340,341,348-350,367,382,383,398,
                  399
L-asparaginase, 395-402
Bis-chloroethyl nitrosourea (BCNU), 134,135,137,300,320,360-366
Bladder, 31,67,93,198,216,217,241,251,321,332,391
"Bone", 253
Brain tumors, primary, 67,136,158,159,300,309,310,343,363,364
Breast, 7,27,32,33,83,85,102,103,116,136,138-140,197,199-202,230,
                  241,243,244,260,261,275,282,284,285,300,302,303,320,322,339,
                  342,343,344,387
Burkitt's lymphoma, 50,105,145
Busulfan, 83,112-129,239,379
Carcinoid,
Cervix, 19,30,31,60-62,83,94,108,136,155-157,198,220,221,241,250,
                  251,300,312,313,391
Chlorambucil, 81-98,114,115,213
CLL, 19,20,30,57,58,82,89-91,115,118,119,252,264,301,342,343,350,
                  351,398
CML, 20,58,59,83,91,92,113,114,119-124,239,240,252,301,379,387,398
Colon, 6,7,8,27,34,83,85,102,116,140,141,198,202-206,241,245,246,
                  260,262,263,275,282,288,300,303,320,324,339,362,387,391
Cortisone, 339,340,342
Cyclophosphamide, 5,25-80,82,83,84,101,102,115,137,197,198,240,281,
                  300,320
Cytosine arabinoside, 227,237
Daunorubicin, 228,367-372
Dibromomannitol, 114,379-381
Dimethyl triazeno imidazole carboxamide, 102,137,373,374